ANNALS
OF LIFE INSURANCE MEDICINE
1964 VOLUME II

EDITORIAL COMMITTEE:
B. A. BRADLOW, JOHANNESBURG
J. E. CLARKE, MELBOURNE
EUGENE V. HIGGINS, NEW YORK
H. JECKLIN, ZURICH
J. C. SINCLAIR, TORONTO
E. TANNER, ZURICH
HARRY E. UNGERLEIDER, NEW YORK

EDITOR:
SWISS REINSURANCE COMPANY ZURICH

WITH 84 FIGURES

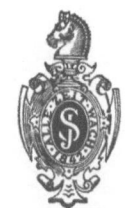

SPRINGER-VERLAG

BERLIN · GÖTTINGEN · HEIDELBERG · NEW YORK

© by Springer-Verlag
Berlin · Göttingen · Heidelberg 1964
Softcover reprint of the hardcover 1st edition 1964
Library of Congress Catalog Card Number 62 – 18597

ISBN 978-3-642-85616-7   ISBN 978-3-642-85614-3 (eBook)
DOI 10.1007/978-3-642-85614-3

Title No. 4067
Printed by Konrad Triltsch, Graphischer Großbetrieb, Würzburg

Contents

Extra Mortality and Expectation of Life

H. Jecklin

The expectation of life of an individual becomes a significant statistical measure only when it is related to a particular mortality table. A mortality table of the type generally used in life assurance work starts with a fictitious population of newborn persons and records, for each year of age, the number of survivors as well as the number of those who die before attaining the next higher age. Death is considered the only cause of decrement. The table is derived from statistical observation and is based on the fundamental assumption that the probabilities of death for the various ages do not change with time. It follows that such a table (sometimes referred to as a period table) does not allow for what are known as secular changes in mortality.

The expectation of life may be regarded as a mean value which, on the basis of the mortality table used, indicates the number of years during which an individual member of a particular age group will, on the average, remain alive. The mathematical statistician looks upon the expectation of life as an "expected value" showing the mean duration of the future lifetime associated with any particular age. Incidentally, the expectation of life should not be confused with the probable duration of life: the latter measures the period within which the number of survivors of a given age falls by exactly one half. Besides these measures we have the concept of the most probable duration of life which is, however, mainly of academic interest and, consequently, rarely encountered in modern literature. The most probable duration of life is fixed at that age in the mortality table (after the first year of life) at which the number of deaths is a maximum. Examples of these three measures, computed from the Mortality Table for the Swiss male population, 1948—1953, are as follows:

Age	Expectation of life	Probable	Most probable
		duration of life	
Years	Years	Years	Years
0	66.36	71.67	76.25
15	54.84	57.55	61.25
30	41.01	43.94	46.25
45	27.45	28.58	31.25
60	15.69	15.68	16.25

The expectation of life is particularly useful for the comparison of mortality tables relating to different periods in order to demonstrate the increasing length of human life that results from the secular fall in mortality rates. Specimen values of the expectation of life, based on a number of Swiss population mortality tables (Males) are as follows:

Age	Period			
	1876−80	1929−32	1941−50	1948−53
	Expectation of life			
Years	Years	Years	Years	Years
0	40.6	59.3	64.0	66.4
20	38.8	45.4	48.8	50.2
40	24.8	28.6	31.0	31.9
60	12.2	13.9	15.1	15.7
80	4.1	4.6	4.9	5.2

It is obvious that decreases in mortality rates must lead to increases in the expectation of life. It is also well known that mortality rates have decreased rapidly during recent decades. However, the decreases are not the same for all countries and races and, in any particular population, the decreases differ for the various age groups. The largest decreases have occurred at the ages of infancy and adolescence. These increases in longevity are attributed to improvements in sociological conditions, the progress of public health and, in particular, the advances of medical science and practice which make it possible successfully to combat many diseases, eliminate epidemics and thus to preserve human life. But it must be pointed out that no success has been, or is likely to be, achieved in materially extending the maximum length of human life. All that has been achieved is an increased expectation of life for each age group which really amounts to an increase in the number of survivors at high ages. But if, biologically, an age of about 100 years must be regarded as the limit of the human lifespan it might follow from the above remarks that an increase in mortality rates at high ages could be expected. Furthermore, it is interesting to reflect that the above-mentioned causes of decreasing mortality, whilst undoubtedly the most important, are not the only ones. The secular trend has been one of falling mortality rates for as long as records exist, in other words, this trend commenced before the present era of medical progress. And this trend that has been in existence for so long has also been noticed in distant countries, more particularly in the East where the sociological structure differs widely from our own. Almost fifty years ago, Professor E. CZUBER, a world authority on actuarial science and population theory, called the decrease in mortality rates one of the most remarkable phenomena [1]. Yet the factors mentioned above have strongly accelerated the decrease in mortality in the technically advanced countries. It thus becomes a legitimate question whether the lowest limit will not be reached soon if, in fact, it has not been reached already. In recent decades the decreases in mortality rates have shown an almost linear trend; were this to continue we would soon be faced by the absurdity of negative mortality.

As stated before, mortality and expectation of life are closely associated; if mortality rates fall, expectation of life rises, and vice versa. The association is not, however, as simple as might be surmised. The same change in the expectation of life may result from quite different changes in mortality rates. When the mortality table is fixed, there is only one value of the expectation of life for each age. Conversely, if the numerical value of the expectation of life is known, no inference can be drawn as to the nature of the mortality table. For the expectation of life is a mean value and such a value does not show the individual values which have contributed to its formation. To make it even more plain for the non-mathematician, the two series 1, 3, 5, 7, 9 and 3, 4, 5, 6, 7 have the same arithmetic mean or average, namely 5.

Yet the question how the expectation of life is affected when the corresponding mortality rates are changed is not only theoretically reasonable but also of practical interest. The usual procedure in insuring substandard risks is to increase the probabilities of death taken from the mortality table that is used for the insurance of standard risks. As a rule the normal mortality rates are increased by a fixed percentage, corresponding to the severity of the impairment. This is known as the method of constant multiplicative extra mortality. It would be useful to known by how many years the expectation of life is decreased when the mortality rates are increased by a specific percentage. In individual cases this can be ascertained by calculation, but this would be a laborious process. On the other hand, it is known that a mortality table can be represented as an analytical function, i.e. by a mathematical formula, best of all with the aid of what, after its discoverer, is called a Makeham function. However, as soon as the normal mortality rates are increased and an attempt is made to compute the expectation of life of the increased risk as a function of the expectation of life of the normal risk, one is led to formulas that are difficult to handle and, consequently, useless for practical purposes.

The theoretically inclined might be tempted to make especially simple mathematical assumptions in order to bring about an analytical representation of the mortality table. Such an attempt might take the form of assuming — without regard for the realities of the situation — that the probability of death is constant, i.e. independent of age. If q_x denotes, as usual, the probability of a person aged x dying within one year, the relationship $q_x = k =$ constant would hold, with $0 < k < 1$. If l_x stands for the number living at age x, then

$$l_{x+1} = l_x \cdot (1-k)$$

and, consequently,

$$l_0 \cdot (1-k)^x = l_x.$$

This formula expresses the so-called law of mortality of DORMOY, a law that postulates a series of decrements constructed in the same way as a table of discount factors, as used in the theory of compound interest. Indeed, the constant k corresponds to what in the mathematics of finance is called d, the rate of discount, i.e. the rate of interest, payable annually in advance. This analogy shows that the mortality law of DORMOY is quite unsuitable for the representation of any mortality rates that can be used in practice. For such a mortality table will reach zero at around age 100, in contradistinction to the compound discount factors which, whilst asymptotically tending to zero, do not reach that value within a finite number of years. Let us, nevertheless, use DORMOY's law and assume that the probability of death is increased by a specific percentage. If k and $k^{(\alpha)}$ signify, respectively, the normal and increased probabilities of death, we can write

$$k^{(\alpha)} = k\,(1+\alpha)$$

which shows that $100\,\alpha$ is the extra mortality, expressed as a percentage of normal mortality.

It now becomes necessary to introduce some precision: when we speak of the expectation of life for age x we have in mind the so-called "complete" expectation of life $\overset{\circ}{e}_x$; the values of this function are tabulated in many mortality tables; they are calculated as follows:

$$\overset{\circ}{e}_x = \frac{1}{l_x}\sum_0^\infty l_{x+t} - \frac{1}{2} = \frac{1}{l_x}\sum_1^\infty l_{x+t} + \frac{1}{2}$$

There is no reason why one should not also consider those modifications of the expectation of life which are equivalent to annuity values at zero rate of interest, payable in advance, $\ddot{e}_x$, and in arrear, e_x, namely

$$\ddot{e}_x = \frac{1}{l_x}\sum_0^\infty l_{x+t} \quad\text{and}\quad e_x = \frac{1}{l_x}\sum_1^\infty l_{x+t}.$$

The value e_x is also known as the curtate expectation of life. It is obvious that $\ddot{e}_x = e_x + 1$ and, consequently,

$$\overset{\circ}{e}_x = \tfrac{1}{2}\,(\ddot{e}_x + e_x).$$

It can now be shown easily, for we only have to evaluate the sum of a geometric progression, that the expectation of life is constant, i.e. independent of age, when DORMOY's law holds. It has already been shown that

$$l_{x+t} = l_x\,(1-k)^t$$

hence
$$\ddot{e}_x = \frac{1}{l_x}\sum_0^\infty l_x\,(1-k)^t = \sum_0^\infty (1-k)^t = \frac{1}{k} = \text{constant},$$

$$e_x = \frac{1}{l_x}\sum_1^\infty l_x\,(1-k)^t = \sum_1^\infty (1-k)^t = \frac{1-k}{k} = \text{constant}.$$

If, in the case of a substandard risk, we put $k^{(\alpha)} = k\,(1+\alpha)$ we obtain

$$\ddot{e}_x^{(\alpha)} = \frac{1}{l_x^{(\alpha)}}\sum_0^\infty l_x^{(\alpha)}[1-k\,(1+\alpha)]^t = \frac{1}{k\,(1+\alpha)}$$

$$e_x^{(\alpha)} = \frac{1}{l_x^{(\alpha)}}\sum_1^\infty l_x^{(\alpha)}[1-k\,(1+\alpha)]^t = \frac{1-k\,(1+\alpha)}{k\,(1+\alpha)} = \frac{1}{k\,(1+\alpha)} - 1$$

$$\overset{\circ}{e}_x^{(\alpha)} = \frac{1-k\,(1+\alpha)}{k\,(1+\alpha)} + \frac{1}{2} = \frac{1}{k\,(1+\alpha)} - \frac{1}{2}.$$

In the case of $\ddot{e}_x^{(\alpha)}$ we thus obtain the surprisingly simple relationship:

$$\ddot{e}_x^{(\alpha)} = \frac{1}{1+\alpha} \ddot{e}_x.$$

From the practical point of view an expectation of life that is independent of age is obviously nonsensical. The expectation of life is the same as the mean future lifetime and it is clear from first principles that its value must essentially depend on the attained age. It follows that the above simple formula cannot be applied with accuracy to any mortality table that is used in practice. As an isolated occurrence, the formula has unfortunately appeared in medico-actuarial literature [2], and it must, therefore, be emphasized that this leads to entirely incorrect results. It can be proved mathematically that the formula thus rejected gives correct results only if DORMOY's law holds. This, however, is inapplicable to human mortality which is a further reason for rejecting as unsound the application of the above formula.

Elsewhere, the author has published an approximation formula [3] which expresses the expectation of life for a substandard risk (the enhanced rates of mortality bearing a constant ratio to the normal rates) as a simple function of the expectation of life of a normal risk of the same age. However, the medical underwriter does not like to apply mathematical formulas, no matter how simple. We, therefore, have examined the question whether it is not possible to find a solution which, even though a straight-forward rule of thumb, yet produces sufficiently accurate results. Such a solution does in fact exist.

It is generally known that MAKEHAM's law of mortality represents a refinement of an earlier formula devised by GOMPERTZ. When GOMPERTZ' formula is used it is possible to equate annuity values on two joint lives of equal age to an annuity value on a single life of a higher age. If, instead of probabilities of death, we use forces of mortality, calculations based on twice the normal mortality are the same as calculations involving two normal lives of equal age. Taking this fact as a starting point and bearing in mind that the expectation of life may be regarded as an annuity value, at zero rate of interest, it must be possible to approximate the expectation of life of a substandard risk (assuming the normal rates of mortality to be increased by the application of a constant factor) as the expectation of life of a standard risk of an appropriately increased age. If h stands for this increase in age we have the equation

$$\overset{\circ}{e}_x^{(\alpha)} = \overset{\circ}{e}_{x+b}.$$

We shall try to interpret this formula. In terms of GOMPERTZ' law the probability of death can be represented, almost accurately, in the form

$$q_x = bc^x$$

where b and c are constants. For a risk subject to extra mortality α this formula becomes

$$q_x^{(\alpha)} = (1+\alpha)\, bc^x.$$

If the extra mortality is equivalent to an age increase h of the normal risk, we obtain

$$(1+\alpha)\, bc^x = bc^{x+h}$$

hence

$$(1+\alpha) = c^h$$

and

$$h = \frac{\log (1+\alpha)}{\log c}$$

It appears that when GOMPERTZ' law holds, the increase in age is entirely independent of the age. In the case of modern mortality tables the constant c almost universally has a value of about $1\cdot1$. The factor $1/\log c$ can thus be taken, roughly, as 25. We thus have as a rule of thumb

$$h = 25 \log (1+\alpha)$$

which is best written in the form

$$h = \frac{100}{4} \log (1+\alpha).$$

If one adopts the usual procedure of taking the mortality of the normal risk as 100% and, similarly, expresses the extra mortality as a percentage, then the last-mentioned formula enables one directly to read off from a table of logarithms the increase in age that corresponds to any particular extra mortality. Starting with 100, the total (percentage) mortality of the risk is to be taken as the numerus; the required increase in age is simply one quarter of the first two digits of the mantissa of the corresponding logarithm. If, for instance, the extra mortality is 75%, the numerus becomes 175 and the first two digits of the mantissa are 24, which gives an increase in age of $h = 6$ years. In this manner the following table is constructed:

Extra mortality expressed as a percentage of normal mortality (100 α)	Corresponding age increase h expressed in years
25	2.4
50	4.4
75	6.1
100	7.5
125	8.8
150	9.9
175	11.0
200	11.9
250	13.6
300	15.1

For reasons that will be stated later, it is recommended that each of the foregoing values of h be increased by half a year.

Conversely, if the increase in age is known, the corresponding extra mortality may be estimated. If, for example, $h = 7$ then $4 \times 7 = 28$ will be taken as the first two digits of the mantissa of a logarithm. The numerus is 190 and the extra mortality is 90%.

We thus have solved the problem of estimating the expectation of life when the degree of extra mortality is known. All we have to do is to ascertain the expectation of life of a normal risk whose age is increased by h years. Using, as an example, the expectation of life of the male population of Switzerland for the period 1948—1953, the following table results:

Age (Years)	Expectation of life (expressed in years) corresponding to an extra mortality of				
	0% (normal)	50%	100%	150%	200%
20	50.2	45.6	42.8	41.0	39.2
30	41.0	36.4	33.7	31.9	30.1
40	31.9	27.5	24.9	23.2	21.6
50	23.2	19.3	17.1	15.7	14.3
60	15.7	12.4	10.6	9.5	8.5
70	9.5	7.1	5.9	5.2	4.6

Our simple rule for the conversion of extra mortality into an age increase, and vice versa, is not only applicable in respect of the expectation of life but can also be used with advantage in fixing the extra premium payable for a substandard risk. One of the merits of the rule is that it produces reasonably good results even in the case of endowment assurances with high maturity ages and in the case of whole life assurances, i.e. in those cases where other well-known approximations fail [4]. The success of our rule can be viewed as a vindication of the method of enhanced ages. Generally speaking, underwriters do not like to deal with substandard risks by increasing the age but prefer to quote percentage increases in mortality. The doctor, on the other hand, may find the concept of a percentage increase in mortality somewhat abstract whereas an increase in age conveys to him a concrete picture of the situation.

Finally, we still have to make a concession to theoretical accuracy. What has been stated above is based on the assumption that the mortality table can be represented by GOMPERTZ' formula. In actual fact this is rarely the case; for an adequate representation MAKEHAM's more complex formula is needed. In the case of MAKEHAM's formula the extra premium for the increased risk (assuming again a uniform percentage increase of normal mortality) is also obtained by an increase in age but there is also an addition, independent of age, to the premium [5]. This last-mentioned addition is, however, small; in the case of endowment assurances the addition amounts to less than one twentieth of one percent of the sum assured. Instead of working out this small addition, it is permissible, as a quid pro quo, slightly to overstate the increase in age. This is the reason for our above suggestion that the age increase should be further augmented by half a year.

References

[1] Czuber, E.: Mathematische Bevölkerungstheorie. Leipzig-Berlin: Verlag Teubner 1923, p. 282.

[2] Sarre, H., und P. von Dittrich: Ergebnisse der inneren Medizin und Kinderheilkunde. Herausgegeben von L. Heilmeier, R. Schoen und B. de Rudder, neue Folge, Band 13. Berlin-Göttingen-Heidelberg: Springer 1960, p. 373.

[3] Jecklin, H.: Genäherte Bestimmung der mittleren Lebensdauer erhöhter Risiken. Blätter der deutschen Gesellschaft für Versicherungsmathematik V, 37 (1960).

[4] — Genäherte Prämienbestimmung bei Versicherungen anomaler Risiken mit hohem Endalter. Mitt. Vereinigung schweizer. Vers.-Math. 62, 195 (1962).

[5] Saxer, W.: Versicherungsmathematik. Zweiter Teil. Berlin-Göttingen-Heidelberg: Springer 1958. Anhang von H. Jecklin, p. 236 et seq.

Reference may also be made to the following recent paper:

Jäkel, H. K.: Über funktionale Zusammenhänge zwischen Sterblichkeitsvariationen und mittlerer Lebenserwartung. Blätter der deutschen Gesellschaft für Versicherungsmathematik VI, 163 (1963).

Maximum Utilization of the Life Table Method in Analyzing Survival *

S. J. CUTLER, M.A. · F. EDERER, B.S.

Measurement of patient survival is necessary for the evaluation of treatment of usually fatal chronic diseases. This is particularly true for cancer. The American College of Surgeons, recognizing this, requires the maintenance of a cancer case registration and follow-up program for approval of a hospital cancer program [1]. Acceptance of survival as a criterion for measuring the effectiveness of cancer therapy is also attested to by the very large number of papers published every year reporting on the survival experience of cancer patients.

Although the proportion of patients alive 5 years after diagnosis (5-year survival rate) is the most frequently used index for measuring the efficacy of therapy in cancer, an increasing number of investigators are reporting on the manner in which patient populations are depleted during a period of time, e.g., survival curves. A popular and relatively simple technique for describing survival experience over time is known as the actuarial or life table method. Whereas the method and its uses have been admirably described by a number of authors [2—6], one important aspect has received relatively little attention. A principal advantage of the life table method is that it makes possible the use of all survival information accumulated up to the closing date of the study. Thus, in computing a 5-year survival rate one need not restrict the material to only those patients who entered observation 5 or more years prior to the closing date. We will show that patients who entered observation 4, 3, 2, and even one year prior to the closing date contribute much useful information to the evaluation of 5-year survival.

Let us consider a group of patients entering observation continuously beginning with Jan. 1, 1946. Sometime early in 1952, we decide to analyze the survival experience of these patients to obtain a 5-year survival rate. We choose Dec. 31, 1951, as the closing date, i.e., the follow-up status and survival time of each patient is recorded as of that date.

Of the patients entering the study during the 6 years ended on Dec. 31, 1951, only those diagnosed in 1946 were exposed to the risk of dying for at least 5 years[1]. The exposure time for patients entering in each of the calendar years is shown in Table I.

---

* Published in Journal of Chronic Diseases.

[1] In this example, date of entry into the study is defined as date of diagnosis. In practice, other reference dates, such as date of initiation of a particular course of therapy, may be used.

It might be supposed, intuitively, that the patients who entered observation from 1947 to 1951 are of no value in computing a 5-year survival rate as of Dec. 31, 1951, since each of these patients was under observation for less than 5 years.

Table I.

Calendar year of diagnosis	Years of exposure to risk of dying
1946	5 to 6
1947	4 to 5
1948	3 to 4
1949	2 to 3
1950	1 to 2
1951	Less than 1

This, however, is not true. MERRELL and SHULMAN [5] have pointed out that patients for whom less than the required number of years survival information is available should not be discarded from the analysis. WILDER [7] has demonstrated that, through maximum utilization of the life table method, it is possible to compute reliable 5-year survival rates for a large series even when the longest possible exposure time is just short of 5 years [1]. The primary objective of this paper is to show how partial survival information can be included in the life table and to show how much is gained by doing so. Data from the Connecticut Cancer Register are used for illustrative purposes [2].

The anatomy of the life table [3]

Table II provides the basic facts, as of Dec. 31, 1951, concerning 126 male patients with localized cancer of the kidney, diagnosed during the period 1946 through 1951. The cases are divided into 6 cohorts, one for each year of diagnosis. The columns of Table II are described here.

Column 1. Years after diagnosis (x to x + 1). — This column gives the time elapsed from the date of diagnosis in intervals of one year, i.e., 0—1, 1—2, etc. For example, a patient who was diagnosed Jan. 20, 1946, and died on Oct. 5, 1948, died during the third year after diagnosis, i.e., during interval 2—3. The number of patients that left observation during each interval is entered in the appropriate column (3, 4, or 5), according to the reason for removal from observation.

Column 2. Alive at beginning of interval (l_x). — The entry on the first line of this column indicates the number of cases alive at diagnosis, i.e., the initial number of patients in the cohort.

---

[1] In the series reported by WILDER, the range of exposure time was from one day to, but not including, 5 years.

[2] We wish to thank Dr. MATTHEW H. GRISWOLD, Director Division of Cancer and Other Chronic Disases, Connecticut State Department of Health, for his courtesy in making these data available.

[3] We borrowed the phrase "anatomy of the life table" from PEARL's [2] excellent textbook *Biometry and Medical Statistics.*

Table II. *Survival data for single year cohorts*
(126 Male Connecticut residents with localized kidney cancer; diagnosed 1946—1951 and followed through Dec. 31, 1951)

Years after diagnosis (1) x to $x+1$	Alive at beginning of interval (2) l_x	Died during interval (3) d_x	Lost to follow-up during interval (4) u_x	Withdrawn alive during interval[1] (5) w_x
Patients diagnosed in 1946 (1946 cohort)				
0—1	9	4	1	—
1—2	4	—	—	—
2—3	4	—	—	—
3—4	4	—	—	—
4—5	4	—	—	—
5—6	4	—	—	4
Patients diagnosed in 1947 (1947 cohort)				
0—1	18	7	—	—
1—2	11	—	—	—
2—3	11	1	—	—
3—4	10	2	2	—
4—5	6	—	—	6
Patients diagnosed in 1948 (1948 cohort)				
0—1	21	11	—	—
1—2	10	1	2	—
2—3	7	—	—	—
3—4	7	—	—	7
Patients diagnosed in 1949 (1949 cohort)				
0—1	34	12	—	—
1—2	22	3	3	—
2—3	16	1	—	15
Patients diagnosed in 1950 (1950 cohort)				
0—1	19	5	1	—
1—2	13	1	1	11
Patients diagnosed in 1951 (1951 cohort)				
0—1	25	8	2	15

[1] Alive at closing date of study.

Column 3. Died during interval (d_x). —

Column 4. Lost to follow-up during interval (u_x)[1]. — In this column we enter the number of patients whose survival status as of the closing date, Dec. 31, 1951, was unknown. The length of observation for each patient lost to follow-up is the time elapsed from date of diagnosis to data last known to be alive. Thus, a patient observed for 3 years and 4 months is entered on the fourth line, i.e., interval 3—4.

In applying the life table method it is usually assumed that *subsequent to date of last contact,* the survival experience of lost cases was similar to that of cases remaining under follow-up. In contrast, complete omission of lost cases

---

[1] We are using the letter "u" to represent "untraced" cases, rather than the letter "l" which comes to mind as a symbol for "lost" cases, because "l" is a standard life table notation for "alive at beginning of interval".

from the analysis is equivalent to assuming that from *date of diagnosis* the survival experience of lost cases was similar to that for cases with complete follow-up information.

Column 5. Withdrawn alive during interval (w_x). — In this column we enter the number of patients known to have been alive on the closing date, Dec. 31, 1951. The interval during which these patients withdrew from observations depends on their date of diagnosis. For example, all patients diagnosed in 1949 and alive on Dec. 31, 1951, are recorded as withdrawals from observation during the third year after diagnosis, interval 2—3. Note that, for each cohort in Table II, zeros (symbolized by dashes) are entered in this column for all intervals but the last.

Although only one of the cohorts (1946) provided survival information for a full 5 years, we used the available information on all 6 cohorts. Table III was obtained by pooling all the information in Table II, summing cell by cell. For example, by summing the entries on the first line of Column 3 for each yearly cohort in Table II, we obtained the total of 47 cases who died within one year of diagnosis, shown in Table III.

Table III. *Combined life table and computation of 5-year survival rate*
(126 Male Connecticut residents with localized kidney cancer diagnosed 1946—1951 and followed through Dec. 31, 1951)

Years after diagnosis	Alive at beginning of interval	Died during interval	Lost to follow-up during interval	Withdrawn alive during interval	Effective number exposed to the risk of dying (col. 2 − ½ col. 4 − ½ col. 5)	Proportion dying (col. 3 − col. 6)	Proportion surviving (1 − col. 7)	Cumulative proportion surviving from diagnosis through end of interval ($p_1 \cdot p_2 \cdot \ldots \cdot p_x$)
(1) x to $x+1$	(2)[a] l_x	(3)[a] d_x	(4)[a] u_x	(5)[a] w_x	(6) l'_x	(7) q_x	(8) p_x	(9) P_x
0—1	126	47	4	15	116.5	0.40	0.60	0.60
1—2	60	5	6	11	51.5	0.10	0.90	0.54
2—3	38	2	—	15	30.5	0.07	0.93	0.50
3—4	21	2	2	7	16.5	0.12	0.88	0.44
4—5	10	—	—	6	7.0	0.00	1.00	0.44[c]
5—6[b]	4	—	—	4				

    a Columns 2 through 5 of this table were obtained by summing, cell by cell, the survival data of the 6 yearly cohorts of Table II.

    b This line is not needed for computing the 5-year survival rate; it is included here merely to complete the account of the initial 126 patients. Four were alive at the closing date of the study.

    c Five-year survival rate.

In practice, the data for the pooled cohort of 126 cases would be tabulated directly, as in Table III, rather than by summing tabulations for 6 individual cohorts. We used the latter procedure to show how much information each of the cohorts contributed to the pooled data. For example, by comparing Tables II and III, we find that of the 5 patients known to have died in the second year after diagnosis (Table III, Line 2, Column 3), one was diagnosed in 1948, three in 1949, and one in 1950. Similarly, of the 18 patients diagnosed in 1947, 6 were alive 4 years after diagnosis; of the 21 patients diagnosed in 1948, 7 were alive 3 years after diagnosis. Thus, each cohort contributes some information to our knowledge of patient survival during a period of 5 years after diagnosis. A statistical measure of the gain in precision resulting from this procedure will be discussed later. First, however, we will explain how the basic data summarized in Columns 1 through 5 of Table III are used to compute survival rates.

Computation of survival rates

The first step in preparing a life table is to distribute the deaths, losses, and withdrawals with respect to the interval in which they left observation[1]. This information is summarized in Columns 3, 4, and 5 of Table III. The sum of the entries in Columns 3, 4, and 5 equals the total number of cases in the study, which is entered on the first line of Column 2 (126 cases). Successive entries in this column are obtained according to the formula:

$$l_{x+1}=l_x-(d_x+u_x+w_x).$$

For example, the number alive at the beginning of the second year (60) was obtained by subtracting from the number alive at the beginning of the first year (126), the sum of the deaths, losses, and withdrawals during the first year (47 + 4 + 15).

The life table is completed by a series of four computations for each follow-up year (Columns 6 through 9).

Column 6. Effective number exposed to risk of dying (l_x'). — It is assumed that patients lost or withdrawn from observation during an interval were exposed to the risk of dying, on the average, for one-half the interval[2]. For example,

---

[1] For a detailed account of the mechanics of recording and tabulating survival data, see BERKSON and GAGE [1], pp. 4—5.

[2] The computing procedure given here is based on the assumption that, for cases withdrawn alive and cases lost to follow-up, survival subsequent to date of last contact is similar to that for cases with complete follow-up information. For cases withdrawn alive, this assumption introduces no bias, because there is no reason to believe that patients alive on the closing date are different from patients observed for a longer period. However, for cases lost to follow-up, this assumption may introduce a bias.

Patients lost to follow-up were alive when last observed, and whether their survival experience is better than, worse than, or equal to the survival of patients remaining under follow-up is highly speculative. For example, cancer patients may be lost to follow-up for a variety of reasons. Faradvanced cases may leave their usual place of residence to enter the household of a relative; successfully treated patients may stop reporting to the tumor clinic, because they feel that no further medical care is required. It is therefore important to keep the proportion of cases lost to follow-up at a minimum. Survival rates based on a series in which a substantial proportion of patients have been lost to follow-up are of highly questionable value, because it is impossible to determine the extent to which they are biased.

Some investigators, such as PATERSON and TOD [8] recommend that lost cases be counted as dead "to avoid undesirable uncertainty ... although (it) may result in a slight bias against the efficacy of treatment". Other investigators, such as RYAN and his colleagues [9] omit lost cases

of the 25 patients diagnosed in 1951, 15 were alive on Dec. 31, 1951 (withdrawn alive). It is reasonable to assume that the date of diagnosis for these 15 patients was roughly equally distributed during the calendar year 1951 and that, on the average, each patient was observed for one-half year.

The effective number exposed to risk is obtained by subtracting from the number alive at the beginning of the year, one-half the sum of the number lost and withdrawn during the year. Thus,

$$l_x' = l_x - (u_x + w_x)/2.$$

Column 7. Proportion dying during interval (q_x). — This is also referred to as the probability of dying during the interval. It is obtained by dividing the number of deaths by the effective number exposed to risk:

$$q_x = \frac{d_x}{l_x'}.$$

To express as a percentage, multiply by 100.

Column 8. Proportion surviving the Interval (p_x). — This is referred to alternately as the probability of surviving the interval, or the survival rate. It is obtained by subtracting the proportion dying during the interval from unity:

$$p_x = 1 - q_x.$$

To express as a percentage, multiply by 100.

Column 9. Cumulative proportion surviving from diagnosis to end of interval (P_x). — This is generally referred to as the cumulative survival rate. It is obtained by cumulatively multiplying the proportion surviving each interval:

$$P_x = p_1 \times p_2 \times p_3 \times \ldots p_x \, {}^1.$$

Note that successive entries in this column give the 1-year, 2-year, 3-year, 4-year, and 5-year cumulative survival rates (Table III). The successive cumulative survival rates are plotted in drawing a survival curve.

Although the computations illustrated in Table III were carried out in intervals of one year after the date of diagnosis, the life table may be set up in terms

---

from the analysis of survival. The latter procedure involves the assumption that *from date of diagnosis* the survival experience of lost cases is similar to that of cases with complete follow-up.

We prefer the first of the several possible assumptions regarding lost cases, namely that subsequent to date of last contact their survival is similar to that for cases with complete follow-up. The complete omission of lost cases from the computation of survival rates discards available information. The assumption that lost cases died immediately after the date of last contact is contrary to fact. Registry experience with intensive field investigation of lost cases, which resulted in recovery of some, indicates that such patients often live for several years beyond the initial date of last contact [10].

Although cases withdrawn alive and cases lost to follow-up are treated alike in the computations described here, we distinguish between the two in the life table for reasons mentioned: (1) it is important to be aware of the number of cases lost to follow-up because of their potential bias, and (2) other computational methods may treat the two groups differently.

¹ This formula as based on the assumption that the various interval probabilities are statistically independent.

of days, weeks, months, years, etc. In fact, the life table may be organized in intervals of varying length. For example, one might record experience during the first year in monthly intervals, and the experience thereafter in annual intervals. This type of presentation may be desirable when a large proportion of deaths occur during the first year. The method of computing survival rates described here may be used whatever the size of the intervals.

Gain in utilizing experience of cohorts with partial follow-up

The standard error provides a measure of the confidence with which one may interpret a statistical result. Thus, the standard error of the survival rate indicates the extent to which the computed rate may have been influenced by sampling variation [1]. For example, by adding and subtracting twice the standard error to and from the computed survival rate, one obtains an approximate 95 per cent confidence interval. This means that in repeated observations under the same conditions the true survival rate will lie within a range of two standard errors on either side of the computed rate, an average of 95 times in 100.

Thus, the computed 5-year survival rate for male patients with localized cancer of the kidney is 44 per cent. The standard error, computed according to the method explained in the Appendix, is 6 per cent. It is therefore likely that the true 5-year survival rate is not smaller than 32 per cent and not larger than 56 per cent.

Admittedly, the computed rate does not yield a very firm estimate of the true survival rate, but we must bear in mind that it was based on a series of only 126 patients and only 9 of these patients were diagnosed a full 5 years prior to the date of study. Furthermore, whereas the survival rate based on all information available on these 126 patients provides at least a rough idea of the true rate (one-third to one-half), discarding the information on the cohorts with partial follow-up information would result in an extremely unreliable estimate. This is explained in the discussion that follows.

The computing method applied to the total series of 126 cases, illustrated in Table III, can be applied to any selected portion of the group. We have therefore used it to compute a series of 5-year survival rates based on successively larger patient cohorts. A 5-year survival rate was computed for the 9 patients diagnosed in 1946, all of whom had a 5-year exposure time. We then added the

---

[1] The 126 cases of localized cancer of the kidney are in effect a sample from a population of male patients with localized kidney cancer.

An illustration of sampling variation may be drawn from baseball. A 0.250 hitter may, in four times "at bat", get one hit. Frequently, though, he will get no hits or two hits. And not too infrequently he will get three hits. If we watch a game and see a player get two hits in four times "at bat", it is difficult for us to judge how good a hitter this player really is. We have to watch this player for many games before we can get a reliable estimate of his batting average.

Survival rates are similar to batting averages in the sense that they are relative frequencies, i.e., the numerator is part of the denominator. For each hit there must be at least one time "at bat", and for each death there must be at least one case exposed to the risk of dying.

18 patients diagnosed in 1947, who had a 4-year exposure time, and computed a 5-year survival rate based on the available information for these 27 patients. This procedure was continued until the known experience of all 126 patients was utilized in estimating the 5-year survival rate. The successive rates and their corresponding standard errors are shown in the uppermost section of Table IV.

Table IV. *Five-year survival rates and their standard errors for five groups of cancer patients, showing the reduction in standard error with increases in cohort size*

Cohort	Number of cases diagnosed	5-year survival rate	Standard error of 5-year survival rate	Per cent reduction in standard error of 5-year survival rate
Kidney, localized				
1946	9	0.53	0.171	—
1946—1947	27	0.46	0.098	43
1946—1948	48	0.43	0.075	56
1946—1949	82	0.43	0.064	63
1946—1950	101	0.45	0.063	63
1946—1951	126	0.44	0.060	65
Kidney, regional				
1946	11	0.18	0.116	—
1946—1947	23	0.33	0.101	13
1946—1948	30	0.28	0.091	22
1946—1949	39	0.25	0.074	36
1946—1950	43	0.23	0.069	41
1946—1951	47	0.24	0.070	40
Breast, localized				
1946	225	0.64	0.033	—
1946—1947	454	0.64	0.025	24
1946—1948	695	0.64	0.023	30
1946—1949	963	0.64	0.022	33
1946—1950	1,227	0.65	0.022	33
1946—1951	1,490	0.65	0.021	36
Breast, regional				
1946	208	0.42	0.035	—
1946—1947	443	0.38	0.025	29
1946—1948	708	0.39	0 021	40
1946—1949	967	0.39	0.020	43
1946—1950	1,239	0.39	0.020	43
1946—1951	1,531	0.39	0.020	43
Lip				
1946	61	0.71	0.060	—
1946—1947	109	0.65	0.048	20
1946—1948	169	0.68	0.042	30
1946—1949	224	0.68	0.040	33
1946—1950	283	0.68	0.040	33
1946—1951	332	0.67	0.039	35

The 1946 cohort of 9 cases yielded a 5-year survival rate of 53 per cent, with a standard error of 17 per cent. The large standard error tells us that this is a very unreliable estimate; the true rate is probably between 19 and 87 per cent [1],

---

[1] These are the 95 per cent confidence limits: 53=2(17).

a very wide range. The combined experience of the 1946 and 1947 cohorts yielded a survival rate of 46 per cent, with a standard error of 10 per cent. Thus, the

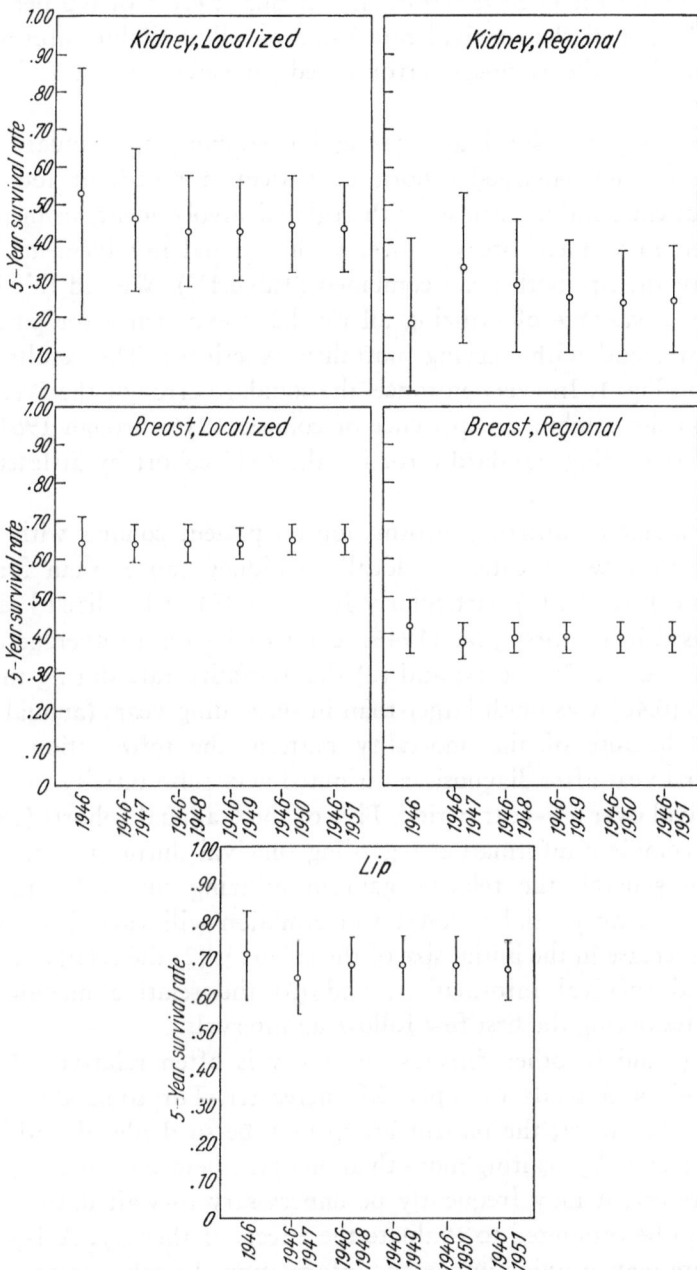

Fig. 1. Decrease in the 95 per cent confidence interval for the 5-year survival rate as cases with less than 5 years' exposure to the risk of dying are added. (The 95 per cent confidence interval is obtained by adding ±2 standard errors to the survival rate.) Source: Table IV

addition of information on cases with 4 full years of exposure reduced the standard error from 17 per cent to 10 per cent, a relative decrease of 43 per cent.

The addition of the available information on cohort 1948 (3 full years of exposure) reduces the standard error to 7.5 per cent, etc. The utilization of all available information on all the cohorts results in a standard error of 6.0 per cent. Thus, the standard error of the survival rate based on all available information is 65 per cent less than the standard error based on cases with a full 5 years of exposure.

We then computed survival rates and corresponding standard errors for series of successively enlarged cohorts of patients for each of four additional groups of patients: kidney cancer with regional involvement, in men; localized breast cancer, in women; breast cancer with regional involvement, in women; and cancer of the lip, both sexes combined (Table IV). We did this in order to illustrate the advantage of utilizing all available experience for patient groups of varying size and with varying mortality experience. The results are shown graphically in Fig. 1. In every instance, the standard error of the 5-year survival rate based on the combined experience of cohorts 1946 through 1951 is smaller than the corresponding standard error for the 1946 cohort by at least one-third.

The advantage of utilizing information on patient cohorts with less than 5 years of exposure was greater for localized kidney cancer than for the other groups. This is because: (1) particularly few cases (9) of localized kidney cancer were diagnosed in the first year (1946), compared with an average of 23 cases in each of the subsequent years; and (2) the mortality rate during the first year of follow-up (0.40) was much larger than in succeeding years (annual average of 0.07). Thus, because of this mortality pattern, the information on survival during the first year after diagnosis contributed very substantially to the information on survival over a 5-year period. Five of the 6 annual cohorts (1946—1950) contributed complete information regarding survival during the first year after diagnosis. In general, the relative gain in utilizing survival information on patient cohorts with partial follow-up information will vary directly with: (1) the relative increase in the initial size of the cohort [1]; (2) the relative completeness of the added survival information; and (3) the relative magnitude of the mortality rates during the first few follow-up intervals.

In cancer, and in other diseases, mortality is often relatively high shortly after diagnosis and tends to taper off thereafter. For some diseases, such as lung or stomach cancer, the patient group may be so depleted within one year that little is gained by waiting more than one year before evaluating therapeutic results. Therefore, it may frequently be unnecessary to wait until a 5-year survival rate can be computed to evaluate the effects of therapy. A 1-year, 2-year, or 3-year rate may provide important information. In other instances, survival data for only 5 years may be inadequate, because of significant changes in the mortality pattern at a later time [11].

---

[1] See the Appendix for a discussion of effective sample size.

Discussion

A category of patients with relatively few new cases per year was intentionally chosen as the principal example to illustrate the advantage of utilizing all available information for the computation of survival rates—only 126 cases of localized kidney cancer in men were diagnosed in 6 years. This was done because it is frequently desirable to describe the survival experience of relatively small groups of patients. For example, if we were interested in evaluating the survival experience of patients with localized breast cancer treated by surgery in combination with radiation, we would find that in any one year the number of patients receiving the combined therapy is small. As an illustration, only 25 of the 225 cases diagnosed in Connecticut in 1946 were treated by the combined therapy. Similarly, if survival is to be evaluated for a specific subgroup with respect to age, the number of cases per year would usually be small. Therefore, in order to increase the reliability of survival rates computed for various patient groups of clinical interest, it is important to utilize all available information.

It is of paramount importance to use all available survival information in computing survival rates if the rates are going to be used as criteria in a clinical trial. For example, a 3-year survival rate may have been selected as a criterion in a clinical trial. It may be possible to determine which of the several treatments being tested yields the best survival before all patients have been followed to death or for a full 3 years. Thus, inferior treatments would be discontinued at the earliest possible point.

Summary

We have illustrated the life table method for computing survival rates with 5-year survival data for cancer patients, emphasizing the advantage gained by including survival information on cases which entered the series too late to have had the opportunity to survive a full 5 years. The advantage is measured in terms of reduction in standard error of the survival rate. For the five series of patients in this paper, the reduction in standard error ranged from one-third to two-thirds.

References

[1] Manual for cancer programs. Bull. Am. Coll. Surg. 38, 149 (1953).

[2] PEARL, R.: Introduction to Medical Biometry and Statistics. Philadelphia and London: W. B. Saunders Company 1923.

[3] HILL, A. B.: Principles of Medical Statistics. New York: Oxford University Press 1956.

[4] BERKSON, J., and R. P. GAGE: Calculation of Survival Rates for Cancer. Proc. Mayo Clin. 25, 270 (1950).

[5] MERRELL, M., and L. E. SHULMAN: Determination of Prognosis in Chronic Disease, Illustrated by Systemic Lupus Erythematosus. J. CHRON. Dis. 1, 12 (1955).

[6] GRISWOLD, M. H., C. S. WILDER, S. J. CUTLER, and E. S. POLLACK: Cancer in Connecticut, 1935—1951. Hartford: Connecticut State Department of Health 1955, pp. 112—113.

[7] Wilder, C. S.: Estimated Cancer Survival Rates Confirmed. Conn. Hlth Bull. **70**, 217 (1956).

[8] Paterson, R., and M. C. Tod: Presentation of the Results of Cancer Treatment. Brit. J. Radiol. **23**, 146 (1950).

[9] Ryan, A. J., et al.: Breast Cancer in Connecticut, 1935—1953. J. Amer. Med. Ass. **167**, 298 (1958).

[10] Griswold, M. H.: Personal communication.

[11] Cutler, S. J., M. H. Griswold, and H. Eisenberg: An Interpretation of Survival Rates: Cancer of the Breast. J. nat. Cancer Inst. **19**, 1107 (1957).

[12] Greenwood, M.: Reports on Public Health and Medical Subjects, No. 33, Appendix 1, The "Errors of Sampling" of the Survivorship Tables. London: H. M. Stationery Office 1926.

Appendix

Computing the standard error of the 5-year survival rate. — The method for computing the standard error of the 5-year survival rate was developed by Greenwood (see ref. [12]) and is also described by Merrell and Shulman (see ref. [5]). The formula is

$$s_5 = P_5 \sqrt{\sum_{x=1}^{5} \frac{q_x}{l'_x - d_x}} = P_5 \sqrt{\frac{q_1}{l'_1 - d_1} + \frac{q_2}{l'_2 - d_2} + \cdots + \frac{q_5}{l'_5 - d_5}},$$

where s_5 is the standard error of the 5-year survival rate. In general, the standard error of the k-year survival rate is

$$s_k = P_k \sqrt{\sum_{x=1}^{k} \frac{q_x}{l'_x - d_x}}.$$

Columns 10 and 11 of Appendix Table I show how the calculation of the standard error of the 5-year survival rate is carried out as a continuation of the computation of the survival rate[1]. The first 9 columns are a replica of Table III. (1) Subtract d_x from l'_x for each line (Column 10); (2) divide q_x by $l'_x - d_x$ for each line (Column 11); (3) total the entries in the first 5 lines of Column 11: 0.0187; (4) take the square root of this number: $\sqrt{0.0187} = 0.137$; (5) multiply the result by P_5: $0.137 \times 0.44 = 0.060$. This is the standard error of the 5-year survival rate.

The standard error of survival rates for end-points other than 5 years is computed similarly. For example, to compute the standard error of the 3-year survival rate, the first three entries in Column 11 must be totaled, the square root taken, and multiplied by P_3.

Effective sample size. — The concept, *effective sample size*, provides another way of assessing the benefit of including in the life table cases with partial survival information. The concept relates to the fact that the reliability of a statistical result depends on the size of the sample, i.e., the number of cases observed. For example, the standard error of a survival rate, P, when all cases have been followed until death or for the required time interval (i.e., no losses from observation or withdrawals alive prior to the cut-off date) is given by the binomial formula

$$s = \sqrt{\frac{P(1-P)}{l_1}}, \tag{1}$$

where l_1 is the sample size, i.e., the initial number of cases. In formula (1), the standard error is inversely proportional to the square root of the sample size.

Let us consider the 1946—1951 localized kidney cancer cohort (Appendix Table I), for which the survival rate is 0.44, and its standard error, 0.060. Of the initial 126 cases in this cohort, a substantial number were withdrawn alive less than 5 years after diagnosis. We now ask how large a cohort, with a 5-year survival rate of 0.44 and with all cases followed to death or for a

---

[1] The standard error computed in this illustration is, itself, only an estimate of the true standard error. An, since it is based on relatively small numbers of cases, it is not a very reliable estimate. For example, had there been, due to sampling variation, one death in the last interval, rather than none, the computed standard error would be 0.0216 rather than 0.0187.

Appendix Table I. *Computation of the 5-year survival rate and its standard error*

(Data from Table III)

Years after diagnosis (1) x to $x+1$	Alive at beginning of interval (2) l_x	Died during interval (3) d_x	Lost to follow-up during interval (4) u_x	Withdrawn alive during interval (5) w_x	Effective number exposed to the risk of dying (col. 2 − ¹/₂ col. 4 − ¹/₂ col. 5) (6) l'_x	Proportion dying (col. 3 − col. 6) (7) q_x	Proportion surviving (1 − col. 7) (8) p_x	Cumulative proportion surviving from diagnosis through end of interval $(p_1 \cdot p_2 \cdot \ldots \cdot p_x)$ (9) P_x	(col. 6 − col. 3) (10) $l'_x − d_x$	(col. 7 ÷ col. 10) (11) $q_x/(l'_x − d_x)$
0—1	126	47	4	15	116.5	0.40	0.60	0.60	69.5	0.0058
1—2	60	5	6	11	51.5	0.10	0.90	0.54	46.5	0.0022
2—3	38	2	—	15	30.5	0.07	0.93	0.50	28.5	0.0024
3—4	21	2	2	7	16.5	0.12	0.88	0.44	14.5	0.0083
4—5	10	—	—	6	7.0	0.00	1.00	0.44[a]	7.0	0.0000
5—6[c]	4	—	—	4						
										0.0187[b]

[a] Five-year survival rate.

[b] This is the sum of the five entries in Column 11. The square root of this number, when multiplied by the 5-year survival rate, yields the standard error of the 5-year survival rate: $s=(0.44)\sqrt{0.0187}=(0.44)(0.137)=0.060$.

[c] See footnote [a], Table III.

Appendix Table II

	Sample size		
	1946–1951 cohort[a]	Effective sample size	1946 cohort[b]
Kidney, localized	126	68	9
Kidney, regional	47	37	11
Breast, localized	1,490	516	225
Breast, regional.	1,531	595	208
Lip	332	145	61

[a] Since the cut-off date was Dec. 31, 1951, cases diagnosed in 1947 or later were eligible for less than 5 years of observation.

[b] Actual number of cases eligible for 5 years of observation.

full 5 years, would have a standard error equal to 0.060. To answer this question, we solve equation (1) for l_1, placing a circumflex over the l_1 to indicate that this is a hypothetical value:

$$\hat{l}_1 = \frac{P(1-P)}{s^2}. \qquad (2)$$

Substituting $P=0.44$ and $s=0.060$, we obtain

$$\hat{l}_1 = \frac{(0.44)(0.56)}{0.0036} = 68.$$

The result, 68, is the *effective sample size*, which we interpret as follows. Had we started with about 68 cases (instead of 126) and followed them all until death or survival for 5 years and found that 44 per cent survived 5 years, then the standard error would have been equal to that we actually obtained in our cohort of 126 cases. Thus, the survival rate we obtained is as reliable as one based on 68 cases. This is in sharp contrast to 9 cases which were eligible for 5 years of observation. These three values are compared for the five cancer groups discussed in the text. In each instance, the effective sample size based on the 1946—1951 cohort is substantially larger than the number of cases eligible for 5 years of observation (1946 cohort).

The Underwriting of Blood Pressure Abnormalities

E. Tanner · A. Marx · J. Ulrich

Foreword

Blood pressure and build have many associations in the minds of life insurance underwriters. Both attributes are capable of continuous variation. Both are capable of exact measurement. In both cases measurement is inexpensive and can be carried out routinely in the course of a standard life insurance medical examination. Average values for groups of insured lives of the same sex and age are known, and these averages are closely associated with favorable mortality. On the other hand, individuals whose weight or blood pressure differs markedly from the corresponding averages are subject to increased mortality rates. These similarities have tempted certain underwriters to think of blood pressure abnormalities as an impairment that can be evaluated as easily and dependably as can abnormalities of weight or abdominal girth. This attitude can be the more easily understood if it is remembered that, in the Build and Blood Pressure Study 1959, mortality experience for various build and blood pressure groupings was investigated concurrently and, very largely, in respect of the same data.

The idea that life insurance risks can be satisfactorily evaluated on the basis of a limited number of factors is not new. Such an approach is not unreasonable as long as each factor is characteristic for a group of individuals that is homogeneous with respect to the mortality levels associated with it. Where, however, the same findings can be due to widely differing causes and these also differ widely in mortality significance, we must try to secure additional information if we wish to assign each risk to its correct mortality classification.

Blood pressure levels are the result of numerous interrelated factors. Without additional information there is no way of satisfactorily evaluating what may appear to be a hypertensive blood pressure level. The authors of the Blood Pressure Study 1959 were alive to the necessity for investigating the mortality significance of various blood pressure levels when other factors, unfavorable or favorable, are present. Tabulations were produced that show the combined effect of blood pressure and overweight, blood pressure and various "minor impairments", e.g. unfavorable family history, fast pulse rate, slight albuminuria. The favorable effects on mortality of normal electrocardiograms and x-ray studies were also demonstrated by special tabulations.

The observations on which the Blood Pressure Study 1959 is based were made during the period 1935 to 1954. Considerable progress has been made since those years in respect of the diagnosis, prognosis and treatment of hypertensive disease. Today, therefore, the results of the Blood Pressure Study 1959 cannot be the sole basis for the underwriting of blood pressure abnormalities. The results of contemporary research must receive adequate recognition.

Although blood pressure estimates have played an important part in underwriting for many years, there can be no doubt that more should be known among underwriters about the nature of blood pressure, its measurement and variability and the numerous factors that influence the blood pressure level over both short and long periods. A thorough understanding of these matters is essential for intelligent underwriting. Only the underwriter who is familiar with his subject is able to call for adequate information and assess such information correctly. Only he is able to deal with queries which so often arise in connection with underwriting decisions, and particularly so in connection with blood pressure.

The problem arises how non-medical personnel should be briefed on blood pressure underwriting. In the course of preparing its new Rating Manual the Swiss Reinsurance Company recently had to face this problem. A team of medical and non-medical underwriters in the Swiss Re group, with the assistance of certain outside consultants, undertook this task and prepared a new blood pressure underwriting guide. As the methods adopted are in some respects novel and as some information has been brought together that is not always readily available, it is thought that the readers of these Annals will welcome the reproduction of this underwriting guide. The text that follows differs from the text in the Rating Manual only by the omission of notes on accident and disability underwriting and by the addition of a few footnotes in lieu of cross-references to other sections of the Rating Manual which are not reproduced here.

Contents

1. Introduction

The diseases of the cardiovascular system are among the leading causes of death. This is true not only for the general population but also for insured lives. Consequently, both medical practitioners and life underwriters are vitally interested in the early recognition and correct evaluation of every form of cardiovascular disease.

Changes, more particularly increases, in blood pressure are of great significance as an early sign of cardiovascular disease. The correct measurement of blood pressure forms a vitally important part of the underwriting process. Fortunately, this measurement is a comparatively simple procedure and causes little inconvenience to the applicant. These facts have long been known to insurers and the recording of blood pressure has been an essential medical underwriting requirement for many years.

Large-scale studies of the prognostic value of blood pressure levels have been carried out on numerous occasions. The Blood Pressure Study 1959 of the Society of Actuaries is the most comprehensive of these investigations. It covers the experience under 3,900,000 policies issued during the period 1935 to 1953 and observed until termination or policy anniversary in 1954. Although present-day life insurance evaluation of blood pressure is influenced by many recent advances in medical science not yet reflected in the results of the Blood Pressure Study 1959, no life company can afford to ignore this work. The results of this Study have been considered in the preparation of the Blood Pressure Rating Tables on pages 32 and 33.

Very often we must underwrite a blood pressure problem simply on the basis of the ordinary insurance medical examination and the history admitted by the applicant. In such an event, the rating is derived from the basic Blood Pressure Rating Table. However, sometimes additional information of prognostic value is available to the underwriter, either detailed information from the applicant's own physician or additional medical studies, such as electrocardiograms, x-rays, blood studies and repeat blood pressure observations secured by the company. Such additional information makes a more refined estimate of the expected mortality possible. In many instances, this will mean that a rating lower than that indicated in the basic blood pressure table is appropriate. In some cases the contrary is true and the basic rating must then be increased.

The rules set out in this section are presented as an attempt to formulate a solution of the complex problem of underwriting blood pressure risks, in the light of the best statistical data available, supplemented by contemporary medical knowledge.

2. Basic facts on blood pressure in healthy individuals

2.1. *Blood pressure or arterial pressure*

The force exerted on the arterial wall by the flow of blood passing through the arteries. It is created by the contraction of the heart, the elasticity of the arterial wall and the resistance against the blood flow of the smaller terminal arteries.

2.1.1. Systolic pressure measures the maximal force with which the heart contracts and drives blood into the arteries.

2.1.2. Diastolic pressure measures the minimal pressure maintained in the arteries during the relaxation period of the heart beat.

2.1.3. Pulse pressure is the difference between systolic and diastolic pressure. (As subsequent paragraphs will show, abnormalities of pulse pressure are equal in prognostic importance to abnormalities of systolic or diastolic pressure.)

2.2. Measurement

Blood pressure is measured by means of a manometer (sphygmomanometer) which indicates the pressure in terms of the height, expressed in millimeters, of a column of mercury (Hg). While the applicant is seated or in a recumbent position an inflatable cuff is applied to the upper arm to cut off completely the flow of blood in the brachial artery. A stethoscope is then applied over the brachial artery at the bend of the elbow and the pressure in the cuff is gradually reduced. When the flow of blood recommences, tapping sounds are suddenly heard; the pressure at this point is recorded as the systolic pressure. With further deflation of the cuff the sounds become less distinct or occasionally disappear temporarily ("auscultatory gap"), especially at higher pressures.

This is called the second phase. The third phase is characterized by loud tapping sounds. On further deflation these sounds suddenly become soft; this point is known as the fourth phase diastolic pressure. The point at which the sounds disappear completely is called the fifth phase diastolic pressure. Some examiners have a tendency to adjust blood pressure readings to the nearest multiple of 5 or 10. In the interest of accurate assessment, such rounding up or down should be discouraged since it is not difficult to record blood pressure to the nearest even readings, e.g. 118/76, i.e. systolic pressure = 118 mm, diastolic pressure = 76 mm.

2.3. The true diastolic pressure

It is generally accepted that fifth phase readings can be obtained with greater accuracy, and that these more correctly reflect the true diastolic pressure, than fourth phase readings. Fifth phase readings are generally used in underwriting and the Tables in this section are based on such readings. Fourth phase readings are still used occasionally. Where a fourth phase reading is supplied, the fifth phase reading may be estimated by deducting 6 mm. On rare occasions an examiner may report that a complete cessation of sound does not occur. In such a case the point of muffling of sound (fourth phase) should be taken as the diastolic pressure. If even that point cannot be determined, the diastolic pressure should be left indefinite and so indicated, e.g. "150/30?".

2.4. Sources of error

2.4.1. Faulty instruments or technique. The recording of blood pressure by means of the sphygmomanometer is subject to several sources of error, due to faulty instruments or faulty technique. Experienced and conscientious examiners know how to reduce these errors to a minimum. It is essential that only such examiners be entrusted with blood pressure examinations.

2.4.2. Right and left arm differences. In most individuals right arm blood pressure readings do not differ materially from left arm readings. However, even in a healthy individual such differences may arise, e.g. from an abnormality in one of the brachial arteries. Such abnormalities usually affect right arm readings less than left arm readings. Right arm readings are therefore preferred for life insurance purposes. In general the higher reading in either arm is the correct reading.

2.4.3. Abnormal arm circumference. When the circumference of the applicant's arm is unusually large, both the systolic and diastolic readings obtained by the method described in 2.2 may overstate the true pressure; in the case of an unusually small arm circumference, the systolic reading may understate the true systolic pressure. In the absence of specific comment by the examiner or by an attending physician, the underwriter ordinarily is not aware of these circumstances. However, when such a situation is brought to his attention, the case should be referred to the Medical Director for evaluation of the reasonableness of the report and for determination of the appropriate underwriting action.

2.5. Variability of blood pressure, basal and casual pressure

Both systolic and diastolic blood pressure readings fluctuate during the course of each day. They also respond, often by rapid and substantial increases of short duration, to various types of stimulation and stress. Basal blood pressure is defined as the pressure present when all physical, emotional and metabolic activity is reduced to a physiological minimum. An approximation to basal pressure may be obtained by measuring blood pressure before the applicant has had breakfast and before he has risen in the morning. Casual blood pressure readings are those obtained by examination in the course of the day. Casual blood pressure readings are intended to measure, as accurately as possible, the applicant's blood pressure during normal resting state. It is essential, therefore, for the effects of any purely temporary disturbance, such as apprehension about the examination, to be eliminated; this will often necessitate a repeat blood pressure reading towards the end of the examination. Life insurance statistics and rating tables are based on casual blood pressure readings. It must be the underwriter's aim to secure in every case the best possible estimate of the applicant's casual, not basal, blood pressure as casual pressure has a closer relationship to longevity than basal pressure.

2.6. Average blood pressures

2.6.1. Table of average blood pressures. The following table of graduated average blood pressures has been extracted from the Blood Pressure Study 1959.

Ages	Men Systolic (mm)	Diastolic (mm)	Women Systolic (mm)	Diastolic (mm)
15—19	117	71	114	70
20—24	119	73	115	72
25—29	121	75	117	73
30—34	122	76	118	74
35—39	123	77	120	75
40—44	124	78	123	76
45—49	126	78	126	78
50—54	128	79	128	79
55—59	130	79	131	80
60—64	132	80	134	81

2.6.2. Variations resulting from differences in build. The foregoing table shows average blood pressure as a function of only two factors, age and sex. The Blood Pressure Study 1959 shows that by introducing another factor, viz. build, a slightly different scale of average blood pressures is found. As relative weight increases, a rise in both the average systolic and the average diastolic blood pressure is noted. However, since the total variation for weight differences up to 80 to 100 pounds does not exceed 6 mm with respect to average systolic and 4 mm for diastolic pressure, the significance of variation in average blood pressure by weight would seem to have little importance and should not ordinarily be taken into consideration in underwriting individual cases.

3. Hypertension

3.1. Definition of hypertension

Elevation of blood pressure above the normal range is called hypertension or, simply, high blood pressure. It is difficult to fix a specific blood pressure level below which pressure may be regarded as normal and above which it should be regarded as abnormal. In clinical medicine a level such as 145/95 is sometimes adopted as indicating the upper limit of normal and the lower limit of high blood pressure. For life insurance purposes it is preferable to avoid any rigid criterion, particularly so because statistical studies show that even relatively small increases above average values are associated with increased mortality.

3.2. Types of hypertension

Hypertension may be either primary, i.e. due to causes that are either not known or not fully understood, or secondary, i.e. it may result from or be closely associated with an identifiable disease.

3.2.1. Essential hypertension. Primary hypertension is usually termed essential hypertension. Idiopathic hypertension is another synonym. Essential hypertension rarely commences before age 35. Sometimes, but not very often, it commences after age 45. The condition may continue, without complications, for many years. These cases have a more favorable prognosis. On the other hand, essential hypertension may, and often does, lead to arterial degeneration and adversely affect various organs, especially kidneys, heart and brain. At this stage the prognosis rapidly deteriorates. Moreover, it may be impossible to decide whether primary or secondary hypertension is present.

3.2.2. Secondary hypertension. Secondary hypertension may arise at any age. Hypertension commencing before age 35 is almost always secondary, as is a sudden onset of hypertension at any age. The following are some of the possible causes of secondary hypertension:

Diseases of the kidneys, including acute or chronic nephritis and abnormalities of the renal arteries.

Pathology of endocrine glands, including adrenal dysfunction (e.g. Cushing's syndrome), hyperthyroidism and pheochromocytoma.

Diseases or abnormalities of the arteries and arterioles, e.g. periarteritis nodosa, necrosis of renal arteries or arterioles resulting in malignant hypertension.

Coarctation of aorta, arteriovenous aneurysm.

The prognosis of secondary hypertension depends to a great extent on the nature and severity of the primary condition and the duration and severity of the hypertension itself. If the primary condition is curable and effective treatment is instituted, the blood pressure may be lowered to normotensive, or near normotensive, levels. In such cases, unless the blood pressure had reached, for a sufficiently prolonged period of time, such levels as to produce irreversible vascular changes, the prognosis is favorable. In females the prognosis of secondary hypertension is for some unknown reason more favorable than in males.

3.3. The underwriting problem

The foregoing paragraphs illustrate that the term hypertension encompasses a wide range of vascular impairment. Therefore, the primary concern of the underwriter in considering this condition is to establish effective selection criteria and procedures which will enable him to discern in this heterogenous group the more favorable and the less favorable risks, and to assign each to the appropriate substandard classification.

4. Hypertension and mortality. The rating tables

The Blood Pressure Rating Tables on pages 32 and 33 show the additional mortality, expressed as a percentage of basic mortality, for various combinations of age at entry, systolic and diastolic pressure. The age at entry groups are 20—29, 30—39, 40—49, 50—59, 60 and over.

Two figures, representing extra mortality, appear in the various fields of these Tables, a higher figure in heavy type and a lower figure in ordinary type. These figures are to be used in the following circumstances:

The higher figures (which will also be referred to as basic ratings) indicate the extra mortality which may be expected when the blood pressure is adjudged to be the only abnormality. This implies that the remainder of the underwriting picture is entirely favorable and does not call for any additional mortality. It also implies that no additional tests, such as electrocardiographic or roentgenological studies, have been carried out. In general, therefore, the basic ratings indicate the average extra mortality applicable to the vast heterogeneous class of those hypertensive applicants whose hypertension has not been or cannot be fully investigated. The majority of those applications which may be assessed in terms of the basic ratings are for comparatively small amounts where the additional trouble and expense of further investigation is not justified. The basic ratings are in no way intended as a substitute for further investigation in those cases, irrespective of the amount of insurance, where the underwriting facts clearly call for additional information. For example, where the personal history suggests that a rapid increase in blood pressure has taken place, a more thorough investigation of the risk than a simple insurance examination and single blood pressure determination would be required.

The lower figures (which will also be referred to as optimal ratings) indicate the minimal extra mortality that may be assessed in those cases which, in accordance with the underwriting rules in the following sections, are adjudged as most favorable. Such assessment must always be reserved for a decision by the Medical Director. Where only some of the favorable criteria are present, an intermediate assessment is indicated, i.e. the extra mortality to be assessed should be somewhere between the basic and optimal ratings.

5. The underwriting of blood pressure abnormalities—without history of treatment

5.1. Underwriting requirements

5.1.1. Repeat blood pressure examinations

(a) General situations in which repeat examinations are called for:

In the interest of correct underwriting and in view of the considerable variability of blood pressure readings, even over short periods, repeat blood pressure examinations are desirable, sometimes necessary, in a number of situations, for example the following:

(i) There may be an indication that the examining doctor tends to understate or overstate blood pressure readings.

(ii) Certain readings, too important to be ignored, may appear to be erratic, possibly due to lack of experience or care on the part of a medical examiner.

(iii) The blood pressure readings set out in the current medical report may be prima facie inconsistent with other findings or earlier readings.

Moreover, it is clear from section 4. above that where the blood pressure figures available to the underwriter are ratable in terms of the basic ratings, a more favorable assessment cannot be reached unless a really representative level of the blood pressure has been established through repeated examinations.

(b) Special situations in which repeat examinations are called for:

Applicants presenting a history or present findings of hypertension should not ordinarily be accepted without repeat blood pressure examinations if certain aggravating features are present. A few examples follow:

(i) Blood pressure and overweight. If the blood pressure, ratable in terms of the basic ratings, combined with overweight, results in a total rating for these two factors of +100 or more.

Blood pressure: Basic ratings and optimal ratings·Age Groups: 20—29, 30—39, 40—49·This Table should be used as outlined in the explanatory text

Each cell shows the basic rating / optimal rating. Rows are grouped by **Diastolic pressure**; columns are **Systolic pressure**.

Diastolic	Ages	Up to 133	134–139	140–145	146–151	152–157	158–163	164–169	170–175	176–181	182–187	188–193	194–199	200–205
Up to 87	20–29	0 / 0	0 / 0	20 / 0	45 / 0	65 / 10	90 / 30	120 / 60	150 / 100	190 / 150*	230 / 200*	280 / —	340 / —	410* / —
	30–39	0 / 0	0 / 0	20 / 0	35 / 0	55 / 10	75 / 20	105 / 50	135 / 80	175 / 130	215 / 180*	265 / —	325 / —	395* / —
	40–49	0 / 0	10 / 0	20 / 0	30 / 0	45 / 5	65 / 10	95 / 20	125 / 50	165 / 100	205 / 150*	255 / 200*	315 / 250*	385* / 350*
88 to 92	20–29	10 / 0	20 / 0	40 / 0	60 / 10	80 / 20	110 / 50	140 / 80	170 / 120	210 / 160*	250 / 200*	300 / —	360* / —	— / —
	30–39	10 / 0	20 / 0	35 / 0	55 / 10	70 / 20	95 / 40	125 / 70	155 / 110	195 / 150*	235 / —	285 / —	345 / —	415* / —
	40–49	15 / 0	20 / 0	30 / 0	50 / 0	60 / 10	80 / 15	110 / 25	140 / 60	180 / 110	220 / 160*	270 / 210*	330 / 250*	400* / 350*
93 to 97	20–29	50 / 20	45 / 20	65 / 30	85 / 40	105 / 60	135 / 80	165 / 110	195 / 160*	235 / 210*	275 / —	325 / —	385* / —	— / —
	30–39	45 / 10	45 / 20	60 / 30	75 / 40	95 / 50	120 / 70	150 / 90	180 / 120	220 / 170*	260 / 230*	310 / —	370* / —	— / —
	40–49	45 / 20	40 / 10	55 / 15	65 / 15	85 / 20	105 / 30	135 / 35	165 / 55	205 / 95	245 / 150*	295 / 220*	355 / 300*	— / —
98 to 102	20–29	110* / —	100* / 80*	110 / 80	130 / 100	150 / 120	180 / 140	210 / 160*	240 / 190*	280 / 250*	320 / —	370* / —	— / —	— / —
	30–39	105* / —	90* / 50	100 / 50	120 / 50	135 / 70	165 / 100	195 / 130	225 / 180*	265 / 230*	305 / —	355* / —	415* / —	— / —
	40–49	95* / —	80* / —	90 / 50	110 / 50	120 / 60	150 / 80	180 / 100	210 / 120	250 / 135	290 / 170	340 / 250*	400* / 300*	— / —
103 to 107	20–29	275* / —	250* / —	230* / —	200* / —	225* / —	255 / —	285 / —	315 / —	355* / —	395* / —	— / —	— / —	— / —
	30–39	265* / —	220* / —	205* / —	180* / —	210* / —	240 / —	270 / —	300 / —	340* / —	380* / —	— / —	— / —	— / —
	40–49	255* / —	210* / —	185* / —	175* / —	195 / 150	225 / 150	255 / 180	285 / 200	325 / 220	365* / 280*	— / —	— / —	— / —
108 to 112	20–29	— / —	— / —	400* / —	320* / —	350* / —	380* / —	410* / —	— / —	— / —	— / —	— / —	— / —	— / —
	30–39	— / —	— / —	375* / —	310* / —	335* / —	365* / —	395* / —	— / —	— / —	— / —	— / —	— / —	— / —
	40–49	— / —	— / —	350* / —	300* / —	320* / —	350* / —	380* / —	410*. / —	— / —	— / —	— / —	— / —	— / —

* Refer to Medical Director

Two dashes indicate that the case should usually be declined. The combination of a rating and a dash means that acceptance, at such rating, may be granted in exceptional circumstances.

Blood pressure: Basic ratings and optimal ratings · Age Groups: 40—49, 50—59, 60 and over · This Table should be used as outlined in the explanatory text

Each cell is shown as **basic rating / optimal rating**.

Diastolic pressure	Ages	\ \ \ \ \ \ \ \ \ \ \ \ \ Systolic pressure												
		Up to 133	134–139	140–145	146–151	152–157	158–163	164–169	170–175	176–181	182–187	188–193	194–199	200–205
Up to 87	40—49	0 / 0	10 / 0	20 / 0	30 / 0	45 / 5	65 / 10	95 / 20	125 / 50	165 / 100	205 / 150*	255 / 200*	315 / 250*	385* / 350*
	50—59	0 / 0	0 / 0	15 / 0	25 / 0	35 / 0	40 / 0	70 / 10	100 / 40	140 / 60	180 / 80	230 / 140*	290 / 220*	360* / 300*
	60 and over	0 / 0	0 / 0	10 / 0	20 / 0	25 / 0	30 / 0	50 / 0	80 / 20	120 / 40	160 / 70	210 / 120	270 / 180*	340* / 250*
88 to 92	40—49	15 / 0	20 / 0	30 / 0	50 / 0	60 / 10	80 / 15	110 / 25	140 / 60	180 / 110	220 / 160*	270 / 210*	330 / 250*	400* / 350*
	50—59	20 / 0	15 / 0	25 / 0	40 / 0	50 / 0	60 / 10	90 / 25	120 / 45	160 / 80	200 / 120	250 / 150*	310 / 200*	380* / 300*
	60 and over	25 / 0	15 / 0	20 / 0	30 / 0	35 / 0	40 / 0	60 / 0	100 / 20	140 / 40	180 / 75	230 / 125	290 / 190*	360* / 260*
93 to 97	40—49	45 / 20	40 / 10	55 / 15	65 / 20	85 / 20	105 / 30	135 / 35	165 / 55	205 / 95	245 / 150*	295 / 220*	355* / 300*	— / —
	50—59	40 / 10	35 / 0	45 / 0	55 / 0	70 / 10	85 / 20	115 / 30	145 / 50	185 / 90	225 / 130	275 / 170*	335* / 210*	410* / 300*
	60 and over	40 / 20	30 / 0	35 / 0	45 / 0	55 / 0	70 / 0	95 / 0	125 / 25	165 / 50	205 / 90	255 / 130	315 / 200*	385* / 280*
98 to 102	40—49	95* / —	80* / —	90 / 50	110 / 50	120 / 60	150 / 80	180 / 100	210 / 120	250 / 135	290 / 170	340 / 250*	400* / 300*	— / —
	50—59	85* / —	70* / 30	80 / 20	95 / 20	105 / 25	130 / 45	160 / 65	190 / 90	230 / 115	270 / 160	320 / 200*	380* / 280*	350* / —
	60 and over	75* / 75*	60* / 30	70 / 20	80 / 20	90 / 0	110 / 0	140 / 40	170 / 75	210 / 95	250 / 160*	300 / 200*	360* / 220*	300* / —
103 to 107	40—49	255* / —	210* / —	185* / —	175* / —	195 / 150	225 / 150	255 / 180	285 / 200	325 / 220	365* / 280*	— / —	— / —	— / —
	50—59	240* / —	185* / —	160* / 150*	160* / 150*	175* / 160*	205 / 160*	235 / 170*	265 / 200*	305 / 250*	345* / —	405* / —	— / —	— / —
	60 and over	225* / —	165* / 50*	135* / —	145* / —	155* / —	185 / —	215 / 120*	245 / 180*	285 / 220*	325* / 300*	375* / —	— / —	— / —
108 to 112	40—49	— / —	— / —	350* / —	300* / —	320* / —	350* / —	380* / —	410* / —	— / —	— / —	— / —	— / —	— / —
	50—59	— / —	400* / —	325* / —	285* / —	300* / —	330* / —	360* / —	390* / —	— / —	— / —	— / —	— / —	— / —
	60 and over	— / —	325* / —	300* / —	270* / —	280* / —	310* / —	340* / —	370* / —	410* / —	— / —	— / —	— / —	— / —

* Refer to Medical Director

Two dashes indicate that the case should usually be declined. The combination of a rating and a dash means that acceptance, at such rating, may be granted in exceptional circumstances.

(ii) Blood pressure and other circulatory or renal impairment. If the blood pressure, ratable in terms of the basic ratings, is combined with a ratable circulatory or renal impairment.

(iii) Blood pressure and family history. If the blood pressure is ratable +50 or over in terms of the basic ratings, and there also is more than one case, among the applicant's parents or siblings, of degenerative cardiovascular or renal disease or marked hypertension. (Both deceased and living members of the applicant's family should be taken into account.)

(iv) Treatment for hypertension. If there is any evidence of past or present medical or surgical treatment for hypertension. See Section 6.

(c) Points to be observed in obtaining repeat blood pressure examinations.

When it is decided to call for a repeat blood pressure reading, it is essential that the services of a doctor be used who is well known to the company and experienced in conducting life insurance medical examinations. As a rule, it is preferable to use a second examiner, but it is unnecessary and sometimes inappropriate to do so when the first examiner is known to be competent and can be expected to supply casual blood pressure readings, unaffected by purely temporary factors such as anxiety.

When blood pressure readings are repeated, it is best to do so on at least two days. Where this is not possible, more than one reading should be obtained in any event. *Every reading should be reported to the company.* The best time for repeat examinations is the late afternoon.

5.1.2. Reexamination of the urine, both chemical and microscopic, is required when there is any ratable blood pressure and there is, at the same time, any indication or suspicion of past or present renal disease; a record of albuminuria is sufficient indication to justify such a suspicion.

5.1.3. Other requirements. In the case of applications for large amounts of insurance and also in those cases where hypertension is suspected, other tests may be required, at the discretion of the Medical Director. These tests may include electrocardiograms, x-ray examinations, ophthalmoscopic examination (see 5.2.9) and certain laboratory tests.

5.2. Rating

5.2.1. Evaluation of blood pressure for rating purposes. For the reasons explained in the foregoing paragraphs it is unwise to base the final rating on only one blood pressure reading. Where more than one reading is available, a "rating average" should be computed on the following lines:

(a) Usually ignore all blood pressure readings taken more than five years prior to the date of the current medical examination.

(b) Form the averages (arithmetic means) of the blood pressures taken on any one day. These may be called the daily averages.

(c) Form the average (arithmetic mean) of the daily averages for the past three months. This may be called the current average.

(d) On similar lines form the average of all earlier blood pressure readings that are higher than the current average, i.e. those taken during the past five years, omitting those taken during the past three months. This may be called the past average.

(e) Form the rating average by adding two thirds of the current average to one third of the past average. Subject to the reservations set out in paragraph (f) the rating average should be used as a basis for rating the risk.

(f) The foregoing averaging method is recommended because it makes allowance for both the present blood pressure levels and any past elevated readings, but gives greater weight to the current levels. Elevated readings from a period over five years ago are not normally considered significant for rating purposes. They might, however, alert an underwriter to the necessity of rechecking the blood pressure if the current readings obtained are normal and there is a history of more than slight hypertension in the past.

Also, it is important to bear in mind that no method of blood pressure averaging should be used mechanically. Simple averaging of blood pressure readings is no substitute for the astute medical judgment required to evaluate the mortality hazard presented by this very complex physical impairment. If averaging seems to distort the significance of any blood pressure reading or series of readings, such as might be the case when one markedly elevated reading is averaged with several normal, or near normal readings, the method should be discarded and the case referred to the Medical Director for evaluation. Similarly, if any reading or readings in a series are considered to be unreliable, either because of their source or because of the conditions under which they were recorded, they should not be used in forming the rating average.

5.2.2. The use of the rating tables — A list of favorable factors. Attention is once more drawn to the fact that the basic and optimal ratings should be used only in the conditions set out in Section 4. The following is a list of the factors which suggest a favorable prognosis and the combined presence of which justifies the use of the optimal ratings:

Favorable family history (see 5.2.3)

Negative personal medical history (see 5.2.4)

Habits (alcohol, tobacco, drugs) not subject to criticism (see appropriate sections of the Manual) [1]

Build favorable (see 5.2.5)

---

[1] The Rating Manual includes underwriting instructions for alcohol and drug abuse. There is also a brief section on smoking. The adverse effects of smoking, particularly in their interrelationship with other existing pathology, are sufficiently stressed to alert underwriters to the mortality significance of the abuse of nicotine.

No albuminuria (see 5.2.6)

Normal ECG (see 5.2.7)

No clinical or radiological evidence of cardiac enlargement (see 5.2.8)

No eyeground changes indicative of angiospastic or malignant hypertension (see 5.2.9)

Reliable medical findings including reliable blood pressure readings

Evidence that blood pressure readings remain constant or increase slowly and that hypertension is not of very recent origin (see 5.2.12)

Absence of any disease liable to lead to further vascular changes, e.g. diabetes mellitus or gout

Absence of any heart disease, e.g. valvular disease or coronary artery disease.

5.2.3. Family history. For the purpose of assessing the blood pressure risk a family history may be regarded as favorable if no member of the applicant's family has died prematurely from, or been afflicted with, any degenerative cardiovascular disease (e.g. apoplexy, hypertension or coronary artery disease), renal disease or diabetes. If two or more such cases have occurred in the applicant's family, the rating that would have been assessed without such family history should be increased by an addition of +50 to +20. In the context of this paragraph ages over 65 are disregarded. Members of the applicant's family are taken to include parents and siblings.

5.2.4. Personal medical history. The prognosis of hypertension is adversely affected when the personal history includes a record of any of the following conditions:

Disease of the kidneys (whether reported as cured or otherwise)

Rheumatic fever

Any cardiac disorder

Any metabolic disorder (e.g. diabetes mellitus or gout)

A history of cerebral angiospasm or any other type of cerebrovascular accident.

Reference to the Medical Director is necessary where hypertension is associated with any such personal history, except in those cases where it is obvious that the risk must be declined, e.g. when diabetes mellitus is combined with a blood pressure rating (basic rating) of at least +50.

5.2.5. Overweight. Slight overweight does not materially increase extra mortality due to moderate hypertension. Marked overweight increases such extra mortality to a greater extent than is indicated by adding the overweight rating to the blood pressure rating.

An overweight rating not exceeding +20 may be ignored in applying the Blood Pressure Rating Tables. An overweight rating exceeding +20 but not exceeding +35 may be applied without additional modification. In that case the blood pressure rating may be based on the optimal ratings only if all the other requirements for favorable consideration are met to the satisfaction of the Medical Director.

An overweight rating of +40 or over should be increased by one half of the basic rating. A credit of −50 may, however, be granted if there is electrocardiographic or roentgenological evidence that the heart is not enlarged.

5.2.6. Albuminuria. Where hypertension exists, the finding of albumin in the urine is an important and usually reliable sign of renal disease. Refer to the sections on urinalysis, nephritis and other renal impairments; this will show that many such cases must be declined [1]. In the most favorable cases the blood pressure rating should be assessed in terms of the basic ratings and the rating for albuminuria added. When, however, albuminuria calls for a rating of +30 up and blood pressure calls for a rating of +50 up, the sum of the ratings should be increased by half the sum of the two ratings.

5.2.7. Electrocardiogram. Sustained hypertension often leads to left ventricular strain and, subsequently, left ventricular enlargement. The electrocardiogram is the most sensitive aid in diagnosing these conditions. See Electrocardiogram, page H2 [2]. The combination of ratable blood pressure and electrocardiographic evidence of disease of the heart is a serious combination which necessitates rejection or a substantial addition to the basic ratings. See also 5.2.8 and 6.4. Refer to Medical Director.

5.2.8. Size of heart (See also 5.2.7). The presence of ratable blood pressure combined with clinical or roentgenological evidence of cardiac enlargement is of serious prognostic significance. All such cases should be referred to the Medical Director. Generally speaking, the basic ratings should be increased, in the case of slight enlargement, by not less than +75, while more than slight enlargement usually necessitates declinature. See also Heart Enlargement page H15 [3], especially for definitions of degrees of cardiac enlargement.

5.2.9. Eyeground changes: Classification and prognostic significance. The retina and the blood vessels of the circulation can be observed through the ophthalmo-

---

[1] A large number of sections of the Rating Manual deals with renal and urinary impairments. The interrelationship between such impairments and hypertension is emphasized wherever the context so requires.

[2] The electrocardiographic criteria (according to BRADLOW and ZION), as stated in the Rating Manual, for the presence of left ventricular strain or enlargement are as follows: Left ventricular enlargement and strain is indicated when there is: High voltage in V leads a) RV 5—6 more than 26 mm., b) SV 1 or 2 + RV 5 or 6 more than 35 mm., c) RV 6 taller than RV 5. High voltage in limb leads a) R 1+S 3 more than 25 mm., b) RaVL more than 11 mm. (in horizontal hearts), c) RaVF more than 20 mm. (in vertical hearts). Delayed intrinsicoid deflection in V 5—6 (0.05 to 0.07 sec.). ST-T depression in V 5—6 and in limb leads with upright QRS. The presence of but one of the foregoing criteria is not necessarily indicative of enlargement or strain. In general, the more of these criteria present, the more likely the diagnosis is to be correct.

[3] The relevant section of the Rating Manual deals, inter alia, with the significance of cardiac enlargement and its measurement, especially by x-ray studies, and also gives ratings for x-ray and clinical evidence of enlargement.

scope. Hypertension, whether essential or secondary, is often associated with certain pathological changes in the appearance of the eyegrounds. Several classifications of these changes have been defined. For prognostic purposes (which includes life insurance underwriting) the following modification of the classification after KEITH-WAGENER is particularly valuable:

Stage I

Minimal narrowing, straightening and sclerosis of the retinal arterioles are the only ophthalmoscopic abnormality. It is difficult to decide whether these minimal changes are caused by hypertension or arteriosclerosis, especially if there is no marked elevation of blood pressure.

Stage II

This is characterized by congestion of veins and a thickening and dulling of vessel reflexes ("copper wire" appearance), localized and generalized narrowing of the arterioles, changes (also known as A-V nicking) at the arteriolar-venous crossings, scattered round or flame-shaped, but small, hemorrhages and very small hard exudates. This stage is associated with essential hypertension; an elevation of blood pressure must be expected when Stage II retinal changes are present. These changes are virtually irreversible. Their presence does not preclude using the optimal ratings, provided the Medical Director is satisfied that no other aggravating factors are present.

Stage III

This stage is characterized by angiospastic retinopathy, as evidenced by localized arteriolar spasms, hemorrhages, exudates, "cotton wool patches", retinal edema. Sclerotic changes of the arterioles may be present but need not be very marked. For evaluation see remarks under Stage IV.

Stage IV

This stage is similar to Stage III, with the addition of a neuroretinopathic sign called papilledema. Stages III and IV are indicative of angiospastic or malignant hypertension. Blood pressure therapy renders many of the Stage III and Stage IV changes reversible. Applicants showing Stage III and IV changes must usually be declined.

Some of the eyeground changes described above are visualized by the illustrations on pages 39 to 42. It should be noted that Fig. 2 (Fundus arterioscleroticus) should be viewed also with reference to the underwriting instructions on arteriosclerosis.

5.2.10. Variations in blood pressure

(a) Labile hypertension

Applicants whose blood pressure fluctuates over short periods from near average to comparatively high values sometimes develop permanent hypertension. In a few cases malignant hypertension may ensue, a disease which calls for rejection. Many cases of labile hypertension must be postponed. Reference to the Medical

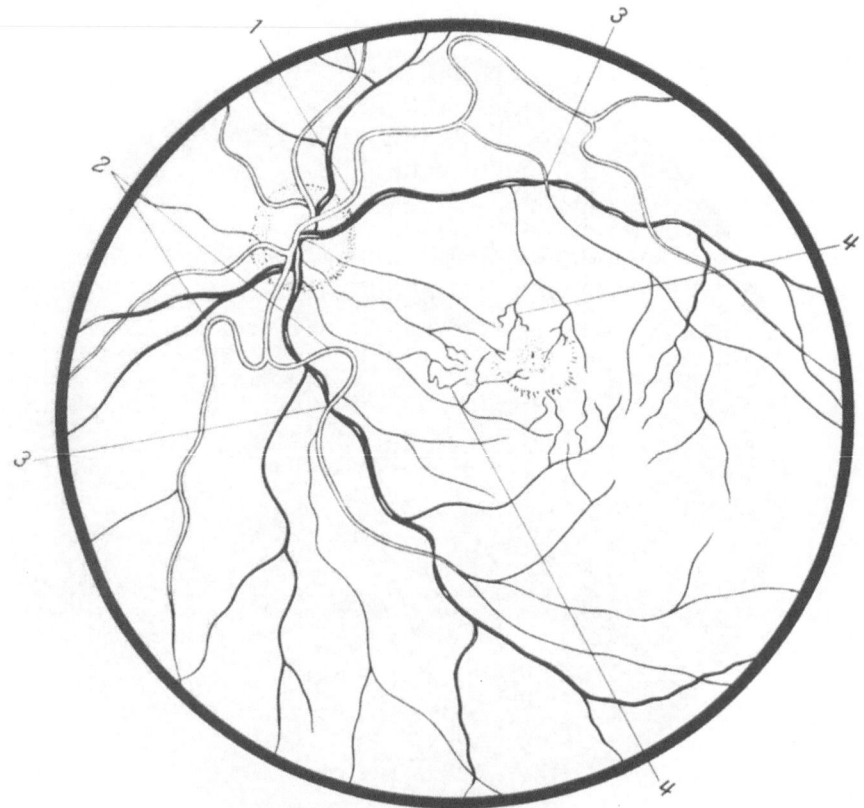

Fig. 1 b. Fundus hypertonicus. Stages 1—2. (1) Retinal arterioles congested. "Copper wire" appearance. (2) Arterioles tortuous. Walls regular, not thickened. (3) Marked indentations of veins at arteriolar-venous crossings. (4) Veins tortuous; corkscrew appearance (Quist' sign)

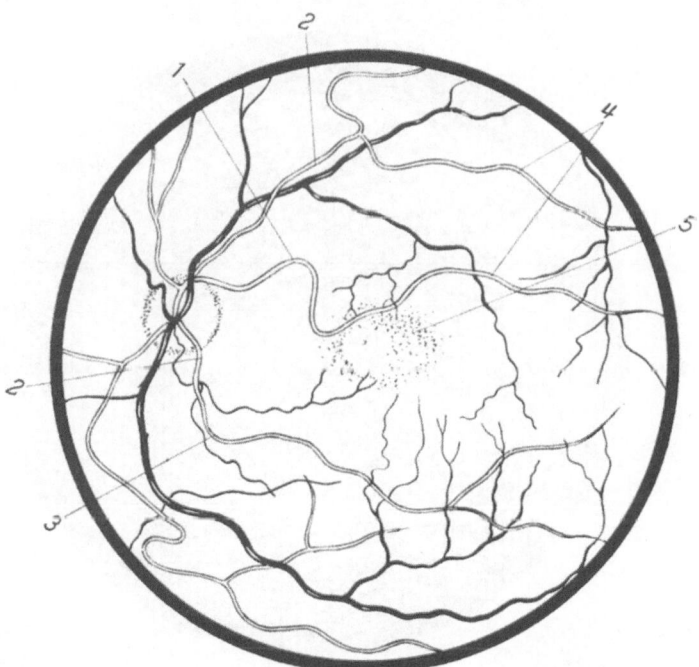

Fig. 2 b. Fundus arterioscleroticus. Stage 2. (1) Retinal arterioles less tortuous than at Stage 1. This is due to the phenomenon described under (2). (2) Thickening of arterial wall with irregular width of lumen. (3) Localized narrowing of arterioles. (4) Generalized narrowing of arterioles. (5) Pigmentation and depigmentation of choroid (choriocapillaris)

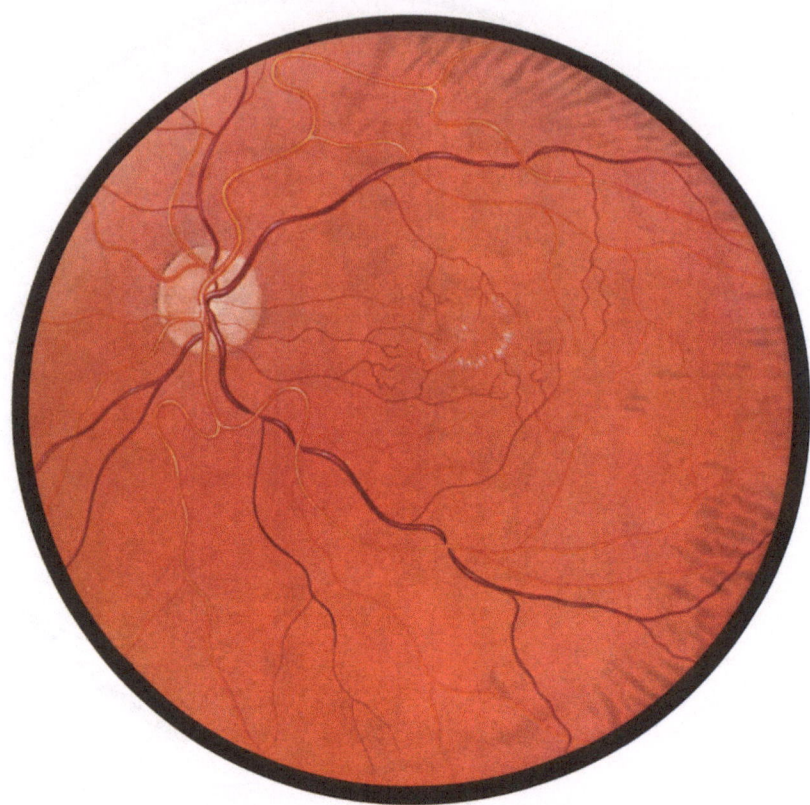

Fig. 1 a. Fundus hypertonicus. Stages 1—2

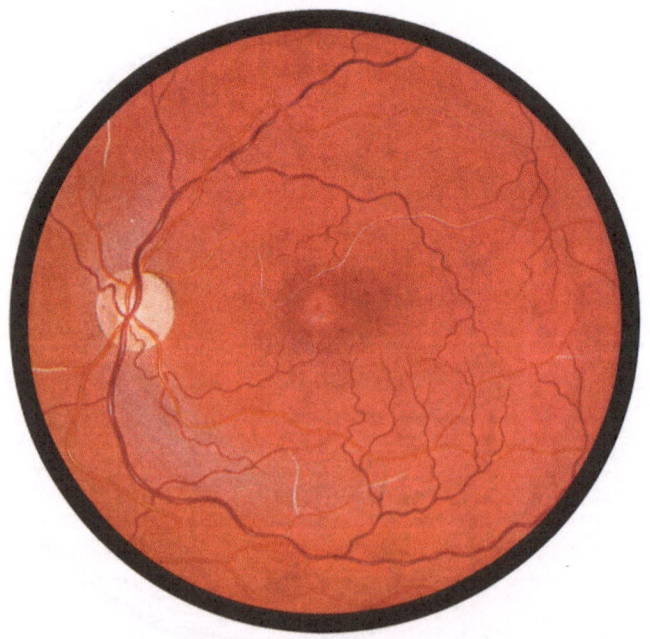

Fig. 2 a. Fundus arteriosclerosis. Stage 2
From Thiel "Atlas der Augenkrankheiten", 6th Edition · Georg Thieme Verlag · Stuttgart 1964

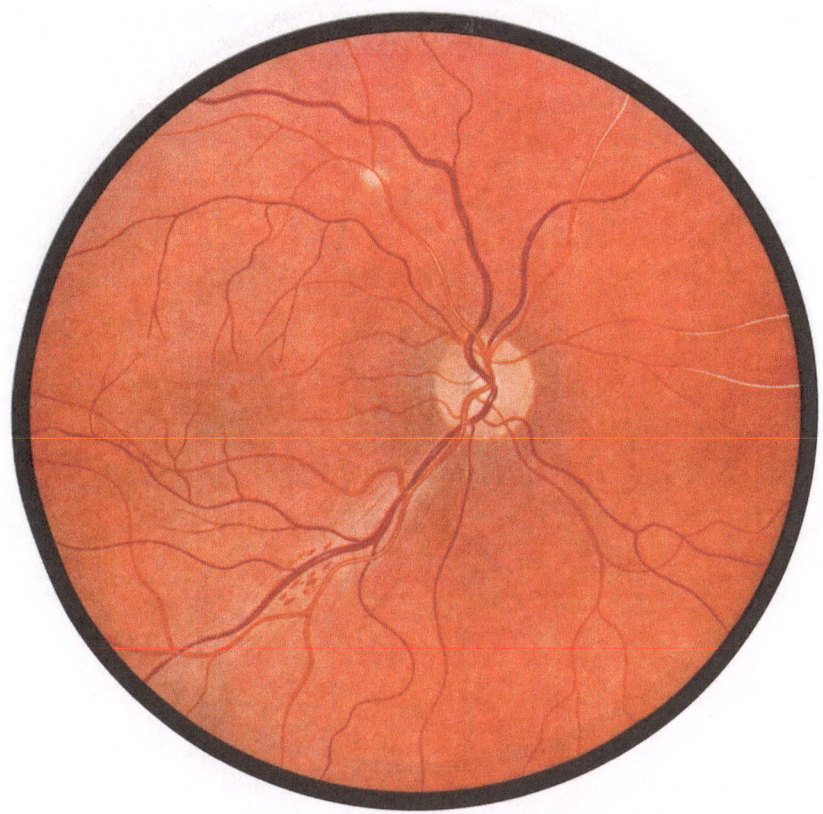

Fig. 3 a. Retinopathia angiospastica. Early stage

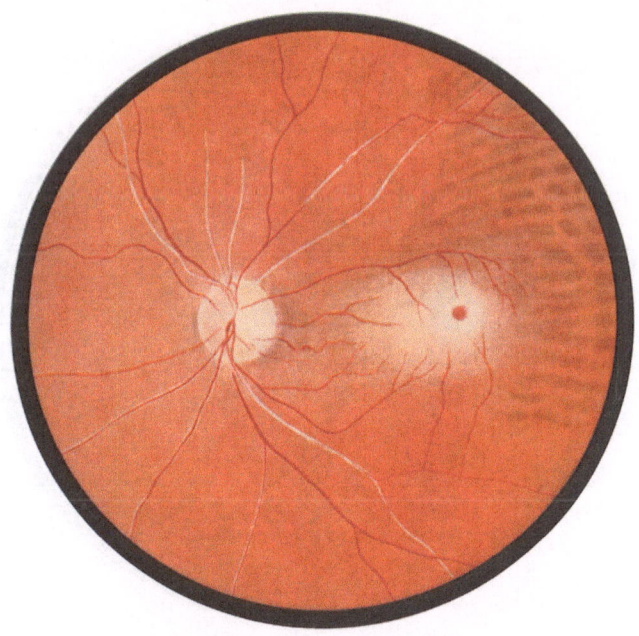

Fig. 4 a. Retinopathia angiospastica. Advanced stage
From Thiel "Atlas der Augenkrankheiten", 6th Edition · Georg Thieme Verlag · Stuttgart 1964

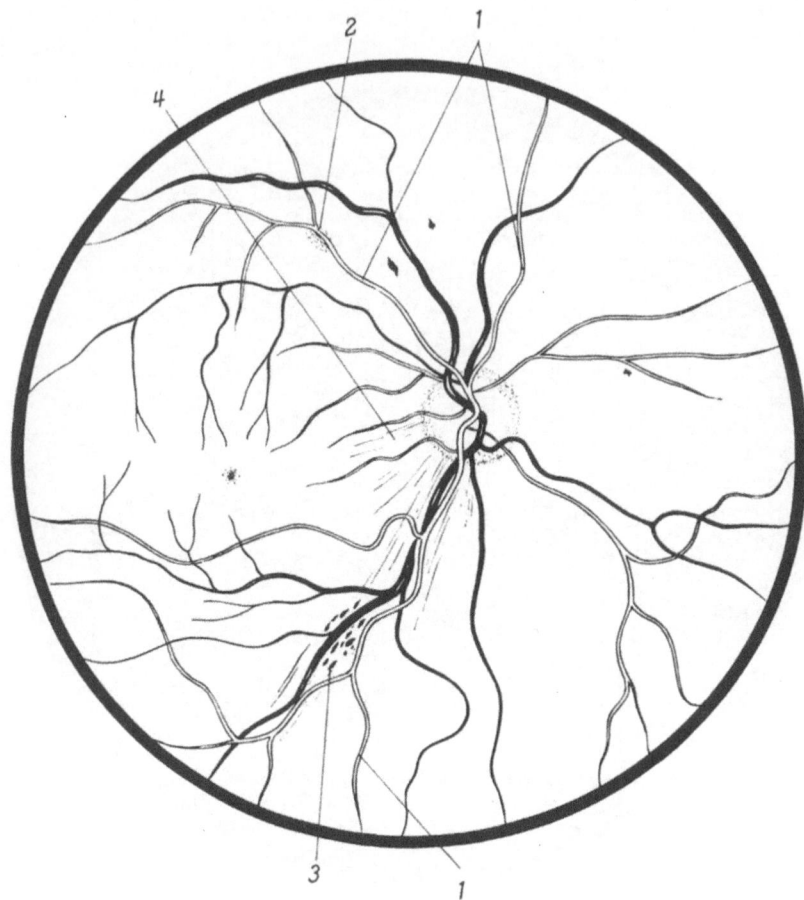

Fig. 3 b. Retinopathia angiospastica. Early stage. Stage 3: (1) General arteriolar constriction. (2) "Cotton wool patches". (3) Fine hemorrhages. (4) Beginning retinal edema

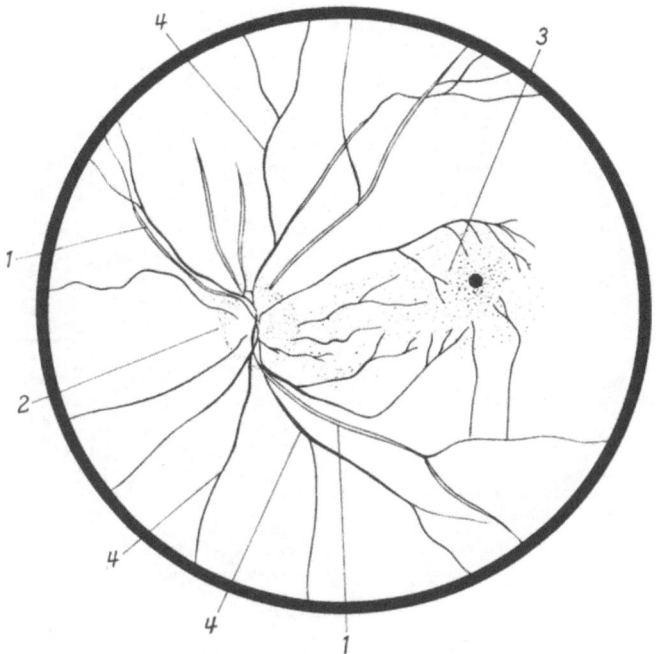

Fig. 4 b. Retinopathia angiospastica. Advanced stage. Stage 4: (1) Advanced arteriolar constriction (silver wire appearance), lumen partially obliterated. (2) Marked papilledema. (3) Ischemic retinal edema. (4) Spasm of the veins.

Director is always necessary. In the most favorable cases the Rating Tables may be used, with the reservation that a minimum rating of +50 be applied.

(b) Reduction in blood pressure

Material reductions (30 mm or more systolic, 10 mm or more diastolic) in ratable blood pressure over short periods (at most six months) may give rise to a suspicion that serious disease is present, or that medical treatment has been instituted. These cases should be referred to the Medical Director (see also 5.2.14).

(c) Malignant hypertension

As stated in (a) above, malignant hypertension should be declined. This disease is characterized by (i) rapidly increasing and very high blood pressure values, (ii) tendency to renal insufficiency and (iii) pronounced changes in retinal vessels (see 5.2.9).

5.2.11. Pulse pressure abnormalities

(a) Wide pulse pressure

A pulse pressure of 60 mm or over suggests the need for a more careful investigation as it may be a sign of aortic valve insufficiency, arteriosclerosis or hyperthyroidism. Ascertain cause and rate accordingly.

(b) Narrow pulse pressure

A pulse pressure of 30 mm or less may indicate heart failure or aortic stenosis. If associated with elevated or normal diastolic pressure it may indicate hypertension under medical treatment.

Underwriting action depends on the cause of the low pulse pressure; many cases will need postponement or rejection.

5.2.12. Duration of hypertension

(a) Hypertension of recent origin

Since hypertension is usually a progressive, and sometimes a rapidly progressive condition, caution must be exercised when evaluating cases of recent onset or recent discovery of high blood pressure. It is preferable to be able to observe the course of the condition for some months or years to judge the rate of progression. Accordingly, when an applicant has not been under medical observation for a reasonable period of time (three to six months) and currently has hypertension requiring a debit of +150 or more (basic ratings) the case should be postponed for three to six months. Milder cases of recent onset may be accepted with the concurrence of the Medical Director.

(b) Hypertension of long standing

Where ratable hypertension is known to have existed for ten or more years, particular care should be taken to exclude any aggravating factors such as those outlined in 5.2.4. Refer to Medical Director.

5.2.13. Female risks. If none of those factors which tend to increase the significance of hypertension are present, female hypertensive applicants may be

assessed in terms of the optimal ratings. Investigations of the risk should be carried out on the same lines as in the case of male applicants.

5.2.14. Low blood pressure. Low blood pressure, also known as hypotension, may be a normal physiological finding and does not usually call for special attention unless the systolic pressure is below 100 mm and/or the diastolic pressure is below 60 mm. When the systolic or diastolic or both readings are below these limits the Medical Director should be consulted.

Marked hypotension may be found in a number of pathological conditions, e.g. cardiac failure, myocardial infarction, Addison's disease and hypothyroidism. Low blood pressure may also be induced by drugs, e.g. an overdose of antihypertensive preparations or tobacco intoxication. See also 5.2.11. Rate for cause.

6. The underwriting of blood pressure abnormalities—with history of treatment

6.1. Surgical treatment

Several surgical procedures have been devised to bring about a control of certain forms of secondary hypertension. The following are the principal surgical procedures; it is apparent that underwriting action must depend on the underlying cause:

Excision of pheochromocytoma or aldosterone-producing tumors of the adrenal gland	See Adrenal Glands, Page A7 [1] and Pheochromocytoma, page P6 [1]
Lumbodorsal sympathectomy (ganglionectomy, splanchnicectomy)	Rate as hypertension, medically treated
Adrenalectomy	Usually decline

6.2. Medical treatment

In recent years many types of drugs capable of reducing blood pressure have come on the market and effective methods of medical treatment of hypertension, based on the use of antihypertensive (or hypotensive) drugs have been, and are being developed. Considerable progress has been made in this field and many cases of hypertension have been brought under control, with correspondingly improved prospects of longevity. But there have also been many disappointments. No longterm follow-up studies are as yet available and the assessment of the mortality hazard of applicants who have undergone antihypertensive treatment

[1] The recommended underwriting action is to defer until one year after operation and then to accept, at suitable ratings, only if the tumor is known to have been benign and there are no sequelae.

is, consequently, still in an experimental stage. (Even the most recent insurance studies afford no guidance on this problem as effective treatment with antihypertensive drugs was not widely applied when the relevant observations were made.) As much has still to be learned about the causation of hypertension and as the modus operandi of many of the antihypertensive preparations is not yet fully understood, it must be expected that the experimental stage in underwriting will continue for a long time. It must also be noted that the effect of treatment often has been most striking in those patients whose pretreatment blood pressure levels were beyond the limits of insurability while patients with lower blood pressure levels may derive comparatively less benefit from treatment.

Successful medical treatment also depends on the cooperation of the patient. Patients often find sustained cooperation difficult because (a) many antihypertensive drugs have unpleasant side effects, (b) treatment may have to be undertaken on a long-term basis, and may often have to be modified, (c) the number of tablets to be taken may be large. The quality and persistence of the patient's cooperation is thus a major factor in underwriting.

The fact that medical treatment may reduce high blood pressure readings to normal or nearly normal levels is used by certain applicants to suppress a personal history of hypertension. The underwriter must be alert to this possibility. — See 6.4. It is apparent that so complex a group of risks cannot be underwritten except in consultation with the Medical Director. It is also obvious that many of these risks will have to be declined and that a large proportion of those that can be accepted cannot receive any credit for their treatment. However, as the following rules will show, worthwhile credits can be granted to a well-defined section of medically treated hypertensives.

6.3. Underwriting requirements

6.3.1. Additional information. The following requirements are in addition to those set out in 5.1:

It is recommended that the application should include a question to the following effect:

> Have you at any time received treatment for high blood pressure or have you at any time taken drugs known for their effect in reducing blood pressure? (If so, state full particulars.)

When it is known that such treatment has taken place, the following particulars should be ascertained from the applicant's attending physician:

> The date on which hypertension was first noticed. The highest and average level of blood pressure at that time.
>
> The nature and degree of any retinal abnormalities noted at that time.
>
> The date on which antihypertensive treatment was instituted.
>
> The type of treatment, including designation and dosage of drugs, used during the various stages of treatment.

The effects of treatment, including representative blood pressure readings and dates of such readings.

Whether treatment still continues.

If treatment was discontinued, when and for what reasons it was stopped.

A specimen form of an Attending Physician's Questionnaire [1] incorporating the relevant questions is included in the Manual.

6.3.2. Other requirements. ECG and chest x-ray for inspection by the Medical Director are normally required. (The chest x-ray may in suitable cases be replaced by a report on a fluoroscopic examination on the applicant's chest.)

6.4. Indications of drug-induced reductions in blood pressure

As stated in 6.2 some applicants suppress the fact that they receive or have received medical treatment for high blood pressure. When there is any suspicion that such treatment has been given and, in particular, that current readings may be affected by treatment, it becomes necessary for the underwriter to proceed with extreme caution. It is known that antihypertensive substances are, in the main, excreted by the kidneys. In principle, therefore, it should be possible to demonstrate the presence of these substances in the urine, if in fact they have been taken. Methods of detection are being developed but they are not yet sufficiently simple and inexpensive to play a major part in underwriting. For the time being, therefore, underwriters and Medical Directors depend on the clues that clinical data may provide. Although not conclusive in themselves, such clues sometimes justify a suspicion that antihypertensive drugs have been administered, and so induce the underwriter either to investigate more thoroughly or decline or postpone the risk. It must not be thought, however, that a careful examination of the clinical picture always provides such clues. In many cases of medically treated hypertension the results of the physical examination provide no clue.

The following is a list — necessarily incomplete — of some of the clues which may lead to a suspicion that the blood pressure level may have been lowered by drugs (where necessary, advice regarding appropriate underwriting action is also supplied):

(a) Blood pressure readings were markedly elevated in the past but current readings are normal or nearly so.

(b) The blood pressure is normal but there is x-ray or ECG evidence of left ventricular strain or hypertrophy or the eyegrounds shows Stage II changes (see 5.2.9).

(c) Marked postural changes in blood pressure are often due to antihypertensive treatment. Some antihypertensive drugs have little effect on the blood pressure in the recumbent position but materially reduce pressure in the upright

---

[1] The recommended form of questionnaire closely follows the suggestions in the text.

position. The advantages of measuring blood pressure in both positions are obvious.

(d) Bradycardia (i.e. a pulse rate of 56 or less per minute) may be induced by certain drugs. This sign is particularly suggestive when accompanied by a collapsing pulse in the upright position.

(e) A swelling of the mucous membrane of the nose may suggest the use of reserpine or drugs of similar composition. This is not a very noticeable symptom. However, if this does come to the attention of the underwriter, and there are other signs or suspicions of antihypertensive treatment, the matter should be examined more carefully.

(f) Nausea, giddiness, vomiting, headaches and tachycardia can be caused by the drug Hydralazine.

(g) Antihypertensive drugs may affect the systolic and diastolic pressures to different degrees. Often the reduction of the systolic pressure is more pronounced than that of the diastolic pressure so that not only is the pulse pressure reduced but also the ratio of systolic to diastolic pressure. When marked departures from average pulse pressure values are noted, consideration should be given to whether the blood pressure readings are being affected by antihypertensive drugs. This question will arise especially when cardiac function appears to be unimpaired.

6.5. Rating principles

6.5.1. Duration of treatment.
Treatment must have continued for at least six months. Reasonable assessment of the effect of treatment is not possible on the basis of a shorter period of treatment.

6.5.2. Factors determining the rating

(a) The pretreatment blood pressure level. All available figures should be considered and an average formed on the lines set out in 5.2.1.

(b) The current blood pressure level. Again all available figures should be considered and an average formed on the lines set out in 5.2.1.

(c) The entire clinical picture as disclosed by the medical evidence, including in particular any permanent damage already suffered as a result of hypertension. The nature of treatment and age of the applicant and his cooperativeness should be considered. Overindulgence in alcohol, tobacco and food should be regarded as factors increasing the hazard.

6.5.3. Rating

(a) If the highest pretreatment blood pressure level is above 220/114, decline.

(b) If the highest pretreatment blood pressure level is below 220/114 but the average pretreatment blood pressure still falls outside the Basic Rating Table and the current blood pressure level is above 140/90, decline.

(c) If the highest pretreatment reading is below 220/114 but the pretreatment blood pressure level still falls outside the Basic Ratings Table while the current blood pressure is 140/90 or lower, rate +200 up. The minimum rating of +200 applies to the most favorable cases only.

(d) If the pretreatment blood pressure level falls within the limits of the Basic Rating Table, extra mortality should be so assessed and the ratings so obtained should, where applicable, be reduced by the percentages shown in the following Table:

Systolic blood pressure	Current blood pressure average		
	Diastolic blood pressure		
	Under 90	90 to 96	Over 96
Under 140 . .	50 %	40 %	0
140 to 155 . .	30 %	20 %	0
Over 155 . .	0	0	0

The Prognosis of Chronic Nephritis

H. SARRE

In principle, chronic nephritis was considered by VOLHARD to be incurable. Its inalterable course led, over the years or decades, to cirrhosis of the kidneys and to death. However, we must assume from our present knowledge of the disease that nephritis is curable even after a considerable period of time. In a survey of 90 patients, ADDIS observed cures after 2 years in 18% of the cases and after 5 years in a further 8%: this was achieved with special dieting and care, of course (see Table 1). With chronic nephritis, modern clearance tests (Inulin and PAH clearance), repeated over a period of years in many cases, have given a constant, almost normal or slightly limited clearance for many years, and in other cases gradual normalisation of the inulin and PAH clearance[1], that is, a slow or partial cure with residual proteinuria, residual hypertension, etc. (See REUBI 1960 and SARRE 1962.) It was possible to demonstrate these cures from chronic nephritis not only by the clearance findings but also by renal biopsy.

Table I. *Period from commencement to cure of glomerulonephritis* (by ADDIS)

Years	No. of cases	
0 to 0.5	21	
1.0	27	~ 82% cured
1.5	12	
2.0	12	
3.0	5	
4.0	2	
5.0	2	~ 18 % cured
6.0	2	
6 to 10.0	5	8 % cured

What is the *life expectation* for cases of chronic nephritis?

In order to assess cases it must be appreciated that chronic nephritis can take two forms: 1. vascular development, 2. nephritis with nephrotic complications.

The *vascular development* is characterised by increasing blood pressure over the years, with little albumen in the urine and possibly the appearance of microhaematuria. Renal insufficiency only occurs in the final stages.

Nephritis with nephrotic complications is characterised chiefly by the high proteinuria (4 to 10%) and the development of a nephrotic syndrome (hyper-

---

[1] The inulin clearance test has a normal range of 100 to 150 ml./min.; the PAH (p-amino-hippurate) clearance test has a normal range of 500 to 830 ml./min.

proteinaemia, dysproteinaemia, cholesterinaemia or edema). Here also it is generally only in the final stages that renal insufficiency occurs. It is not usual to find a marked increase in the blood pressure.

This distinction drawn by VOLHARD roughly corresponds to the American classification made by ELLIS: ELLIS I = vascular development, ELLIS II = nephritis with nephrotic complications.

It has been known for a long time that some patients suffering from chronic nephritis can live for years in good general condition ("kompensiertes Dauerstadium").

Together with ELLINGER, I compared the chronic nephritis cases of the Freiburg Polyclinic for the years 1949—1959 with older records of the Frankfurt clinic (from the Volhard and Nonnenbruch era). The cases of chronic nephritis

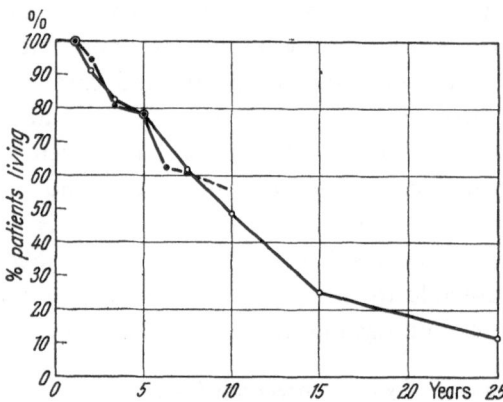

Fig. 1. Chronic nephritis (both forms). Survival period from commencement of disease (164 cases, O—O Freiburg, ●—● Frankfurt)

(77 in all) at the Frankfurt clinic in the years 1930—1945 were evaluated according to the personal medical history, while the 87 more recent cases of the Freiburg Polyclinic were in some instances evaluated according to the personal medical history and in others re-examined, their further development up to 1959 being determined by means of questionnaires. It was possible to assess 87 cases of chronic nephritis of both forms. The results are given in Fig. 1, which shows the proportion of survivors *at differing periods after the commencement of the disease.* The figures for deaths in the first year have been omitted in order to exclude early moribund cases. The survivance curve demonstrates the existence of chronic nephritis with a very long survival time in some cases. (The only cases evaluated were those where the date of commencement of acute nephritis could be clearly ascertained or where it was possible to state accurately when proteinuria, etc., was first observed. For this reason the actual survival times are probably rather longer.)

The curve for the Freiburg cases also shows that only a half of the patients had died after 10 years and that 12% were still alive after 25 years. One of our patients, a doctor, who had suffered from nephritis since 1908, eventually died of uremia in 1958: his professional activities were in no way impaired by his disease. (In a study by DUTZ and associates, covering 21 cases of the ELLIS I type, 15 had died after 10 years, i.e. 71%; of his 11 cases of ELLIS II type, 45%. The figures are, however, too small to justify extensive conclusions.)

It is interesting to observe that the survivance curve (Fig. 1) shows an exponential decline. If it is plotted semilogarithmically a straight line results. It can thus be seen that about 7% of the patients still surviving will die each year. This is strange since one would actually have assumed an increasing mortality rate for these chronic nephritis sufferers. A very similar course is found with essential hypertension (SARRE and LINDNER 1948).

The cases of the Frankfurt clinic are also shown in Fig. 1. These could only be followed up for a period of 7 years but they take approximately the same course as the Freiburg cases, apart from certain deviations which may be a result of less accurate evaluation.

We then divided the Freiburg records into 41 *vascular* cases and 27 *with nephrotic complications* (Fig. 2). In a similar way to DUTZ, we found at first a somewhat poorer development in the vascular forms and later some improvement, but the differences are not significant. The survivance curve of Fig. 1 (both forms together) is just as good as that of the cases of very slight hypertension which we investigated with LIND-

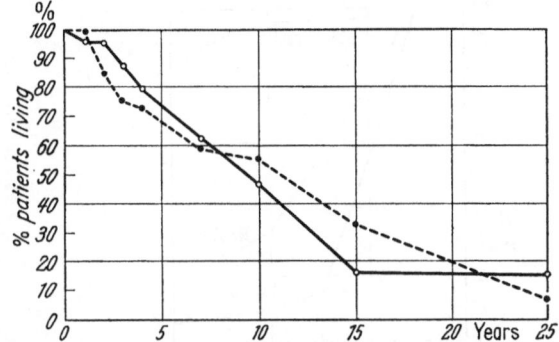

NER some years ago (SARRE and LINDNER 1948). At that time we found that there was stil a 70% survival after 6 years for the group with diastolic pressure below 90 mm Hg. and the group which showed very slight changes in the oculi fundi (THIEL I). This corresponds approximately to the aforementioned survivance curve for all patients with chronic nephritis.

Fig. 2. Same cases as fig. 1, but showing separately the development of vascular (— — —) and nephrotic (o—o) forms

Importance of the blood pressure: The blood pressure, and especially the diastolic pressure, is most important in the life prognosis for chronic nephritis sufferers. In a former work we collated various diastolic blood pressure values with reference to the life expectation of sufferers from chronic nephritis and drew a graph of the number of survivors. It was found that 5 years after the *first examination* of chronic nephritis patients with a diastolic blood pressure below 90 mm Hg., 95% still lived. Of those with a diastolic pressure between 90 and 108 only 32% were still alive and for cases where the diastolic pressure was over 110 mm Hg. the survival was 12%. There were also the cases which died within one year of the first examination but these were discounted in order to exclude the clinic's moribund patients: these would only have falsified the general picture of chronic nephritis sufferers (Fig. 3). It must be emphasized that the survivance curves in Fig. 3 represent a record of *first examinations;* therefore they should not be compared with Figs. 1 and 2 of readings made upon *commencement of the disease.* Since the vascular form mostly involves successive increases in the degree of high blood pressure and kidney insufficiency, the differing paths of the curves in Fig. 3 are attributable to the fact groups 2

and 3 probably contained more advanced cases of chronic nephritis than
group 1. Thus the shorter expectation of life is not a result of the increasing
blood pressure alone, but also of the progressive reduction in renal tissue. These
two processes are parallel both in duration and in pathogeny. Consequently
some patients with chronic nephritis die not from uremia but from cardiac
insufficiency or apoplexy.

The *increase in blood urea* (normal 20—40 mg %) or non protein nitrogen in
the blood can, within limits, be associated with a good life prognosis for chronic
nephritis patients. Fig. 4 clearly shows this. It indicates the average survivance
period in relation to the amount of blood urea at the time of first examination
(107 cases). From the table it may be seen that groups with a moderate blood urea

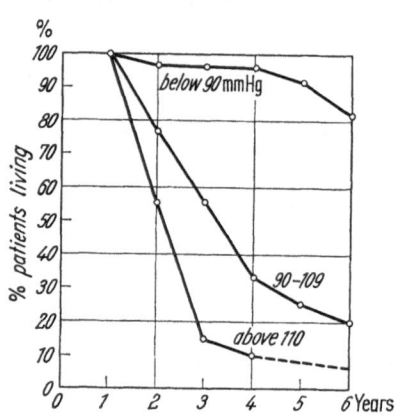

Fig. 3. Life expectation with chronic nephritis, according
to diastolic blood pressure. Percentage survival up to
6 years from commencement of observations (not from
commencement of disease!) (119 cases of chronic nephritis
in vascular form)

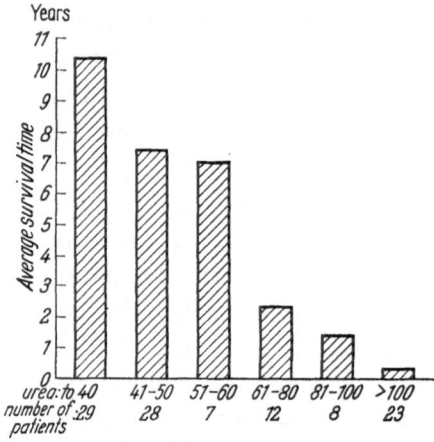

Fig. 4. Average survival time in relation to serum urea
findings upon first examination (107 patients)

increase (41—50, 51—60 mg % blood urea) have a relatively high life prognosis
even of 7.3 and 7.0 years. However, a sharp decline in the life expectation is evident if the blood urea content is more than 60 mg % (Fig. 4). For groups 1, 2 and 3
the significance, calculated by the X^2 method, is high compared with group 4
(P 0.001.). With groups 4—6 it is also high (P 0.001), and likewise with groups
5—6 (P 0.001).

A slight blood urea increase may therefore be associated with a relatively long
survival period. This phenomenon is connected with the fact that a rise in the
blood nitrogen values increases the elimination of nitrogen, causing a normal
decrease in waste products ("compensating retention", SARRE 1959). *60 mg %
blood urea* can be described as the *critical limit*. Nowadays endogenous creatinine
is generally considered to be more reliable, since the blood urea content can be
greatly influenced by the average albumin supply. Detailed investigations by
MERTZ, SARRE and CREMER (1962) indicate a linear relationship between non
protein nitrogen and the plasma concentration of endogenous creatinine. On the

average, 40 mg % non protein-N corresponds to a creatinine value of 2 mg %, 60 mg % non protein-N corresponds to 4 mg % creatinine, 80 mg % non protein-N corresponds to 5.8 mg % creatinine, but with an average dispersion of ± 22 mg % non protein-N! (i.e. a creatinine value of 2.0 can be the equivalent of both a "normal" non protein-N-value of 18 and also a pathological value of 62 mg %!). This illustrates how much more reliable the plasma creatinine estimation is in the assessment of these cases.

Nephritis with nephrotic complications and so-called lipoid nephrosis ("membranous nephritis").

The life prognoses from sufferers from so-called lipoid nephrosis (= *membranous nephritis*) and nephritis with nephrotic complications (ELLIS II) have improved with the introduction of antibiotics and cortisone derivatives into therapy.

Here too we must differentiate between two fundamental forms: 1. nephritis with nephrotic complications and 2. so-called lipoid nephrosis (= membranous nephritis), where there is no clue to nephritis (microhaematuria, elevated blood pressure, renal insufficiency). In adults, instances of the first form are, of course, the more numerous by far. However, the prospects of curing or improving the condition of nephritis with nephrotic complications remain, by the nature of the disease, less bright than for lipoid-nephrosis.

In 1962, ADAMS and associates made an exhaustive survey of a total of 1105 patients to investigate successes achieved in the treatment of the nephrotic syndrome in children and adults. Table 2 shows the results of long-term therapy with corticoids, which is the current practice. The salient feature of this table is the great difference between successes with children and with adults, and we believe this is indeed largely due to the fact that most of the children had lipoid-nephrosis whereas the adults had nephritis with nephrotic complications.

Table II. (by ADAMS *et al.*, 1962)

No. of patients	Short-term therapy	Long-term therapy		
	Total 508	Total 597	Children 333	Adults 120
A. Complete remission . . .	13%	43%	54%	19%
B. Incomplete remission . .	10%	22%	20%	23%
C. Partial effect (only loss of edema) . . .	48%	16%	9%	29%
D. No effect	23%	17%	13%	29%

If we compare these findings with our own figures in 44 cases with nephrotic syndromes over a survey period of 6 years, we find that our cases show somewhat better results as regards cures and improvements than do ADAMS' findings for adults. By dividing our cases into lipoid nephrosis on the one hand and the remaining nephrotic syndrome (mostly nephritis with nephrotic complications) on the other, we perceive the great difference in therapeutic success of steroid treatment of these two main forms of nephrotic syndrome even though adults are involved in both groups (Fig. 5). With lipoid-nephrosis, complete remission occurred in 58% of the cases, but with the other nephrotic syndrome (nephritis with nephrotic complications), it took place in only 12% of cases. In the first group the mortality was 0%, and in the second group 12%.

When one considers that in 1939 OERTEL reported on re-examinations a 25% mortality rate for sufferers from typical nephrosis and a 55% mortality for nephritis with nephrotic complications, one can judge the progress which has been made in modern treatment of the nephrotic syndrome.

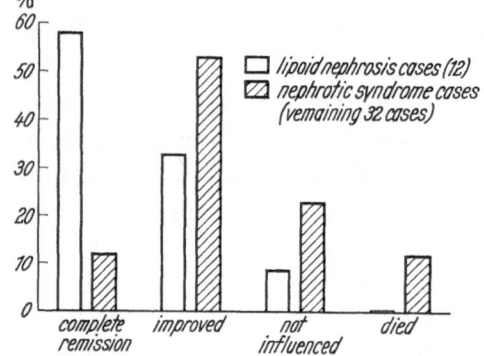

Fig. 5. Success of long-term therapy with corticosteroids (survey over 6 years). Own cases (adults)

In conclusion it should be emphasized that modern clearance tests, especially the estimation of inulin- and PAH-clearance together with clinical findings, permit an accurate diagnosis which was just not possible in VOLHARD's time. One point is that it is now possible for us to separate residual conditions and partial cures from cases of chronic nephritis, especially if we carry out a clearance test two or more times at intervals of a few months. Moreover, we can confirm that many cases of chronic nephritis are fully or partially curable. Finally, we can of course distinguish between acute and chronic nephritis (see SARRE 1962 for details of differential diagnoses). The prognosis of long-term compensated chronic nephritis is favourable over years and decades as the statistics have shown. As I have demonstrated elsewhere, it can exist for many years without impairing the capacity for work. There are many cases where the patient does not even notice it provided the blood pressure has not reached a high level and the function of the kidneys is normal or is only reduced by very gradual degrees (serum urea under 60 mg %). I have discussed elsewhere the working performance and capacity of these cases over the years (SARRE: Der Nierenkranke im Berufsleben 1962). Proteinuria usually has no influence on working capacity if it is not so advanced (generally over 6 gm. per 1000 c.c. Esbach or 8—10 gm. per day) that a nephrotic syndrome with hypoproteinaemia, dysproteinaemia or edema occurs. However, these nephrotic conditions can be influenced so effectively by corticosteroids and other agents, as has been shown, that the capacity for work is often maintained for a long time.

Summary

Even though some patients with chronic nephritis are, as we know now partly or completely curable, the majority of cases are not completely cured. Our own figures for 87 cases of chronic nephritis show that 50% of these cases die within

10 years and the other 50% in some cases have a surprisingly long life expectation. 12% were still alive after 25 years. The prognosis for the form with nephrotic complications was formerly rather less favourable than for the vascular form but the life expectation has been so improved by modern therapy with corticosteroids and antibiotics that it is now almost better than for the vascular form. The decisive factors in the life prognosis are the blood pressure readings, especially the diastolic pressure, and the level of serum urea or nonprotein nitrogen. Reference is made to figures showing the percentage of survivors of chronic nephritis from 1 to 25 years after the commencement of the disease and the average survival time in relation to serum urea findings on the one hand and diastolic blood pressures on the other. In addition there is a report on the results of re-examinations of cases of nephritis with nephrotic complications and also cases of lipoid nephrosis (=membranous nephritis), both diseases showing a marked improvement as a result of modern therapy.

References

ADAMS, D. A., D. BERNSTEIN, and M. H. MAXWELL: Clinical uses of adrenal steroids. Issued by J. Brown and C. M. Pearson. New York: McGraw-Hill Book Co. 1962.

ADDIS, TH.: Glomerular Nephritis. New York: McMillan Co. 1950.

DUTZ, H., J. WENDLER und M. HERBST: Dtsch. Gesundh.-Wes. 1956, 937.

ELLINGER, M.: Doktordissertation, Freiburg 1960.

ELLIS, A. W.: Lancet 1942 I, 34.

HELLMANN, M.: Pediatrics 23, 4 (1959).

LANGE, R.: Dtsch. med. Wschr. 1959, 1442.

MATEER, P.: Am. J. Dis. Child. 93, 310 (1957).

MERTZ, D., H. SARRE und Z. CREMER: Klin. Wschr. 1962, 889.

OERTEL, E.: Dtsch. Arch. klin. Med. 185, 357 (1939).

REUBI, F.: Nierenkrankheiten. Bern: Hans Huber 1960.

SARRE, H.: Nierenkrankheiten. Stuttgart: G. Thieme 1959.

— und H. MAHR: Dtsch. med. Wschr. 1952, 522.

— und E. LINDNER: Klin. Wschr. 1948, 102.

—, J. GAYER und K. ROTHER: Dtsch. med. Wschr. 1957, 1093.

— Der Nierenkranke im Berufsleben. Handb. d. gesamten Arbeitsmedizin Vol. III. München: Urban und Schwarzenberg 1962.

— Dtsch. med. Wschr. 1962, 833.

— In: Das nephrotische Syndrom. II. Symposion d. Ges. f. Nephrologie. Stuttgart: G. Thieme 1963.

SCHALLER, B.: Doktordissertation, Freiburg 1960.

VOLHARD, F.: Die doppelseitigen hämatogenen Nierenerkrankungen. Handb d. inneren Medizin. 2. Aufl. VI, Teil 1 und 2. Berlin: Springer 1931.

A survey of Heart Disease in Africa, with Particular Attention to Southern Africa

B. A. Bradlow, M.D. (Rand.), M.R.C.P. (Lond.), M.R.C.P. (Edin.)

"Ex Africa semper aliquid novi". (Pliny)
("From Africa always something new!")

The multiracial population of the African continent provides a unique source of study in regard to environmental, genetic and epidemiological factors in the aetiology of disease in general, and is of particular interest to the cardiologist. The study of geographical pathology in the natural laboratory provided by this vast continent is of particular importance at the present time, because of the rapid development and emergence from the primitive state of the African populace. Nationalism and industrialism have, since the end of the Second World War, created a number of new states, the people of which show an increasing interest in the way of living common to the Western world.

This awakening and the increasing education of previously primitive people is bound to create new opportunities for life insurance companies, but will bring along with it new and difficult problems in life underwriting because of impairments previously virtually unknown to life insurance companies. It is for this reason that this paper has been written. It is of interest that in Johannesburg which is the most modern and advanced city in Africa, whereas only a decade ago, a negligible proportion of the African population held life insurance policies, at present 12 per cent of the African population of the native townships attached to the city hold life insurance policies [1]. This percentage will undoubtedly increase rapidly.

The major part of this paper will be devoted to Africa south of the Zambesi River, with which part of the continent the author is more familiar, but problems of the whole continent will be mentioned in passing. This area includes part of the present Central African Federation, Mozambique, Angola, The Republic of South Africa and the associated territory of South West Africa and the British Protectorates of Swaziland, Bechuanaland and Basutoland. North of this area is the "Bantu line" which stretches across Africa from the Gulf of Guinea on the West to Tanganyika in East Africa. South of this line the larger part of the population is Bantu or mixed Negro-Hamite, while north of it are the Negroes, Hamites, Nilotes, Arabs and others (Fig. 1).

Table I. *The five different cultures of South Africa with the population figures for each group*

Five cultures		
1. White English speaking 1.2 Mill. ⎫		
2. White Afrikaans speaking 1.8 Mill. ⎭	3	Million
3. Bantu (Africans)	11	Million
4. Cape Coloured (mixed origin) ⎫ sub-group Malays 35,000 ⎭	1.5	Million
5. Asiatics (mainly Indian)	0.5	Million
Total	16	Million

(Negligible: — Bushmen 1500   S. W. A.
Hottentots almost extinct)

In the Republic of South Africa there are at present at least 5 cultures. The numerical composition is shown in Table I. The primitive Bushmen of the Kalahari desert who are probably related to the pigmies of Central Africa are almost extinct and, like the Hottentots who are probably a mixture of Bushman and Hamitic elements, are numerically negligible. At present very little is known of them.

By far the largest group are the Bantu negroids who migrated southward from the Equator. Many still lead very much of a primitive tribal existence, but they are now becoming rapidly urbanized and form the main labour force. They remain economically the poorest of the main racial groups.

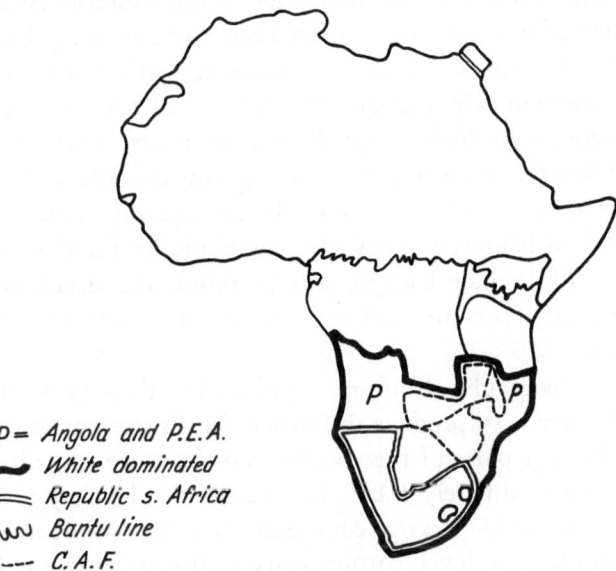

p = *Angola and P.E.A.*
➥ *White dominated*
= *Republic s. Africa*
∿ *Bantu line*
--- *C.A.F.*

Fig. 1. Map of Africa showing the Bantu line, and the main territories constituting Southern Africa

The Cape Coloureds, the largest aggregation of whom live in the Cape Province, but are nevertheless found throughout the Republic, constitute an intermediate group between the African and White groups, both epidemiologically and economically. The Cape Coloured race originated in miscegenation between the original Hottentots, the slaves imported from West Africa, and the East Indies, the White settlers and the Bantu. Their home language is Afrikaans and their culture veers more towards that of the White than the Black races. A proportion of the Cape Coloureds known as Cape Malays have retained their identity, religion (Moslemism) and customs, but not their language. While many

Coloureds are labourers, some are artisans or small tradesmen and a few have entered professions.

The Asiatics are predominantly Indians and are congregated mainly in Natal. There is a small number of Chinese. The Indians were imported about one century ago to work in the sugar cane fields and comprise labourers, waiters, a small professional class and merchants. They are highly westernized and many of them are well educated. They still however retain the culture and religions of the East.

The most highly developed section of the South African population is the white section, whose origins are mainly from the continent of Europe, particularly Holland, the United Kingdom, Germany and, through the Huguenot immigrants, France. They have populated South Africa since 1652 and are subdivided into a larger Afrikaans-speaking group and a slightly smaller English-speaking group. Even in these two groups minor differences of disease incidence occur. The white group has been responsible for the rapid development of South Africa. It has, for example, built large westernized cities like Johannesburg which started as a mining camp in 1886 and has today become the third largest city in Africa after Cairo and Alexandria, with a total population of over 1 million people, of whom about 390,000 are of European extraction. Their standard of living is as high as can be found in any part of the world, and they control industry, commerce and mining and constitute the professional class almost in its entirety. However not all are wealthy, and many are unskilled and semi-skilled labourers. They also constitute by far the greatest proportion of artisans.

With these backgrounds in mind, the diversity of disease patterns due to genetic, economic, cultural and dietary differences will be more readily explicable.

Geographical differences also play their part, and, as explained later in this chapter may produce differences in disease patterns of the same ethnic group in different parts of the country. For instance, the altitude of Johannesburg, which is approximately 5,800 feet above sea level, possibly plays some part in different incidences of conditions like patent ductus arteriosus and, on a more problematic level, coronary artery disease between Johannesburg and the coastal cities.

Certain physiological peculiarities of the various populations require discussion.

At one time it was considered, on the strength of results of an investigation with injection techniques in autopsy specimens of hearts, that a third primary division of the left coronary artery, and preponderance of the right coronary artery were unusually common in the Bantu compared to the White, and this was considered to be the reason for the immunity of the Bantu to atheroma and coronary artery disease [2]. A better intercoronary anastomosis was said to result from such an anatomical difference but further investigations have not confirmed any significant difference in the major coronary artery pattern in the different races [3]. Nor has there been any proof of a suggestion that the intima of the coronary arteries shows any racial differences. However, latter observers confirmed the presence of a better coronary anastamotic blood supply in the Bantu but this cannot explain the lessened degree of atheromatous disease of the coronary vessels [45, 46].

Differences in serum levels of cholesterol exist in the various racial groups. These may be dietary or due to some other cause, but as the theories would occupy a complete and lengthy monograph only the facts need presentation. In Uganda at age 40, the mean serum cholesterol in African men was 145 mg.% whilst in Asians (Indians) it was 248 mg.% which corresponds well with the incidence of coronary artery disease in the two groups [4]. The latter disease is almost non-existent in Africans in Uganda, but is a major problem in Asians [4]. This low serum cholesterol in Bantu and Negroes has been corroborated by studies in South Africa [5, 25, 156] and Nigeria [6]. In Cape Town, the mean serum cholesterol was found to be 168 mg.% in the Bantu, 195 mg.% in the Cape Coloured, and 242 mg.% in the European [7].

Racial differences in blood coagulation have also been shown to exist. Lower plasma prothrombin and serum-factor-VII levels as well as better prothrombin consumption and higher plasma levels of antihaemophilic globulin have been shown to be present in the Bantu as compared to Europeans. The Bantu also generate more plasma thromboplastin, and fibrinolytic activity is faster than in White controls [8]. These differences may mean a diminished thrombotic tendency in the Bantu, but this is speculative as yet, especially as cerebral thrombosis is as common in South African Bantu as in the European despite the difference in the incidence of coronary artery disease [9].

Electrocardiographic studies in normal Bantu have shown special features similar to those seen in lesser degree in American negroes [10, 104]. These changes would be regarded as extremely abnormal in white people, but are compatible with normal health, and are not uncommon in mine labourers working underground and doing heavy work. Autopsy studies after accidental death in such cases has not revealed any cardiac pathology [11]. Effort tests have also not shown ischaemic changes. The abnormal E.C.G. has been described in most parts of Africa among the Bantu, Negro, and Nilotic population, and is familiar to physicians as far afield as Tanganyika, Kenya [115, 118] Southern Rhodesia and the Republic of South Africa [12, 13, 14] and has also been noted to occur in Gabon in French Equatorial Africa [103]. Three main patterns occur but the variations are innumerable. The first pattern is said to be similar to the "juvenile pattern" of the European, and consists of inverted T waves in the praecordial leads, with an upward convexity of the ST segment. The T waves may be inverted in leads V1 to V4 or in midpraecordial leads only (e.g. V3—V4) or in the left praecordial leads or even in all praecordial leads (Figs. 2, 3, 4, 5, 6). A second pattern has considerably raised ST segments ending in a slow rising proximal limb and abrupt descent of the distal limb of the T wave. The third

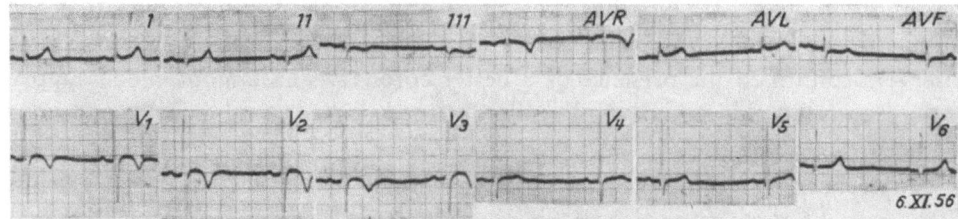

Fig. 2. Persistent "juvenile" pattern (so-called) in normal Bantu

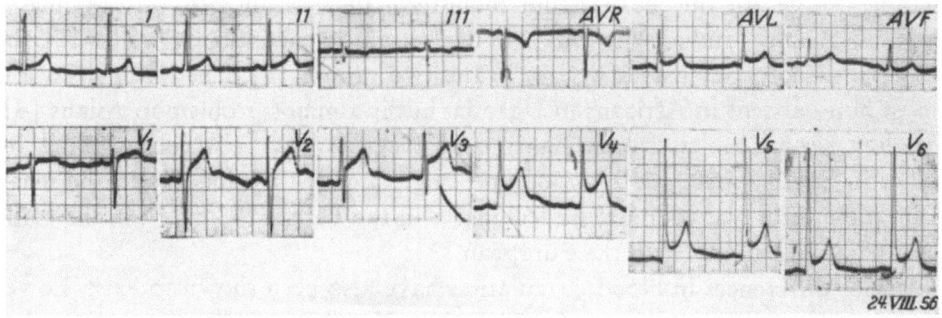

Fig. 3. Typical raised ST segments and high voltage in a normal Bantu male

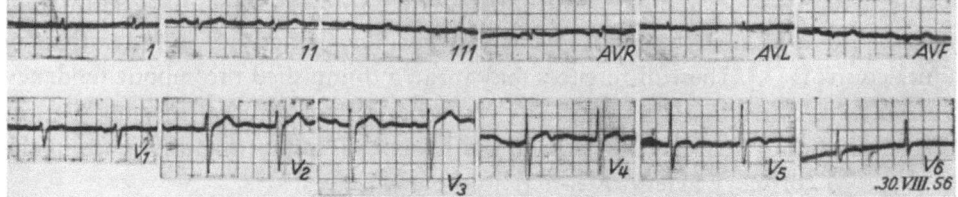

Fig. 4. Midpraecordial T wave inversion in a normal Bantu male

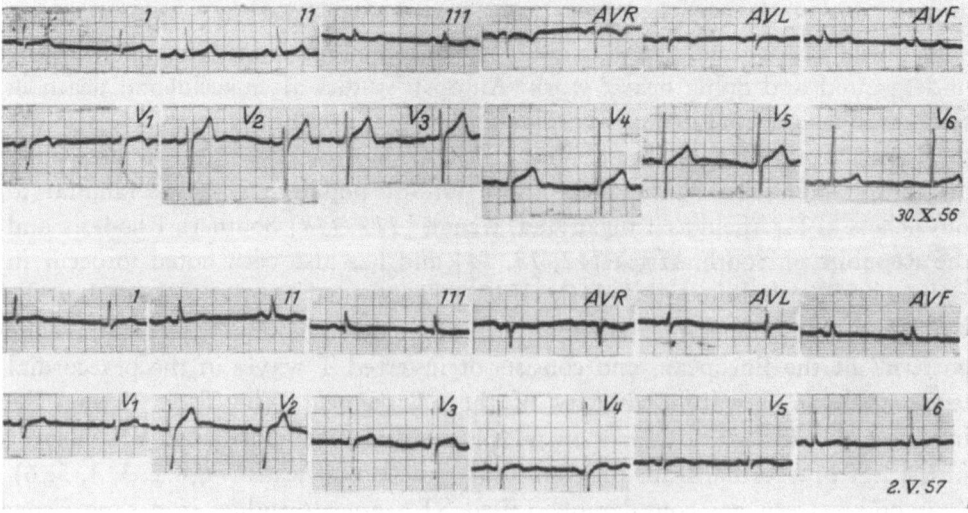

Fig. 5. Two E.C.G's from the same normal Bantu subject showing further T wave changes after an interval of seven months

pattern is a combination of the first and second patterns. A further feature common to all patterns is an extremely high voltage at times, an R wave of up to 40 mm. in V4 or V5 being not uncommon. The author has noted that the slow

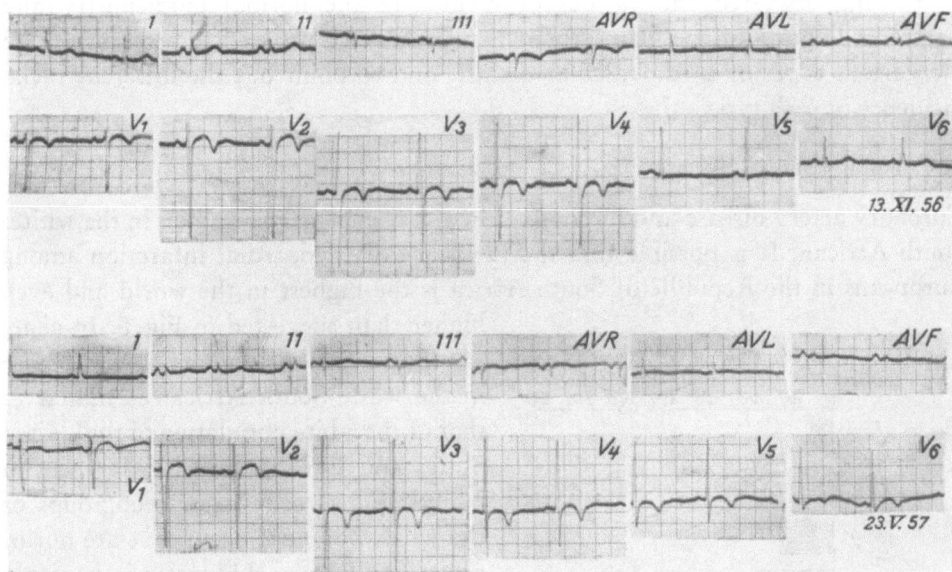

Fig. 6. A further example of so-called juvenile pattern in a normal Bantu male. This shows the extremely high voltage over the chest Leads and extension of T wave inversion to the left chest Leads over a period of six months

ascent of the ST segment to a pointed peak of the T wave with an abrupt descent of the distal limb of the T wave is a common feature in the otherwise normal electrocardiogram of the African and at times may help to identify the racial origin of the subject on whom the record was taken (Fig. 7). The abnormal changes vary from day to day and may disappear with deep inspiration or effort. They are unrelated to the obscure cardiomyopathies so common in the Bantu, and no biochemical abnormality has been shown to be present in subjects with these peculiar E.C.G. patterns. They have not been demonstrated to have any relationship to malnutrition or abnormal liver function tests and their cause remains completely obscure [13, 118] but

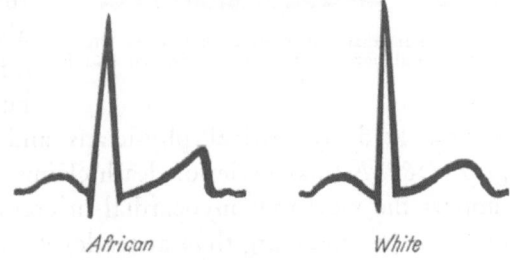

Fig 7. The difference in shape of T wave in White and African (diagrammatic)

the suggestion has been made that these E.C.G. changes may be due to increased vagal tone [11, 12, 115]. The incidence varies in different series from about 20 per cent to almost 60 per cent and is higher in the hospital population [11, 12, 13]. The changes occur in nurses and other similar economic groups as well as in labourers. Furthermore the variants appear to have no relationship to the degree of siderosis, an condition which occurs in over one third of the Bantu population south of the Zambesi river. This condition is due to the large amounts of iron in the food and alcoholic beverages consumed by these people [15].

Having discussed the various differences in the normal biochemistry and electrocardiogram of the main groups it is possible to proceed to a discussion on the various types of cardiovascular disease, and to point out the different racial incidence of each type.

1. Coronary artery disease

Coronary artery disease and its consequences are extremely common in the white-South African. It is possible that the incidence of myocardial infarction among Europeans in the Republic of South Africa is the highest in the world and even higher than suggested in Fig. 8. In general, the pattern of coronary artery disease in the white South African is similar to that of the white population of the United States and Europe. Small differences in incidence between various subgroups of the white populace occur, but are not of great significance. However it is stated that the incidence is higher among the Jews and Africaans-speaking sections, than among those of British origin [16]. In fact, it has been stated that myocardial infarction is more common in Jewish women than in men of British origin in South Africa, although as a rule, men are afflicted very much more frequently than women in any community [17]. It also appears probable that myocardial infarction is more common in Johannesburg than at the coast. This has long been a view held by critical physicians and disputed by others equally critical [157, 158]. A small series of death claims under life insurance policies appear to support the view that myocardial infarction in white people may be more frequent in Johannesburg than at sea level, but as places of residence at the time of death or after issue of the policies were not enquired into, these figures are too unreliable to be quoted.

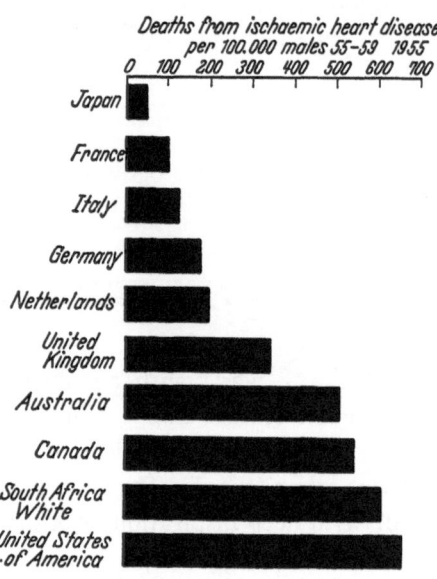

Fig. 8. The International incidence of Ischaemic Heart Disease (1955) (modified from BRONTE-STEWART [40] F Fig. 1)

However, the differences in certain parameters in Johannesburg and at sea level have been analyzed. Table II shows the climatic and population differences in the two cities of Johannesburg and Cape Town. It will also be seen that there is a considerable difference in atmospheric pressure and oxygen saturation of arte-

Table II. *Climatic, population and certain physiological parameters compared in Johannesburg and Cape Town*

	Cape Town	Johannesburg
Altitude:	Sea level	5,900 ft.
Climate:	Winter Rainfall-Cool Humid Summer dry and hot	Winter — dry and cool Summer rainfall — hot Humidity low.
	(Winter: June to August) (Summer: September to May)	
Seasonalinc idence of myocardial infarction	Similar (Winter increase)	
Population	W 280,000 CC 380,000 BA 65,000 AS 9,500 Total 730,000	W 390,000 CC 57,000 BA 623,000 AS 27,000 Total 1,097,000
Tempo	slow	fast
Atmospheric pressure	760 mm. Hg.	609 mm. Hg.
O$_2$ content of blood	19 vols% (95% sat) (20 vols% O$_2$ cap.)	18.7 vols% (91%) (20.3 vols% O$_2$ cap.)
Lung ventilation . .	normal	plus 15
Heart size	identical	
Blood press.	identical	
Smoking . . . . . (20 cig. daily)	HB co equals 5%	HB co equals 5% (Alt. of 12,000 ft.)

rial blood, as well as an increase of 15 per cent in lung ventilation at the higher altitude. These differences account for the inability of even well-trained and acclimatized athletes to perform well at high altitudes in long distance events

Table III. *Pulmonary artery pressure and arterial oxygen saturation at various altitudes. ([154] for figures from Denver, Leadville, and Morococha.) The arterial saturation for Leadville appears to be rather higher than expected, as the Johannesburg figures have been rechecked*

Pulmonary artery Pressure and O$_2$ sat.% at different altitudes.			
	(Alt. Ft)	M.P.A.(mm.Hg)	Art. O$_2$ Sat %
Cape Town (S. A.).	0	13	97
Denver (USA) . .	5,280	16	95
Joh'burg (S. A.). .	5,800	17	91 **
Leadville (USA) .	10,150	25	92
Morococha (Peru) .	14,900	28	78

such as a one mile race. It appears improbable at present that any athlete could run a "four-minute mile" at the altitude of Johannesburg. It is also notorious that unacclimatized sportsmen are incapable of prolonged exertion on first arriving from sea level. Table III shows the increase in mean pulmonary artery pressure and decrease in arterial oxygen saturation as the altitude above sea level increases. These studies appeared to suggest that there may in fact be further significant differences, and for this reason investigations have been started by the Department of Medicine of the University of the Witwatersrand [18, 162]. These are as yet incomplete. Preliminary results are detailed in Tables IV to VI inclusive, and Figs. 8 and 9. Table IV shows the increase in the ventilation

Table IV. *The differences between various blood and gas levels and lung ventilation at an altitude of 5,800 feet (Johannesburg) and at sea level* [164]

	Johannesburg	Sea level
O$_2$ tension.	85 mm. Hg.	105 mm. Hg.
Ventilation aequivalent	2.4 L/min	2.0 L/min
O$_2$ saturation.	92%	97%
Haemoglobin	16.4 G%	15.6 G%
Alveolar p^{CO_2}	35 mm. Hg.	41 mm. Hg.

Table V. *Electrolyte and haemoglobin levels in Johannesburg and Cape Town*

	Johannes- burg (5800′)	S. E.	Cape Town (sea level)	S. E.	Significance "p"
Sodium	138.6	.324	140.4	.361	.02—.05
Potassium	4.09	.030	4.04	.025	. 4—.3
Chloride	105.7	.330	103.1	.584	.01—.001
Bicarbonate	21.82	.984	24.0	.252	.02—.05
Phosphorus	3.81	.112	3.64	.117	. 5—.4
Haemoglobin	16.4	.157	15.60	.181	.01—.001

Table VI. *Blood volumes at two different altitudes* [18]

No. of subjecets	Altitude	Red cell volume (^{51}Cr) (ml./kgm.)	Plasma volume (Risa) (ml./kgm.)	Venous haematocrit (per cent)	Body haematocrit (per cent)	Body venous haematocrit ratio
18	Sea level	30.53 ± 0.694	43.96 ± 0.799	45.83 ± 0.512	40.99 ± 0.358	0.902 ± 0.00965
18	5,740 ft.	35.72 ± 0.817	41.40 ± 0.584	48.11 ± 0.551	46.25 ± 0.549	0.962 ± 0.00830

aequivalent in Johannesburg and the diminished alveolar p^{CO_2} as compared to Cape Town. The diminished alveolar p^{CO_2} may explain the significant differences of sodium, chloride and, in particular, of bicarbonate in normal individuals at the two altitudes as shown in Table V. This table also reflects the increased haemoglobin in the peripheral blood, the reason for which is obvious in Table VI where it is seen that the red cell volume, venous haematocrit and body haematocrit and the body to venous haematocrit ratio are all significantly increased at the higher altitude, while the plasma volume is slightly decreased. Figures 9 and 10 show these differences graphically. The implication that can be deduced from these latter differences in plasma volume and red cell volume and haematocrit is that the viscosity of the blood is increased at the higher altitude, and that clotting is thus more likely, while the work of the heart is increased. It is presumptious to consider that this results in a higher incidence of myocardial infarction at high altitudes, but if in fact such an increased incidence does exist, (and this latter aspect obviously requires investigation) the blood changes may be one of the factors responsible. In the case of Johannesburg and Cape Town however, other factors may result in a possible different incidence of myocardial infarction in the two cities. In Cape Town the tempo of life is slower, and the presence of the sea and Table Mountain more conducive to physical exercise whereas in Johannesburg competition in all fields is keener, resulting in more tension, longer working

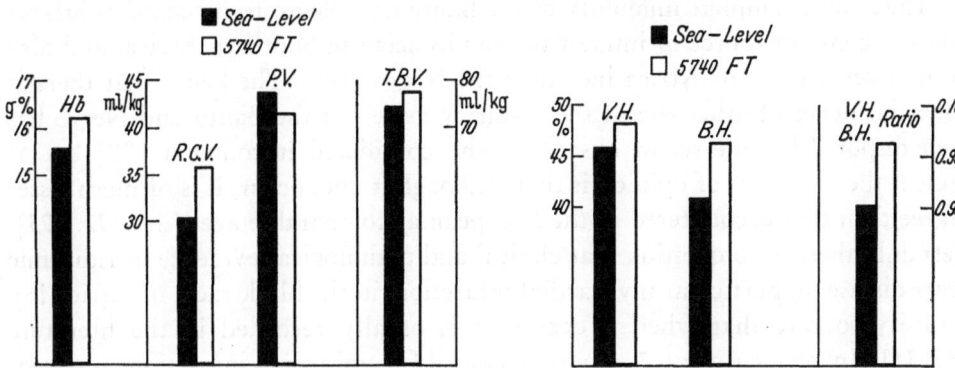

Fig. 9. Blood volumes at different altitudes (Hb=Haemoglobin, in Gm. per cent, R.C.V.=Red Cell volume in ml./kg., P.V.=Plasma Volume in ml./kg., T.B.V.=Total Blood Volume in ml./kg. [162]

Fig. 10. Haematocrit levels at two different altitudes (V.H.=Venous Haematocrit., B.H.=Body Haematocrit) [162]

hours, and less physical exercise. Although, as shown in Table II, the climate differs in the two cities, Johannesburg having a dry atmosphere with a summer rainfall and Cape Town being more humid and having a winter rainfall, the seasonal incidence of myocardial infarction is the same in both cities [49, 50]. The seasons are of course the same in both cities despite the fact that Cape Town is 1000 miles further south. The future studies on such differences in climatic and working conditions should yield a rich dividend in knowledge concerning certain aspects of the aetiology of coronary artery disease.

The Asiatic appears to suffer from coronary artery disease to the same extent as the European in South Africa [17, 19] and probably in Uganda [4, 20]. In Bulawayo in Southern Rhodesia the crude death rate from arteriosclerotic and degenerative heart disease among the Coloured and Asian subjects combined showed a frequency of less than one quarter of that of the European [21]. However, this incidence is undoubtedly too low for the Asian as it is too high for the Coloured, and, being based on municipal statistics of crude death rates, it is not really comparable to the figures for Europeans in the same study as these were based on clinical diagnosis [21]. As in fact the Indian in South Africa has a considerably greater incidence of diabetes mellitus than the European, and diabetes is known to predispose to coronary artery disease, it is natural to expect a high incidence of coronary artery disease among Indians [17, 22]. However, it has been shown in at least one study that atheroma of the coronary vessels in the Indian is of lesser degree and severity in the Natal Indian than in Whites from the same area [24].

The Cape Coloured is intermediate between the European, Asian and the Bantu groups in the incidence of coronary artery disease. In a Cape Town study, whereas 23 per cent of electrocardiograms showing ischaemia were found among the total electrocardiograms recorded on white people, the percentage was 11 cent for the Cape Coloureds, and 2 cent for the Bantu [23] showing the intermediate position of the Coloureds as regards coronary artery disease incidence.

The almost complete immunity of the Bantu and Negro to myocardial infarction is a constant source of interest to the physician in Southern Africa, and also in most other parts of Africa including the Negro areas. The belief that there is a low incidence of atheroma of the coronary vessels in the Bantu and Negro has been disputed by one set of observers who considered it common [28] but at present the consensus of opinion is that, although it does occur, it is of much lesser degree than that encountered in the European at comparable ages [24—32, 103]. Certainly there is no question that clinical and pathological evidence of ischaemic heart disease, in particular myocardial infarction, in the black races of Africa is a curiosity so rare that when it occurs, it is usually recorded in the literature [33, 34]. In one series of 3 reported cases of myocardial infarction, one was associated with severe hypertension without atheroma of the coronary vessels, and one with syphilitic aortic incompetence without involvement of the coronary vessels or their ostia while one was due to atheroma [33]. The literature abounds with confirmatory evidence that myocardial infarction in the African is almost non-existent [4, 6, 21, 23—25, 27, 29—44, 102, 103, 107, 143]. This statement applies to the whole of Africa wherever Bantu or Negro are found. It has sometimes been stated that the low incidence of ischaemic heart disease in the Bantu is the lessened expectation of life so that few individuals live into the "coronary age group" but investigations in the elderly Bantu show clearly that this is not the case, and show that coronary ischaemia is rare in all Bantu age groups [32, 107, 121]. It is however of interest that at Baragwanath Hospital, Johannesburg, in the last 11 years, with an annual admission rate of 30,000 to 50,000 Bantu, 30 cases of myocardial infarction were diagnosed on clinical and pathological evidence [17]. This hospital serves a population of 500,000 people, most of whom are rapidly becoming "Westernized". The majority (19) of the 30 cases occurred in the last four years, and included, among others, cooks, teachers, and other highly paid workers. Four were diabetics although in general diabetes is still a comparative rarity among the Bantu [47]. In all 30 cases the cholesterol or one parameter of a lipogram was raised, even by European standards. Thus, although still extremely rare, it is possible that with the adoption of European standards of living, myocardial infarction is beginning to occur in the Bantu.

The causes of the incredible difference in frequency of ischaemic heart disease in the White and Black races is undergoing intensive investigation. Dietary factors may be important, the South African Bantu consuming maize as his main food with additions of sorghum, beans and pumpkin, occasional meat and often soured milk. The total fat content in the Bantu diet supplies only 18 per cent of the calorie value whereas the Whites obtain 43 per cent of their calories from fats, the total calorie value of both the diets consumed by Black and White being similar [6]. It is of great interest that, in white prison communities in South Africa, myocardial infarction is exceptionally rare, possibly due to less fat in the diet and this applies too to the poorest section of the white population [54]. However genetic factors, physical exercise, smoking habits, hormonal factors and emotional stress have also to be considered in a disease state which is notorious for its multifactorial aetiology. This subject requires a separate monograph and has been adequately discussed elsewhere [119]. It is known that certain lipid fractions such as the triglycerides in the plasma are equally low in both Bantu and White prisoners on low saturated fat diets in South Africa, and that this fraction is equally raised by diets containing a high saturated fat content, but the significance of such observations remains to be seen [120].

Although, in general, atheroma of all vessels including the cerebral vessels is less in the Bantu than in White people, cerebro-vascular accidents, in contrast to the rarity of myocardial infarction, are extremely common, [102] and this paradox may be partly explicable on the basis of hypertension and syphilitic arteritis as discussed later.

Sudden death in the Bantu on the Witwatersrand (Johannesburg) is nearly always attributable to cardio-vascular syphilis whereas in White individuals of the same area, it is nearly always due to cardiac infarction [36]. Similarly, ventricular aneurysms in Europeans are always caused by coronary atherosclerosis, while in the Bantu ventricular aneurysms are not uncommon but are never due to atheroma but are caused by syphilis, tuberculosis, mycotic abscesses and other conditions [36].

2. Hypertension

In the Whites, hypertension appears to have the same incidence and pattern of disease as in their Northern ancestors, and requires no discussion. In England and Wales in 1952, 4 per cent of deaths were classified as being due to hypertension [52], whereas in White South Africans it was 2.65 per cent. This difference is not really significant.

Among the Indian population of South Africa and East Africa, hypertension appears to have much the same incidence and pattern as in the Whites. In the figures supplied by the Bureau of Census and Statistics of the Republic of South Africa, deaths due to cerebro-vascular disease and hypertension are classified separately, and from these figures it appears probable that hypertension is a

slightly more frequent cause of death in the Indian than in the White or
Coloured races [51]. The difference is not really significant but certainly
(Table VII) requires further clinical investigation. Deaths due to cerebro-vascular
disease however appear to be similar in incidence in the White and the Asiatic
(Table VII).

In the Cape Coloured too, the frequency of hypertension is much the same
as in the European and Indian (Table VII) [53]. However the disease seems to
appear at an earlier age especially in the female, and to be more severe than in
the European [53]. Cerebro-vascular accidents are, however, apparently less
frequent as a cause of death among Coloureds compared to Indians and Whites
[17] (Table VII).

Table VII. *The incidence of cerebrovascular disease and hypertension in 3 racial groups (* calculated from figures in [51])*

	White	Asiatic	Coloured
Cerebro-vascular disease . .	11.9	9.2	5.4
Hypertension	2.65	4.5	2.83

* Percentage of deaths (1958). Republic of South Africa.

In the Bantu of South Africa and Southern Rhodesia, hypertension is at least
as frequent and possibly more frequent than in Whites [17, 35, 41, 42, 53, 55, 56,
57, 134]. Hypertension also appears a decade earlier in the Bantu than in the
White race, and the general impression is that malignant hypertension is more
frequent than in the European [60]. From the aetiological point of view essential
hypertension is the most common type in the South African Bantu [59]. Cerebro-
vascular accidents in the Bantu are also common and are a cause of 3 to 4 per cent
of deaths [9, 61, 102]. However syphilis too plays its part in the production of
the frequency of cerebro-vascular accidents.

It appears that hypertension is in fact universally common in Bantu and
Negro Africans, and may be the most frequent cause of heart disease on the
continent [20]. In East Africa and Liberia hypertension among Africans appears
to be less frequent than in other areas, but this requires confirmation [62—67,
71, 105]. In fact hypertension was at one time claimed to be almost non-existent
in East Africa [62, 63, 65]. Death from cerebro-vascular disease in Uganda
natives is also apparently extremely rare, being the cause of only 0.3 per cent of
the total deaths [68]. More recent information from Gabon and Nigeria
however, confirms that hypertension on the African West Coast is of the same
order as that seen in the White races [72, 73, 103].

In the Arab-Egyptians of Egypt, hypertension is apparently almost as
frequent as in Europe, and in the Arab-Berbers of Algeria, the incidence has
risen considerably, especially in the cities [69, 70].

While hypertension among the South African Bantu is less often due to
renal disease than in White subjects in Britain [59 108], in East Africa it is said

to be more often the result of renal disease [64, 111, 112]. This has also been claimed at times for the South African Bantu but is open to considerable doubt [59, 108—110].

It is of interest to compare the frequency and severity of hypertension among the Bantu especially in Southern Africa, with that of the American Negro, who is known to get hypertension twice as frequently as the American White, and to get it at an earlier age, and also in a more malignant form [74, 75, 76, 106]. The disease patterns in the American Negro and Southern African Bantu appear to be similar, and a genetic influence may be the common factor.

3. Cryptogenic or idiopathic heart disease

Heart disease of unknown origin is to the Negro and Bantu African what ischaemic heart disease is to the White man. It is the "heart disease of Africa", and is known by various names. To confuse the issue further, the entity of cryptogenic heart disease in Africa comprises more than one syndrome. Generic terms such as "cardiomyopathy", "cardiopathy" or "primary parietal endomyo-carditis" [78] are frequently used to embrace all forms. A further term used to group all forms is "primary mural endocardial disease" [77]. These diseases have no relationship to the condition of endocardial fibroelastosis [103, 114].

Endomyocardial fibrosis (E.M.F.) appears to have been the form first described in 1946 by BEDFORD and KONSTAM in West and East African native troops [79]. Since then this form has been extensively studied, in particular by DAVIES and his colleagues in Uganda [80, 81, 82]. It is extraordinary that the disease is rare in neighbouring Kenya [83], and virtually unknown further south in Southern Rhodesia and South Africa. It has been reported in the Sudan and probably in West Africa and in the Belgian Congo as well as French Equatorial Africa [103, 104, 139]. In the White races it is extremely rare, but isolated cases have even been reported in Europe and the United States [84—89]. Many of the White patients reported on other continents have at some time lived in Africa [103].

The pathology of E.M.F. consists essentially of enormous fibrosis giving a thick rugose appearance to the endocardium like sugar icing, the fibrosis having a rolled edge. Both ventricles and atria may be affected, especially the inflow tracts of the ventricles involving the papillary muscles, chordae and the posterior cusps of the atrio-ventricular valves. The right ventricle shows a characteristic depressed area over the apex due to the almost complete obliteration of the cavity. Despite a very thick layer of clot over the fibrous tissue, emboli do not occur [90] (Fig. 11).

The clinical picture is almost always that of right heart failure with severe dyspnoea, peripheral oedema, and pain over the enlarged liver together with some left heart failure. In a few cases there are no distinguishing signs of valvular involvement. Most however have signs of valvular disease the majority having a regurgitant apical systolic murmur and occasionally a short or faint diastolic murmur. Some have a palpable systolic thrill. These latter cases present as mitral incompetence, but a smaller number present as tricuspid incompetence or as combined mitral and tricuspid incompetence. Triple rhythm is almost invariable [113]. The pulse pressure is invariably small. In some patients the picture more closely resembles constrictive pericarditis both from the haemodynamic and clinical aspects, even to the presence of a loud third sound, but as a rule cardiac enlargement, and absence of pericardial calcification, as well as a thin pericardium on x-ray after introduction of air, suggest the correct diagnosis of obliterative endocardial fibrosis. Hydropericardium is common.

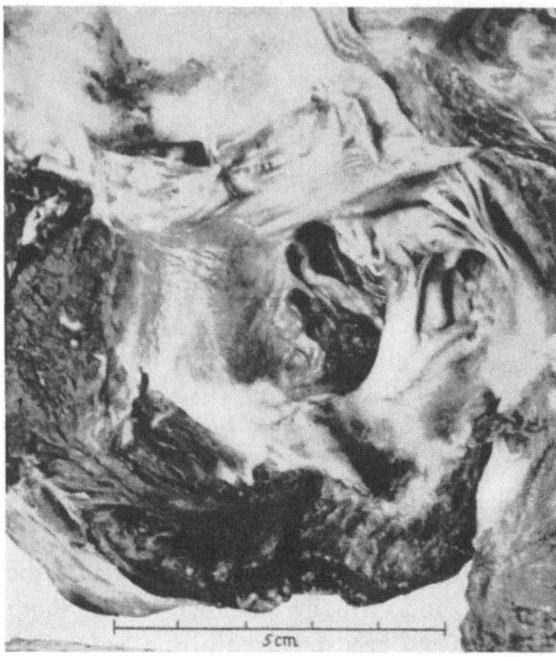

Fig. 11. Endomyocardial fibrosis. Cavity of left ventricle showing the mass of fibrous tissue at the apex and extending up on the posterior wall (Published with the kind permission of Prof. J. N. P. DAVIES and the Editor of the Central African Medical Journal [80]

Roentgenograms show cardiac enlargement in all cases with diminished pulsation and left or right atrial enlargement. The electrocardiogram is usually of low voltage and may show low T waves and incomplete right bundle branch block, but is of little value in diagnosis [90, 113].

The prognosis is poor, and death usually occurs within 20 months of observation, although rare cases may live longer. Remission is unusual, and the response to conservative treatment for heart failure is poor [80, 81].

In Nigeria, ABRAHAMS and BRIGDEN have described an almost identical entity which on clinical and radiological investigation and on cardiac catheterisation, shows pulmonary hypertension [91, 92]. The E.C.G. usually shows sinus rhythm, left atrial and right ventricular hypertrophy. Aschoff-like nodules in the endomyocardium and myocardium as well as a raised antistreptolysin-o titre suggested to these authors that this disease may represent an unusual expression of rheumatic fever, in areas where the latter disease in its usual form is extremely uncommon. They suggested that tropical causes of anaemia, intestinal parasites and protein malnutrition, which are all common in East and West Africa, may be causative factors. It would appear that these observers have described the disease known in Uganda as E.M.F., and that only one clinical entity exists, the aetiology of which is by no means certain. Recent clinical and haemodynamic studies in Uganda confirm the similarity of the Nigerian and East African diseases [113].

In Southern Rhodesia and the Republic of South Africa a different form of cardiomyopathy of non-coronary origin exists [90]. This was first adquately described in the Bantu by GILLANDERS in Johannesburg under the term of "Nutritional Heart Disease" [93, 94]. However it soon became apparent that the disease was not due to malnutrition and that the same disease was indeed described also in Johannesburg as "Cardiovascular Collagenosis" [96] under the mistaken impression that the two conditions were separate entities [90]. The disease is extremely common in South Africa and is the most frequent type of heart disease among Bantu admitted to hospital, at least in the Cape, Natal, Johannesburg and further north in Bulawayo [40, 41, 42, 78, 97, 107, 143, 146]. The disease is by no means confined to the Bantu, but occurs also, though to a far lesser extent, among the well-nourished and, in many cases, prosperous Europeans (Table VIII). It is also more than likely that many cases of cardiomyopathy of

Table VIII. *Incidence of Idiopathic Cardiac Hypertrophy (I.C.H.) compared to that of Myocardial Infarction (M.I.) when the latter is taken to represent 100 per cent, in several series*

	I.C.H.% CF M.I. (= 100%)			
	Race			
Series	White	Bantu	Cape Coloured	Asiatics
BRADLOW (clinical)	3% I.C.H. 22 M.I. 800	—	—	—
SIEW (autopsy)	10% I.C.H. 22 M.I. 226	1400% I.C.H. 85 M.I. 6	225% I.C.H. 10 M.I. 4	—
SCHRIRE (E.C.G.)	1.9%	1,600%	4%	—
SEFTEL (clinical + autopsy) .	—	10,300% I.C.H. 103 M.I. 1	—	—
COSNETT (clinical + autopsy) .	—	—	—	9%

unknown origin occurring elsewhere in the world are the type of cardiac disease under discussion [95, 98, 99, 100, 101]. It is also probable that many cases of "Fiedler's myocarditis" or "Loffler's endomyocarditis" in the European literature belong in this category. However the prevalence of this disease in Africa especially in the Bantu of Southern Africa including Southern Rhodesia, South Africa and Portuguese territories like Mozambique is particularly high, and even the White populace has a greatly increased incidence compared to the White race in Europe or the United States. The disease probably occurs also in other more northern parts of Africa [103]. Many cases occurring in other parts of the world have a history of having resided at some time in Africa.

At autopsy the most constant feature is generalized cardiac hypertrophy, frequently with ante-mortem endocardial thrombosis. For this reason the

condition is most often known in South Africa as "Idiopathic Cardiac Hypertrophy" (I.C.H.) at the present time.

Table IX shows a list of pseudonyms for this entity, many of them, such as
"reversible heart failure", being, for the most part, inaccurate. However some
Bantu cases respond, partially at least, in the initial stages, to improved diets,
and relapse again on inadequate diets, but they are not truly reversible [41, 93].
Undoubted complete recoveries have been reported in a small number of
instances [122, 125]. The discrepancy between the necropsy incidence, [97] in
which I.C.H. ranks only fourth in the causes of death from heart disease, and
the hospital admission rate [41] where it ranks first in the causes of heart
disease in the same hospital, has been said to be due to a number of patients
recovering completely after being discharged from hospital [125] but this is a
facile explanation as it is known that chronically sick Bantu will frequently
return to their homes when death appears to be imminent. In personally fol-
lowed-up cases of I.C.H. in White men, the author has not yet seen a recovery.

Table IX. *Synonyms for Idiopathic Cardiac Hypertrophy or Primary Parietal Endomyocarditis*

I. C. H.
1. Nutritional heart disease
2. Cardiovascular collagenosis with endocardial thrombosis (Becker's disease)
3. Idiopathic cardiac hypertrophy in African children
4. Acute reversible heart failure in Africans
5. Peripartum (post-partum) cardiomyopathy
6. Cryptogenic heart disease
7. Primary mural endocardial disease

In the European cases in South Africa malnutrition plays no part in the
aetiology, and temporary remissions that occur are not influenced by dietary
therapy.

Cases occurring in connection with pregnancy in the Bantu may recover
completely in about half the patients. They usually respond to bed rest with or
without the use of digitalis and diuretics [41, 124]. They are known in Johannesburg as "peripartum cardiomyopathy", as they may present during a period
ranging from the last month of pregnancy to one year after delivery. In the
fatal cases, the pathology differed in no way from idiopathic cardiac hypertrophy
[41, 123]. Twin births were especially high in these patients [123, 124]. These
peripartum cases do not appear to resemble the cardiomyopathy of pregnancy
and the puerperium seen in other parts of the world, as in these cases, which
occur also, although rarely, in White females in South Africa, recovery is
usually complete [95, 126]. However similar cases have been reported occasionally in White people in Europe, and in fair numbers in American Negroes [127,
128, 129].

Idiopathic hypertrophy has also been reported in African children and is of the same pathological type as I.C.H. but is more rapidly progressive, and has not been shown to be related to malnutrition [130].

The disease occurs more commonly in the Cape Coloured than in the European, but is of extreme rarity in the South African Indian. The incidence of the disease compared to that of myocardial infarction which for this purpose is taken as a unit of 100 per cent is shown in different series in South Africa in Table VIII.

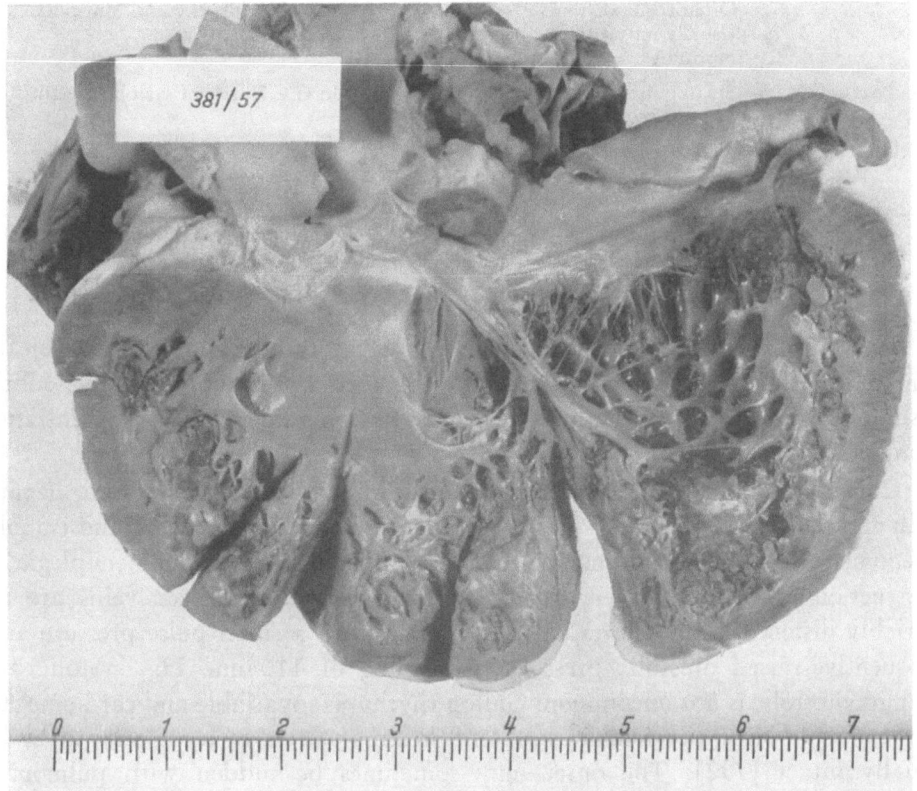

Fig. 12. A case of I.C.H. showing ante-mortem mural thrombosis and subendocardial necrosis with slight fibrosis. The valves are intact. (This picture was kindly supplied by Prof. B. J. P. Becker, Department of Pathology, University of the Witwatersrand.)

At necropsy, the heart invariably shows dilatation and hypertrophy with antemortem thrombosis on the ventricular endocardium, which may show varying degrees of fibrosis or necrosis [96, 131] (Fig. 12). The subendocardial fibrosis is slight, unlike that in E.M.F., and patchy interstitial fibrosis may occur. Primary thrombosis of the large pulmonary arteries is common, and embolism to the lungs and peripheral vessels may be seen [96, 131]. Cases have been described in which neutrophil infiltration of the myocardium was present, and, in a few cases, the appearances may resemble to a slight extent E.M.F. [78]. The differences between E.M.F. and I.C.H. are summarized in Table X.

Table X. *Differentiation between E.M.F. and I.C.H*

Endomyocardial fibrosis (E.M.F.) and idiopathic cardiopathy (I. C. H.)

	E. M. F.	I. C. H.
Distribution . .	E. and W. Africa	S. Africa C.A.F. (Rhod. and Nyas.)
Pathology . . .	Gross endocardial thickening (ventricles). Dilatation and hypertrophy rare. No embolism.	Severe dilatation. Often hypertrophy. Slight to moderate endocardial fibrosis. Embolism frequent.
Clinical	Slow onset of chronic failure. Often triple rhythm. Usually mitral and or tricuspid murmurs	Recurrent C.C.F. very large heart. Always triple rhythm. Murmurs infrequent
Blood pressure .	Small pulse pressure. B.P. normal or low	In C.C.F. rise of systolic pressure
E.C.G.	Not specific. Low voltage	Not specific. ST elevation or depression
Course	Progressive. Fatal in few years	Initial response to treatment. Many relapses. Duration several years, (about 4 years.)

True Loffler's endomyocarditis may also occur rarely in all sections of the community, and is a separate entity, recognized by lung lesions, vasculitis, eosinophilia and a raised erythrocyte sedimentation rate, so that differentiation from I.C.H. is not difficult.

Clinically I.C.H. may present with an insidious onset of dyspnoea, hepatic pain and peripheral oedema. Pleural effusions and ascites may occur and embolic phenomena resulting in pulmonary emboli, with haemoptysis, or hemiplegia or obstruction to a limb artery are extremely common. The neck veins are invariably distended, and the radial pulse small, with a small pulse pressure and, frequently, raised diastolic pressure. A reading of 110 mm. Hg. systolic and 90 mm. diastolic is not uncommon. Gallop rhythm is invariable and cardiomegaly clinically and on X-ray is always present. Murmurs are a rarity as the valves are usually intact [132]. The onset may sometimes be sudden with pulmonary oedema. Cardiac pain on exertion is rare.

The E.C.G. is invariably abnormal. Ventricular extrasystoles, prolonged P—R intervals, conduction disturbances, ST depression, T inversions and arrhythmias may all occur. Pathological left axis deviation with an S2, S3 pattern is not uncommon in the African cases [133]. Figures 13 and 14 show the X-ray, E.C.G. and phonocardiographic appearances of some White patients, whilst Fig. 15 and Table XI show the findings on cardiac catheterisation and illustrate well the pulmonary hypertension. At times the disease may resemble constrictive pericarditis very closely and even require exploratory thoracotomy before the diagnosis can be finalized.

The course may vary from a few weeks to 3 or 4 years, and in rare cases, even up to 5 or 6 years. Remissions occur not infrequently, but although signs of

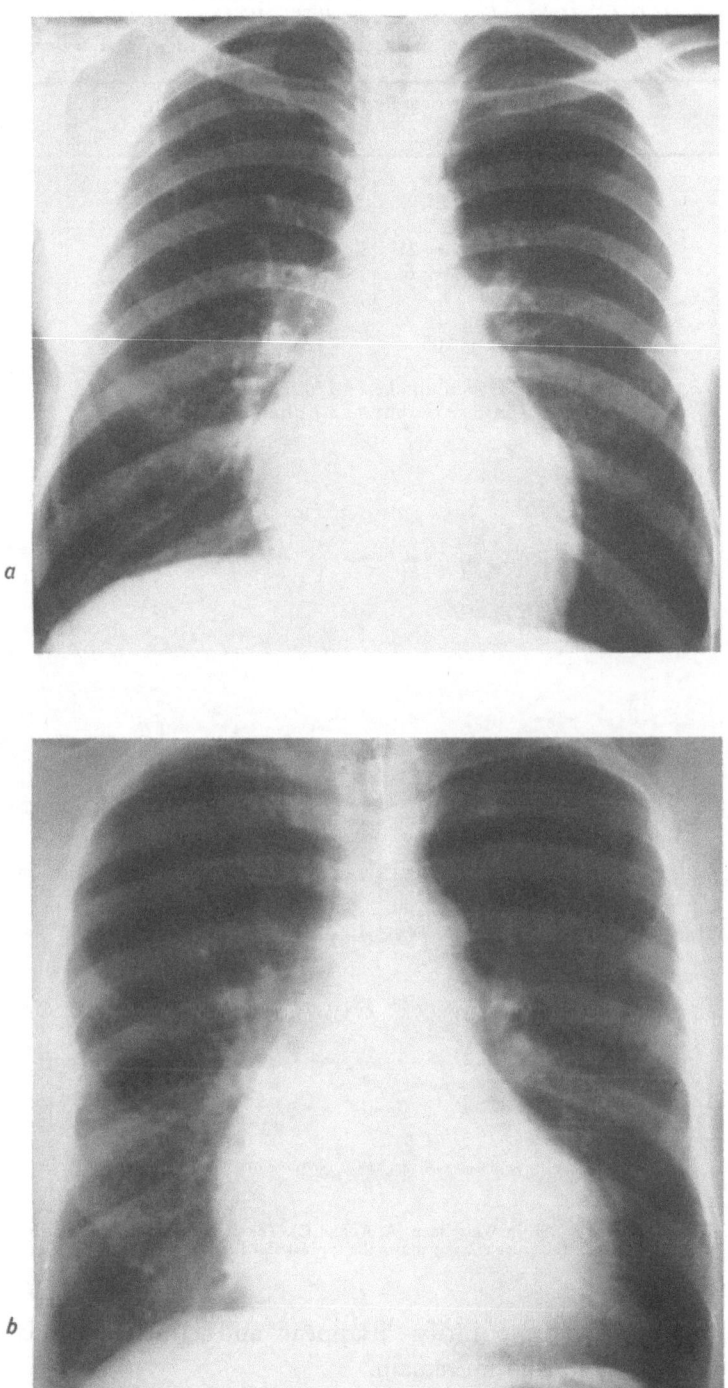

Fig. 13. X-ray appearances of chest in 2 cases of I.C.H. in White men, showing cardiomegaly and lung vasculature suggestive of pulmonary hypertension

Table XI. *Cardiac catheter findings in a case of I.C.H. (same as in Fig. 15) (R.P.A.=Right pulmonary artery, M.P.A.=Main pulmonary artery, R.V.=Right ventricle, Mid.R.A.=Mid. right atrium, High R.A.=High right atrium, S.V.C.=Superior vena cava, B.A.=Brachial artery)*

Site	Pressure (mm.Hg.)			O₂ Saturation %	O₂Content vols %
	Sys.	Dias.	Mean		
R. P. A.	75	25	50	59.0	8.15
M. P. A.	80	25		59.0	8.15
R. V.	80	0—20		58.2	
Mid. R. A.	$A = 21$	$V = 21$			
	$X' = 11$	$Y = 6$	16	58.5	8.08
High R. A. . . .				55.0	7.60
S. V. C.				55.0	
B. A.	155	105	125	89.0	12.29

Oxygen uptake — 176 cc./min
Cardiac output — 3.7 l/min

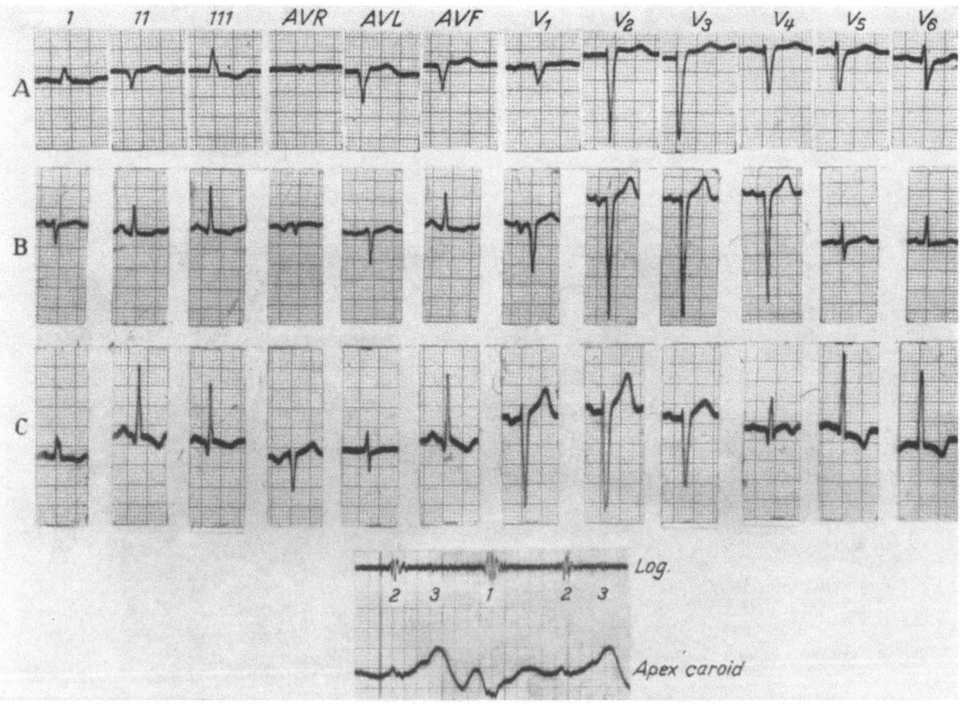

Fig. 14. The E.C.G. in 3 cases of I.C.H. in White men (A, B, and C). The phonocardiogram with the apex cardiogram as a reference tracing shows the typical third heart sound

congestive failure may temporarily disappear and effort tolerance improve, cardiomegaly and gallop rhythm remain.

As yet there is no specific treatment, but digitalis, diuretics and anticoagulants provide some relief, and the latter may be helpful in preventing embolization. Corticosteroids although used, produce no obvious therapeutic benefit.

These cardiomyopathies of Africa, such as E.M.F. and I.C.H. are thus both a puzzle and a challenge.

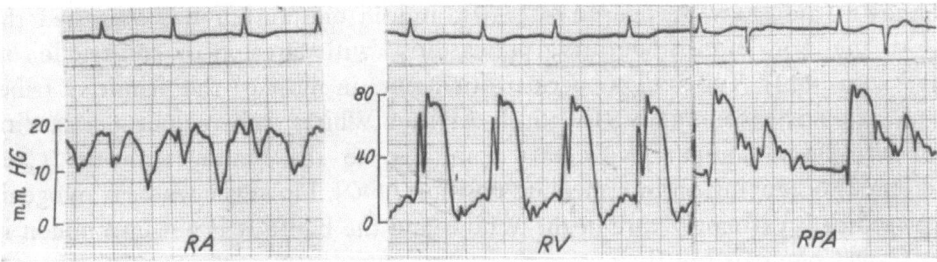

Fig. 15. Cardiac catheter tracings in a case of I.C.H. in a White man (R.A.=Right atrium, R.V.=Right ventricle, R.P.A.=Right pulmonary artery)

4. Rheumatic heart disease

It is a common observation in Africa that rheumatic fever may be difficult to diagnose, joint swellings and rheumatic nodules being less common than in Europe. However rheumatic heart disease is common in most parts, and in certain areas like Algeria the incidence is increasing as civilization spreads among the Arab-Berber population [70]. At the southern tip of Africa, rheumatic valvular disease is more common in the Cape Coloured than in the Whites, and is at least as common in the Bantu as in the Whites. The fact that after the age of 40 years far fewer cases are found in the Cape Coloured and Bantu than in the White populace has raised the suggestion that the disease is more severe in the two dark skinned races [53, 135]. It is also likely that rheumatic valvular disease is not only more severe but usually occurs at a younger age in the Bantu than in the Whites, not only in South Africa but in East Africa and in Nigeria [38, 112, 135, 136, 137, 139]. Rheumatic heart disease is however still far less frequent among the Bantu than cryptogenic heart disease [41, 107].

In the Nilotic people of the Sudan too, the incidence of rheumatic heart disease is rising and the disease appears to appear earlier than is usual among White races [137].

However the incidence varies sometimes even among different tribes in the same area, as in Gabon [103]. The disease is said to be rare in its typical form in Southern Nigeria, but if it occurs it is said to present in the unusual form of endomyocardial fibrosis (E.M.F.) [91]. This latter statement must be accepted with considerable reserve, as in Uganda both rheumatic heart disease and E.M.F. occur.

5. Pericarditis

In the South African Bantu pericarditis is one of the most common types of heart disease [140, 141]. It is usually tuberculous and may present as an effusion or as constrictive pericarditis, or constriction may develop and is probably hastened by antituberculous treatment, even with corticosteroids [141]. In about one third of the pericardial effusions or constrictions in the Bantu, the cause although often thought to be tuberculous, is not really known or proven, and some other as yet unknown cause may be operative [140]. Indeed one author has suggested the use of the term "non-suppurative pericarditis" with effusion or constriction in the Bantu [142]. Tuberculous pericarditis occurs in most of the primitive tribes of Africa fairly commonly. In South African Whites, tuberculous pericarditis and effusion is comparatively rare compared to the Bantu, with the Cape Coloureds occupying an intermediate position [140]. However whereas pyogenic pericarditis is extremely rare in the Whites and the Bantu it is not uncommon in the Cape Coloureds [140].

6. Congenital heart disease

Congenital heart disease is probably of similar incidence in all races although it has at times been considered to be rare in the Bantu, although this is probably incorrect. However one form of congenital heart disease — patent ductus arteriosus — is of interest in that it is considerably more frequent in Johannesburg at an altitude of 6,000 feet above sea level than it is at sea level at least in the White race. This is well known to South African cardiologists, although the exact difference in incidence at the two altitudes has not been adequately studied.

The lowered oxygen saturation at an altitude of 6,000 feet is said to be the responsible factor, and this is borne out by the classical experiments of Dawes on the effects of anoxia on new born lambs in which the ductus remains patent, and by observations from South America [147, 148]. It is thus more than likely that most cases of simple patent ductus arteriosus are in fact "acquired" and not "congenital".

7. Beri-beri heart disease

Heart disease due to thiamine deficiency has a high frequency in the Cape Coloured community due to the high intake of alcohol among those individuals who work in the Western Province of the Cape, which is a great wine-producing centre [143]. Some Cape Coloured labourers receive part of their wages in the form of a daily ration of wine, and in general, wine and spirits are cheap and easy to obtain. Beri-beri in Cape Town accounts for about one half of the causes of "primary myocardial failure" [144]. The disease is probably just as common among White alcoholics and also occurs in the Bantu in the Western Cape Province [145]. The signs and symptoms are those of hyperkinetic heart failure with warm hands, bounding pulse, and a rapid circulation time, unlike the hypokinetic state seen in I.C.H. The electrocardiogram is frequently normal during the height of failure and this in itself suggests the diagnosis [144]. Later, transient ST segment changes and T wave inversions, usually over leads facing the right ventricle and sometimes over the left ventricle, occur as recovery proceeds, and eventually normality of the electrocardiogram returns [144]. A high percentage of cases have signs of peripheral neuritis. Beri-beri heart disease, usually associated with alcoholism, has also been reported in Johannesburg [122] among the Bantu. However despite the high incidence of Kwashiorkor, Pellagra and general malnutrition in Africa, Beri-beri is an uncommon disease in Africa compared to the high incidence in the Far East [145]. There is however no part of Africa in which it does not occur [145].

8. Syphilis

This disease is rare and becoming less common among white populations such as those in South Africa, but is still common among the African inhabitants and is a common cause of sudden death in Johannesburg [36]. It also results in a fair

Table XII. *The general pattern of heart disease and diabetes in several South African groups of diverse race compared with figures taken at random from the Statistical Bulletin of the Metropolitan Life Insurance Company of New York (in the second last vertical column on the right). (W=White race, C.C.=Cape Coloureds, B=Bantu)*

	Capetown 1957 % of C.V.S. EGC. (adults)			Bara. Jhb. 1957 % of C.V.S. (adults)	Joh'burg 1936−56 % of all autopsies (adults)			Durban % all deaths all ages Asiatics	Metro. 56−59 % all deaths per 100,000	S. A. M. % all deaths 56−59
	W	C. C.	B	B	W	C.C.	B			
Pericarditis	1	4	20.5	4.0	4.7	12.5	18.1	—	—	—
Rheumatic	11	20	17	23.3	6.4	7.5	5.6	4.8	1.7	0.43
S. B. E.	—	—	—	1.3	—	—	—	—	—	—
Myo. infarct.	38	21	2	0.36	9.15	1.26	0.265	2.7	17.84	32.29
Other disease of heart	—	—	—					—	1.6	6.6
Idiopathic	1	1	5.5	37.5	0.27	0.84	1	—	—	—
Cor pulmonale	3	4	3.5	10.9	5.5	3.2	2.2	4.0	—	—
Hypertensive	42	48	31	19.6	10.2	4.15	3.1	1.9	2.75	1.12
Congenital	5	6	6	1.1	0.7	0	1.2	—	—	—
Syphilis	0.2	3	3	1.1	0.94	7	5.7	—	...	—
Cerebro vasc Accidents								6.7	1.31	9.94
Diabetes								2.4	2.3	

References: Vertical Column 1 on left is taken from [23]. This refers to adults with cardiovascular disease diagnosed by E.C.G. Column 2 from Baragwanath Hospital [41], Clinical diagnoses in adults with cardiovascular disease. Column 3 from [38]. Column 4 from [19]. Column 5 from the "Statistical Bulletin of the Metropolitan Life Insurance Company". Column 6 on right is taken from figures kindly supplied by the South African Mutual Life Insurance Company for death claims in the years 1956 to 1959 and can be regarded as being predominantly concerned with Whites).

Table XIII. *General pattern of deaths from various causes in South Africa in 1958 and life expectancy at birth as calculated in 1952. (Rh. Ht. Dis.=Rheumatic Heart Disease, Myo. Infarc. =Myocardial Infarction, Hypert.=Hypertension, C.V.A.=Cerebro-vascular accident) From [155]*

	Republic of South Africa 1958 (per 100,000 population)											
	White				Coloured				Asiatics			
	Males		Females		Males		Females		Males		Females	
	NO	%	NO	%	NO	%	NN	%	NO	%	NO	%
Total deaths	987.0	100.0	736	100.0	1825	100.0	1555	100.0	920	100.0	706	100.0
Rh. ht. dis.	3	0.3	3	0.41	6	0.32	14	0.9	12	1.3	16	2.0
Myo. infarc	**250**	**27.0**	**138**	**19.2**	88	**4.8**	62	**4.0**	98	**12.2**	**54**	**7.9**
Other ht dis	7	0.7	3	0.41	9	0.48	6	0.38	6	0.65	1	0.12
Hypert	21	2.3	39	5.32	39	2.1	53	3.4	36	3.9	31	4.7
C. V. A.	**81**	**9.1**	105	**14.51**	73	**4.0**	101	**6.9**	82	**8.9**	54	**7.9**
Diabetes	6	0.6	12	1.6	3	0.15	8	0.5	10	1.1	12	1.7
Pneumonia	59	6.1	48	6.6	**232**	**12.8**	**223**	**15.4**	**153**	**16.7**	**138**	**19.0**
Malignant	146	14.9	123	16.6	86	4.7	76	4.9	30	3.2	24	3.7
Life expect (yr 1952)	64.57		70.08		44.82		47.77		55.77		54.75	

proportion of hospital admissions among the Bantu and Coloureds [38, 41, 42] and causes aortic incompetence, aortic aneurysms and even affects at times the myocardium and may cause aneurysms of the ventricle [38, 41]. It is found throughout Africa, although becoming less frequent than formerly because of better public health and therapeutic measures.

9. Cor pulmonale

In general the causes of this condition resemble those found elsewhere in the world. In some areas such as South Africa where silicosis is still a hazard on the Rand Gold Mines, many cases may be due to this condition but it has no special racial predilection.

In Egypt Schistosoma mansoni infections affect the majority of the population, and in 30 per cent of cases involves the pulmonary vasculature leading to pulmonary hypertension and cor pulmonale [149]. In other areas of Africa especially in the south, Schistosoma haematobium is the more frequent cause of bilharziasis. This parasite involves the urinary tract and in these areas, such as South Africa, cor pulmonale is not commonly due to bilharzia.

10. Rare causes of heart disease in africa

It is said that thyrotoxicosis is rarely seen in Africans, either Bantu or Negro and most physicians would agree with this. There is less agreement on the incidence of subacute bacterial endocarditis which is also said to be rare, but some investigations have shown it to be not uncommon [38, 41, 80, 140]. It may well be that in the African the disease is less easy to diagnose as skin manifestations are difficult to see on the pigmented skin, and splenomegaly from other causes is common. Obstructive cardiopathy or assymetrical hypertrophy of the heart involving the outflow tracts of the ventricles [164] is common in White South Africans but has not yet been reported in the Bantu [163].

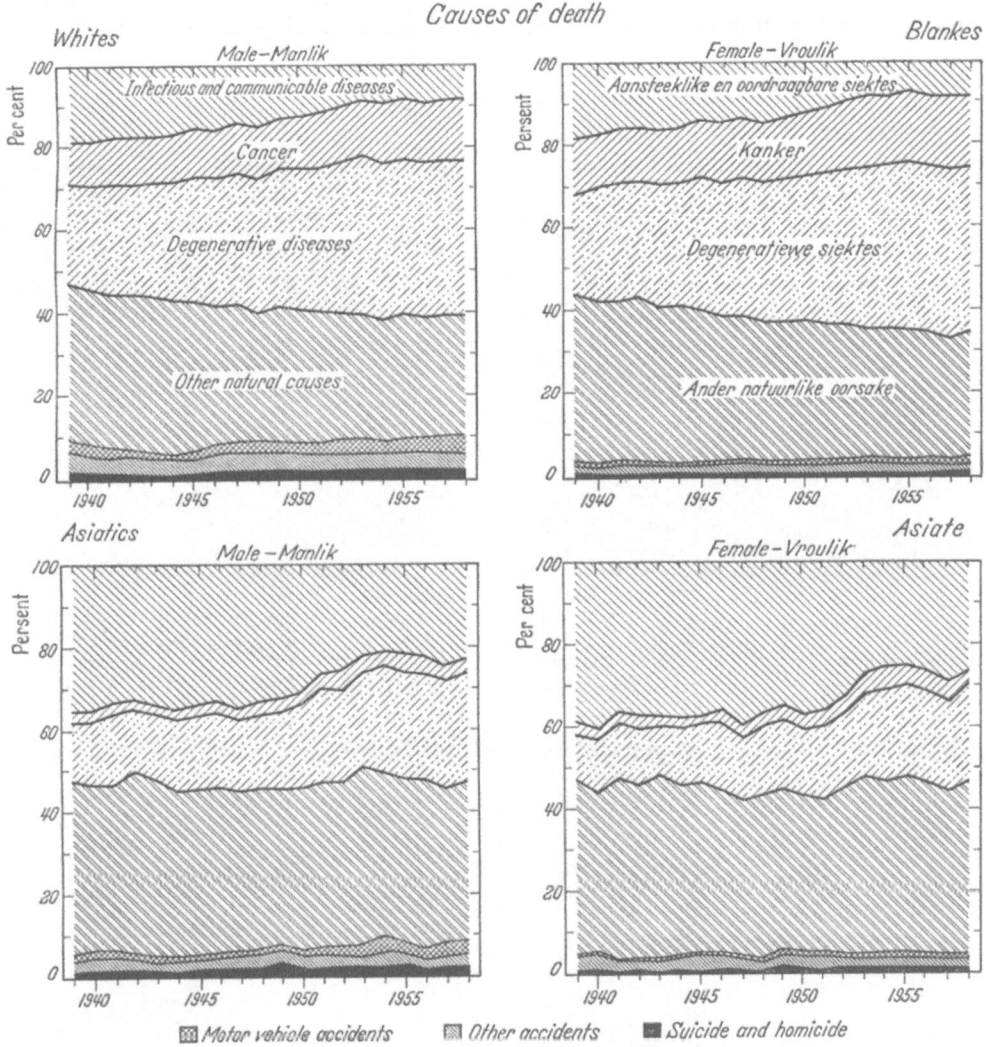

Fig. 16. Causes of death in South Africa in Whites and Asiatics. (In English and Afrikaans)

Tuberculosis involving the myocardium is an extreme rarity in the European, but in the African is not so uncommon and may be a cause of ventricular aneurysms [36, 103].

A rare syndrome, described in young Nigerians, of multiple non-luetic aneurysms of the aorta and its main branches [150] probably occurs also further south in Rhodesia and South Africa [151, 152, 153]. The condition may possibly be the result of a vasculitis of unknown aetiology [150].

11. General position of cardiovascular diseases in pattern of disease in republic of south africa

Table XII shows the general pattern of cardiovascular disease and diabetes in various South African races and one North American group, the latter being life insurance policy holders. Table XIII shows the general pattern of disease of

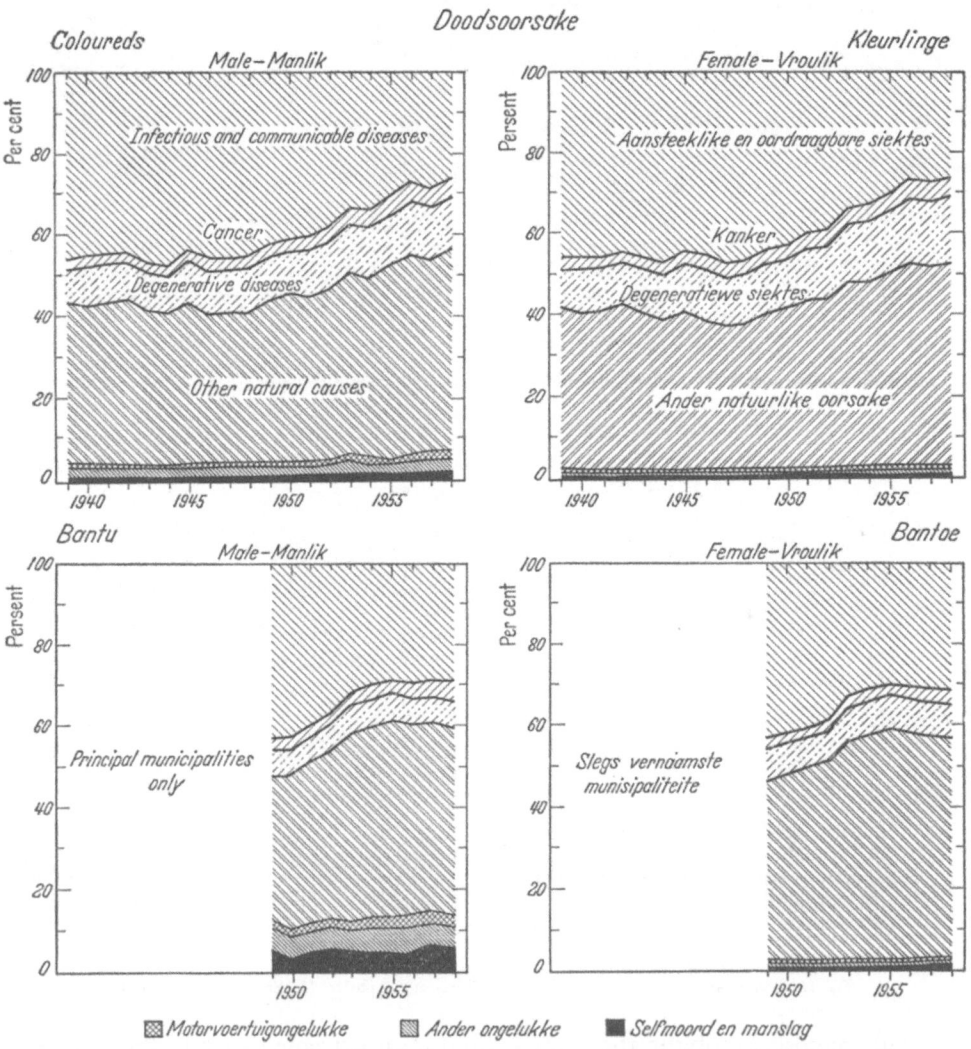

Fig. 17. Causes of death in South Africa in Cape Coloureds, and Bantu. (Figs. 16 and 17 are published with the kind permission of Mr. H. M. STOKER, Director of Census and Statistics, Republic of South Africa and by Mr. S. A. MYBURGH, Government Printer [51].) (For English aequivalent of Afrikaans terms cf. Fig. 16)

various types in three South African racial groups and shows the high incidence of infective diseases among Asiatics and Coloureds compared to the White race. The mortality from various causes has been calculated from official figures and the table includes also the life expectancy for Whites, Coloureds, and Asiatics in 1952. No reliable figures for the African are available as yet, but it may be assumed that his life expectancy is shorter than that of the European, Asiatic or even the Cape Coloured.

The charts (Figs. 16 and 17) show the general disease pattern in graphic form and are published with the permission of the Director of Census and Statistics for the Republic of South Africa.

Conclusion

Africa provides a vast natural laboratory for the study of the aetiology and epidemiology of heart disease. Varying races, customs, altitude and climate all seem to produce new disease syndromes and incidences of diseases different from those met with in Europe and the United States. The potential of this vast continent as regards the knowledge it can produce to the benefit of all mankind has barely been tapped, and it is to be hoped that more resources and personnel will become available in order to utilize the unending variety of material.

Summary

1. Racial differences of heart disease in Africa are discussed together with apparent differences in standards of normality as regards electrocardiograms and serum lipid patterns.

2. The high incidence of ischaemic heart disease in White South Africans, and its virtual absence in the Bantu has been stressed.

3. Heart diseases peculiar to Africa, such as I.C.H. and E.M.F., are described.

4. The difference in altitude found in two South African cities is shown to result in a different incidence of patent ductus arteriosus and in various differences in blood findings. Speculation concerning the possibility of these blood differences causing different incidence of myocardial infarction is discussed.

5. The general pattern of heart disease, and its relationship to the pattern of other diseases in South Africa receives brief mention.

Acknowledgements

Apart from acknowledgements made in the legends for various tables, and figures, the author wishes to acknowledge the generous permission of Dr. S. J. FLEISHMAN for allowing him to publish Figs. 2 to 6, and the Photo Unit of the Department of Medicine of the University of the Witwatersrand for reproducing all the figures and tables in this paper. Table VI and Figs. 9 and 10 are published with the permission of Dr. J. METZ, of the South African Institute for Medical Research.

References

[1] Article in "News Check on South Africa and Africa" [Quoted from "An African Day", published by Market Research, Africa (Pty) Ltd.]: News Check. 1, 7 (1963).

[2] BRINK, A. J.: Coronary vessels in Bantu: Preliminary Report on Coronary Artery Pattern in Adult Bantu. Clin. Proc. 8, 137 (1949).

[3] SINGER, R.: The coronary arteries of the Bantu heart. S. Afr. med. J. 33, 310 (1959).

[4] SHAPER, A. G., and K. W. JONES: Serum cholesterol, diet and coronary heart disease in Africans and Asians in Uganda. Lancet 2, 534 (1959).

[5] VAN QYE, E., and P. CHARLES: Ann. Soc. belge Méd. trop. 32, 297 (1952) cited by BROCK, J. F., and H. GORDON [6].

[6] BROCK, J. F., and H. GORDON: Ischaemic heart disease in African populations. Postgrad. med. J. 35, 223 (1959).

[7] GORDON, H.: Dietary fat and coronary heart disease. Centr. Afr. J. Med. 4, 424 (1958).

[8] MERSKEY, C., H. GORDON, and H. LACKNER: Blood coagulation and fibrinolysis in relation to coronary heart disease, a comparative study of normal White men, White men with overt coronary heart disease and normal Bantu men. Brit. med. J. 1, 219 (1960).

[9] BERSOHN, I.: A holistic conception on the association of patterns of diet and disease in the Bantu. Leech (Johannesburg) 28, 33 (1958).

[10] LITTMAN, D.: Persistence of the juvenile pattern in the precordial leads of healthy adult negroes. Amer. Heart J. 32, 370 (1946).

[11] FLEISHMAN, S. J.: Personal communication (1963).

[12] GRUSIN, H.: Peculiarities of the African's electrocardiogram and the changes observed in serial studies. Circulation 9, 860 (1954).

[13] POWELL, S. J.: Unexplained electrocardiograms in the African. Brit. Heart J. 21, 263 (1959).

[14] FLEISHMAN, S. J., and M. GELFAND: The electrocardiogram in apparently healthy African men. Centr. Afr. J. Med. 8, 356 (1960).

[15] BOTHWELL, T. H., and C. ISAACSON: Siderosis in the Bantu. Brit. med. J. 1, 522 (1962).

[16] BOTHA, M. C.: Abstract of paper read at "Southern Africa Cardiac Congress", Cape Town (1960).

[17] SEFTEL, H. C.: Personal communication (1962).

[18] GOLDBERG, B., N. W. LEVIN, A. RUBENSTEIN, and D. HACK: Personal communication (1962).

[19] COSNETT, J. E.: Illness among Natal Indians. A survey of hospital admissions. S. Afr. med. J. 31, 1109 (1957).

[20] WHITE, P. D.: Notes on cardiovascular disease in Africa. Amer. Heart J. 61, 133 (1961).

[21] SHEE, J. C.: Myocardial Infarction in Southern Rhodesia. Brit. Heart J. 25, 25 (1963).

[22] CAMPBELL, G. D.: The insurability of the Natal Indian with special reference to the incidence and natural history of diabetes: Med. Proc. 7, 395 (1961).

[23] SCHRIRE, V.: The comparative racial prevalence of ischaemic heart disease in Cape Town. Amer. J. Cardiol. 8, 173 (1961).

[24] WAINWRIGHT, J.: Atheroma in the African (Bantu) in Natal. Lancet 1, 366 (1961).

[25] HIGGINSON, J., and W. J. PEPLER: Fat intake, serum cholesterol concentration and atherosclerosis in the South African Bantu. 11. Atherosclerosis and coronary artery disease. J. clin. Invest. 33, 1366 (1954).

[26] SACKS, M. I.: Aortic and coronary atherosclerosis in the three racial groups in Cape Town. Circulation 22, 96 (1960).

[27] BECKER, B. J. P.: Cardiovascular disease in the Bantu and Coloured races of South Africa. IV. Atheromatosis. S. Afr. J. med. Sci. 11, 97 (1946).

[28] LAURIE, W., J. D. WOODS, and G. ROACH: Coronary heart disease in the South African Bantu. Amer. J. Cardiol. 5, 48 (1960).

[29] HANNAH, J. B.: Civilization, race and coronary atheroma: Centr. Afr. J. Med. 4, 1 (1958).

[30] DAVIES, J. N. P.: Pathology of Central African Natives. Mulago Hospital postmortem studies I. E. Afr. med. J. 25, 454 (1948).

[31] EDINGTON, G. M.: Cardiovascular disease as cause of death in Gold Coast Africans. Tr. Roy. Soc. trop. Med. Hyg. 48, 419, 514 (1954).

[32] REEF, H., and C. ISAACSON: Atherosclerosis in the Bantu: The distribution of atheromatous lesions in Africans over 50 years of age. Circulation 25, 66 (1962).

[33] SCHRIRE, V., and C. J. UYS: Cardiac infarction in the Bantu. Amer. J. Cardiol 2, 453 (1958).
[34] GRUSIN, H., and R. V. DANDO: Myocardial infarction in a South African Bantu. Med. Proc. 2, 290 (1956).
[35] SNYMAN, H. W.: The pattern of heart disease in Africa. Med. Proc. 8, 391 (1962).
[36] ELLIOTT, G. A.: The coronary arteries and their diseases in the Bantu. Leech (Johannesburg) 23, 25 (1953).
[37] ELLIOTT, G. A.: Le coronaropatei nei negri Bantu. Minerva med. 1, 465 (1953).
[38] SIEW, S.: Comparative study of the autopsy incidence of cardiovascular disease in the Bantu on the Witwatersrand. Leech (Johannesburg) 28, 61 (1958).
[39] WILLIAMS, A. W., and J. N. P. DAVIES: cited by J. F. BROCK and B. BRONTE-STEWART: Arteriosclerosis in African populations. Minnesota Med. 38, 852 (1955).
[40] BRONTE-STEWART, B.: The epidemiology of ischaemic heart disease. Postgrad. med. J. 35, 180 (1959).
[41] SCHWARTZ, M. B., L. SCHAMROTH, and H. C. SEFTEL: The pattern of heart disease in the urbanized (Johannesburg) African. Med. Proc. 4, 275 (1958).
[42] COSNETT, J. E.: Heart disease in the Zulu especially cardiomyopathy and cardiac infarction. Brit. Heart J. 24, 76 (1962).
[43] BALDACHIN, B. J.: Cardiac disease in African in Matabeleland. A survey based on records of 150 patients. E. Afr. med. J. 36, 542 (1959).
[44] GELFAND, M.: Cardiac and vascular disorders in the African. W. Afr. med. J. 1, (New series) 91 (1952).
[45] PEPLER, W. J., and B. J. MEYER: Interarterial coronary anastomoses and coronary arterial pattern. A comparative study of South African Bantu and European hearts. Circulation 22, 14 (1960).
[46] LAURIE, W., and J. D. WOODS: Anastomosis in the coronary circulation. Lancet 2, 812 (1958).
[47] SEFTEL, H. C., and E. SCHULTZ: Diabetes mellitus in the urbanized Johannesburg African. S. Afr. med. J. 35, 66 (1961).
[48] POLITZER, W. M., B. HARDEGGER, and T. SCHNEIDER: The incidence of diabetes mellitus in one district of Basutoland. S. Afr. med. J. 34, 95 (1960).
[49] BRADLOW, B. A., and M. M. ZION: Seasonal variation of the incidence of myocardial infarction in Johannesburg. S. Afr. med. J. 32, 427 (1958).
[50] SCHRIRE, V.: The seasonal incidence of cardiac infarction at Groote Schuur Hospital, Cape Town. S. Afr. med. J. 32, 429 (1958).
[51] Deaths. South Africa and South West Africa. 1958 and earlier years. Vol. 2. Causes. Pretoria: Government Printer 1961.
[52] PICKERING, G. W.: High Blood Pressure. London: J. and A. Churchill Ltd. 1955.
[53] SCHRIRE, V.: The racial incidence of heart disease at Groote Schuur Hospital, Cape Town, Part II. Hypertension and valvular disease of the heart. Amer. Heart J. 56, 742 (1958).
[54] WALKER, A. R. P., K. L. MORTIMER, P. J. KLOPPERS, D. BOTHA, H. GRUSIN, and H. C. SEFTEL: Coronary heart disease in South African "Poor Whites" and White prisoners habituated to a Bantu type of diet. Amer. J. clin. Nutr. 9, 643 (1961).
[55] ORDMAN, B.: A review of the incidence of hypertension in the Non-European Races. Survey of Blood pressures in the South African Bantu. Clin. Proc. 7, 183 (1948).
[56] BECKER, B. J. P.: Cardiovascular disease in the Bantu and Coloured races of South Africa. I. Incidence, pathology and general features. S. Afr. J. med. Sci. 11, 1 (1946).
[57] GELFAND, M.: The Sick African. 3rd ed. Cape Town: Juta and Co. 1957.
[58] WILLIAMS, A. W., J. D. BALL, and J. N. P. DAVIES: Endomyocardial fibrosis in Africa: Its diagnosis, distribution and nature. Trans. Roy. Soc. trop. Med. Hyg. 48, 290 (1954).
[59] ISAACSON, C., and P. KINCAID-SMITH: Study of the kidney in the Bantu with hypertension. Brit. Heart J. 24, 372 (1962).
[60] UYS, C. J.: The pathology of renal disease in the Bantu on the Witwatersrand; Hypertensive vascular disease. S. Afr. J. Lab. clin. Med. 2, 13 (1956).
[61] LAURIE, W., and J. D. WOODS: Atherosclerosis and its cerebral complications in the South African Bantu. Lancet 2, 251 (1958).
[62] DONNISON, C. P.: Blood pressure in the African native. Its bearing upon the aetiology of hyperpiesia and arteriosclerosis. Lancet 1, 6 (1929).
[63] VINT, F. W.: Post-mortem findings in the natives of Kenya. E. Afr. med. J. 13, 322 (1937).

[64] Williams, A. W.: Heart disease in the native population of Uganda. Part IV. Hypertensive heart disease. E. Afr. med. J. 21, 328 (1944).

[65] Jex-Blake, A. J.: High blood pressure. E. Afr. med. J. 10, 286 (1934).

[66] Shattuck, G. C.: The African Republic of Liberia and the Belgian Congo. Report of the Harvard Expedition to Liberia Harvard University Press. Cambridge 1930. Cited by Schulze, V. E. and E. H. Schwab, Arteriolar hypertension in the American Negro. Amer. Heart J. 11, 66 (1936).

[67] Kröber, F.: Klin. Wschr. 18, 724 (1933) cited by Schrire, V. [53].

[68] Davies, J. N. P.: cited by Bersohn, I. [9], 1958,

[69] Ismai, A.: Aetiology of hyperpiesis in Egyptians. Lancet 2, 275 (1938).

[70] Sarrouy, Ch.. L. Sendra, and B. Diboucher: Considerations on the evolution of heart disease in Algeria. Amer. Heart J. 61, 145 (1961).

[71] Moser, M.: Epidemiology of hypertension with particular reference to racial susceptibility. Ann. N. Y. Acad. Sci. 84, 989 (1960).

[72] Abrahams, D. G., C. A. Alele, and B. G. Barnard: The systematic blood pressure in a rural West African community. W. Afr. med. J. 9, 45 (1960).

[73] Abrahams, D. G., and C. A. Alele: A clinical study of hypertensive disease in West Africa. W. Afr. med. J. 9, 183 (1960).

[74] Shapiro, P. F.: Malignant nephrosclerosis; Pathogenesis. Arch. int. Med. 48, 199 (1931).

[75] Phillips, J. H., and G. A. Burch: A review of cardiovascular diseases in the White and Negro races. Medicine 39, 241 (1960).

[76] White, P. D.: "Heart Disease". 4th edn. New York: The MacMillan Co. 1951.

[77] Chatgidakis, C. B., and J. B. Barlow: Primary mural endocardial disease. A discussion of the condition and a report of a case in a White male aged 54 years. Med. Proc. 7, 377 (1961).

[78] Weber, H. W.: Pariëtale endomiokarditis in die Karl Bremer-Hospitaal. S. Afr. med. J. 37, 149 (1963).

[79] Bedford, D. E., and G. L. S. Konstam: Heart failure of unknown aetiology in Africans. Brit. Heart J. 8, 236 (1946).

[80] Davies, J. N. P.: Endomyocardial fibrosis in Uganda. Centr. Afr. J. Med. 2, 323 (1956).

[81] Ball, J. D., J. N. P. Davies, and A. W. Williams: Endomyocardial fibrosis. Lancet 1, 1049 (1954).

[82] Davies, J. N. P., and J. D. Ball: The pathology of endomyocardial fibrosis in Uganda. Brit. Heart J. 17, 337 (1955).

[83] Turner, P. P., and P. E. C. Manson-Bahr: Endomyocardial fibrosis in Kenya and Tanganyika Africans. Brit. Heart J. 2, 305 (1960).

[84] Penfold, J. B.: Endocardial fibrosis of unknown origin. Lancet 1, 456 (1957).

[85] Smith, J. J., and J. Furth: Fibrosis of the endocardium and myocardium with mural thrombosis. Notes on its relation to isolated (Fiedler's) myocarditis and to Beri-Beri heart disease. Arch. int. Med. 71, 602 (1943).

[86] McKusick, V. A., and T. H. Cochran: Constrictive endocarditis; Report of a case. Bull. Johns Hopk. Hosp. 90, 90 (195)2.

[87] Edge, J. R.: Myocardial fibrosis following arsenical therapy: Report of a case. Lancet 2, 675 (1946).

[88] Fienberg, R., and D. Holzman: Bull. int. Ass. med. Mus. 32, 34 (1951) cited by Ball, J. D., and J. N. P. Davies [81].

[89] Gray, I. R.: Endocardial fibrosis. Brit. Heart J. 13, 387 (1951).

[90] Davies, J. N. P., J. Higginson, M. McGregor, B. J. P. Becker, K. J. Keeley, and B. Van Lingen: Some African cardiopathies. Report of a joint seminar of the Departments of Pathology and Medicine of the University of the Witwatersrand. S. Afr. med. J. 31, 854 (1957).

[91] Abrahams, D. G.: An unusual form of heart disease in West Africa. Lancet 2, 111 (1959).

[92] Abrahams, D., and W. Brigden: Syndrome of mitral incompetence, myocarditis, and pulmonary hypertension in Nigeria. Brit. med. J. 2, 134 (1961).

[93] Gillanders, A. D.: Nutritional heart disease. Brit. Heart J. 13, 177 (1951).

[94] Higginson, J., A. D. Gillanders, and J. F. Murray: The heart in chronic malnutrition. Brit. Heart J. 14, 213 (1952).

[95] BRIGDEN, W.: Uncommon myocardial diseases. The noncoronary cardiomyopathies. Lancet 2, 1179 and 1243 (1957).

[96] BECKER, B. J. P., C. B. CHATGIDAKIS, and B. VAN LINGEN: Cardiovascular collagenosis with parietal endocardial thrombosis. Circulation 7, 345 (1953).

[97] HIGGINSON, J., C. ISAACSON, and I. SIMSON: The pathology of cryptogenic heart disease. Arch. Path. 70, 497 (1960).

[98] FLYNN, J. E., and F. D. MANN: The presence and pathogenesis of endocardial and subendocardial degeneration, mural thrombi and thrombosis of the Thebesian veins in cardiac failure from causes other than myocardial infarction. Amer. Heart J. 31, 757 (1946).

[99] LEVY, R. L.: Idiopathic cardiomegaly. J. chron. Dis. 1, 292 (1955).

[100] DOCK, W.: Marked cardiac hypertrophy and mural thrombosis in the ventricles in Beri-Beri heart. Tr. Ass. Amer. Phycns 55, 61 (1940).

[101] LÖFFLER, W.: The pathogenetic significance of the so-called endocarditis parietalis fibroplastica. Bull. schweiz. Akad. med. Wiss. 2, 287 (1946—1947).

[102] WALKER, A. R. P., and H. GRUSIN: Coronary heart disease and cerebral vascular disease in the South African Bantu. Examination and discussion of crude and age specific death rates. Am. J. clin. Nutr. 7, 264 (1959).

[103] MILLER, D. C., S. S. SPENCER, and P. D. WHITE: Survey of cardiovascular disease among Africans in the vicinity of the Albert Schweitzer Hospital in 1960. Am. J. Cardiol. 10, 439 (1962).

[104] BEHEYT, P.: Analysis of 1081 cases of cardiovascular disease from the Belgian Congo. Proc. Third World Cong. Cardiol., Brussels, 1958; cited by MILLER, D. C., S. S. SPENCER, and P. D. WHITE [103].

[105] MOSER, M., M. HARRIS, D. PUGATCH, A. FERBER, and G. GORDON: Epidemiology of hypertension. II. Studies of blood pressure in Liberia. Amer. J. Cardiol 10, 424 (1962).

[106] ADAMS, J. M.: Some racial differences in blood pressure and morbidity in a group of White and Coloured workmen. Amer. J. med. Sci. 184, 342 (1932).

[107] GELFAND, M.: Heart disease in the elderly African. Brit. Heart J. 23, 387 (1961).

[108] BECKER, B. J. P.: Cardiovascular disease in the Bantu and Coloured races of South Africa. V. Hypertensive heart disease. S. Afr. J. med. Sci. 11, 107 (1946).

[109] LEVIN, N. W.: The presence of hypertension and uraemia in 85 cases of chronic pyelonephritis diagnosed at necropsy. Leech (Johannesburg) 27, 29 (1957).

[110] FRASER, B. N.: Manifestations and aetiology of hypertension in the Coloured and Bantu. Brit. med. J. 1, 761 (1959).

[111] SOMERS, K.: Mecamylamine and Reserpine in the management of severe and malignant hypertension in Uganda. S. Afr. med. J. 33, 515 (1959).

[112] SHAPER, A. G., and A. W. WILLIAMS: Cardiovascular disorders at an African Hospital in Uganda. Trans. roy. Soc. trop. Med. Hyg. 54, 12 (1960).

[113] SHILLINGFORD, J. P., and K. SOMERS: Clinical and haemodynamic patterns in endomyocardial fibrosis. Brit. Heart J. 23, 433 (1961).

[114] THOMAS, W. A., R. V. RANDALL, E. F. BLAND, and B. CASTLEMAN: Endocardial fibroelastosis: A factor in heart disease of obscure aetiology. New Engl. J. Med. 251, 327 (1954).

[115] TURNER, P. P.: The electrocardiogram in fifty normal young adult Kikuyu males. E. Afr. med. J. 36, 555 (1959).

[116] GREENE, C. R., and J. J. KELLY: Electrocardiogram of the healthy adult Negro. Circulation 20, 906 (1959).

[117] WASSERBURGER, R. H.: Observations on the juvenile pattern of adult Negro males. Amer. J. Med. 18, 428 (1955).

[118] SOMERS, K., and A. M. RANKIN: The electrocardiogram in healthy East African (Bantu and Nilotic) men. Brit. Heart J. 24, 542 (1962).

[119] STAMLER, J., D. M. BERKSON, Q. D. YOUNG, H. A. LINDBERG, Y. HALL, L. MOJONNIER, and S. ANDELMAN: Diet and serum lipids in atheromatous coronary heart disease. Etiologic and preventive considerations. Med. Clin. N. Amer. 47, 5 (1963).

[120] ANTONIS, A., and I. BERSOHN: Influence of diet on serum triglycerides in South African White and Bantu prisoners. Lancet 1, 3 (1961).

[121] Walker, A. R. P., and I. W. Simson: Mortality from cerebral vascular and coronary disease among the South African Bantu. (correspondences) Lancet 1, 1126 (1958).

[122] Grusin, H.: Acute reversible heart failure in Africans. Circulation 16, 27 (1957).

[123] Reid, J. V. O.: Postpartal cardiomyopathy. S. Afr. med. J. 35, 165 (1961).

[124] Seftel, H., and M. Susser: Maternity and myocardial failure in African women. Brit. Heart J. 23, 43 (1961).

[125] Keeley, K. J.: Prognosis of "nutritional heart disease" in the Bantu. Report of a case of chronic reversible heart failure. S. Afr. med. J. 34, 1071 (1960).

[126] Gilchrist, A. R.: Cardiological problems in younger women: including those of pregnancy and the puerperium. Brit. med. J. 1, 209 (1963).

[127] Gouley, B. A., T. M. McMillan, and S. Bellet: Idiopathic myocardial degeneration associated with pregnancy and especially puerperium. Amer. J. med. Sci. 194, 185 (1937).

[128] Melvin, J. P.: Post-partal heart disease. Ann. int. Med. 27, 596 (1947).

[129] Hull, E., and E. Hidden: Postpartal heart failure. S. med. J. (Nashville) 31, 265 (1938); cited by Seftel, H., and M. Susser [124].

[130] Altman, H., and H. Stein: Idiopathic hypertrophy of heart in African children: Report of four cases. Brit. med. J. 1, 1207 (1956).

[131] Becker, B. J. P.: Personal communication, 1962.

[132] Klachko, D. M., N. L. Schwarz, and H. C. Seftel: Idiopathic cardiomyopathy simulating organic valve disease. S. Afr. med. J. 35, 728 (1961).

[133] Schamroth, L., and D. Blumsohn: The significance of left axis deviation in heart disease of the African. Brit. Heart J. 23, 405 (1961).

[134] Scotch, N., B. Gampel, J. H. Abramson, and C. Slome: Blood pressure measurements of urban Zulu adults. Amer. Heart J. 61, 173 (1961).

[135] Bradlow, B. A.: Haemoptysis in Mitral stenosis. S. Afr. med. J. 24, 93 and 108 (1950).

[136] Bradlow, B. A., and G. R. Crawshaw: Mitral valvotomy in the younger age groups. S. Afr. med. J. 29, 639 (1955).

[137] Halim, A. M., and J. E. Jacques: Rheumatic heart disease in the Sudan. Brit. Heart J. 23, 383 (1961).

[138] Beet, E. A.: Discussion on paper "Endomyocardial fibrosis in Africa: Its diagnosis, distribution and nature". A. W. Williams, J. D. Ball, and J. N. P. Davies. Trans. Soc. trop. Med. Hyg. p. 290—303, 48, 309 (Discussion p. 306—311) (1954).

[139] O'Brien, W.: Endocardial fibrosis in Sudan. Brit. med. J. 2, 899 (1954).

[140] Schrire, V.: Experience with pericarditis at Groote Schuur Hospital, Cape Town. An analysis of one hundred and sixty cases studied over a six-year period. S. Afr. med. J. 33, 810 (1959).

[141] Baskind, E.: Personal communication from a thesis submitted for the degree of Doctor of Medicine in the University of the Witwatersrand, entitled "Non-suppurative pericarditis with effusion in the Bantu: A clinical study of 20 cases". 1952.

[142] Heimann, H. L., and S. Binder: Tuberculous pericarditis. Brit. Heart J. 2, 165 (1940).

[143] Adams, E. B., and J. Wainwright: (Correspondence) Myocardial disease of obscure aetiology. Brit. med. J. 2, 914 (1958).

[144] Schrire, V., and J. Gant: The electrocardiographic changes associated with Beri-Beri heart disease: An analysis of 50 cases studied at Groote Schuur Hospital Cape Town, during a period of 5 years. S. Afr. J. Lab. clin. Med. 5, 195 (1959).

[145] Williams, T.: "Toward the Conquest of Beriberi." Cambridge: Harvard University Press 1961.

[146] Keeley, K. J.: In seminar on "Some African Cardiopathies". S. Afr. med. J. 31, 854 (1957).

[147] Dawes, G. S.: "Physiological effects of anoxia in the foetal and new-born lamb", in "Lectures on the Scientific Basis of Medicine" Vol. 5. 1955—56 University of London. Athlone Press. Pp. 53—56, 1957.

[148] Marticorena, E.: In "Etiology and anatomy of Congenital heart diseases". Symposium: "Helen Taussig". The IV World Congress of Cardiology. Mexico City, 1962.

[149] El Mofty, A.: "Clinical aspects of Bilharziasis" in "Bilharziasis". Ciba Foundation symposium J. and A. Churchill Ltd., London. Pp. 173—197, 1962.

[150] Abrahams, D. G., and W. P. Cockshott: Multiple Non-luetic aneurysms in young Nigerians. Brit. Heart J. 24, 83 (1962).

[151] GELFAND, M.: Giant cell arteritis with anurysmal formation in infant. Brit. Heart J. 17, 264 (1953).
[152] ISAACSON, C., D. M. KLACHKO, S. WAYBURNE, and I. W. SIMPSON: Aortitis in children. Lancet 2, 542 (1959).
[153] JACOBSON, B.: Some radiological observations in aortitis. Brit. J. Radiol. 33, 523 (1960).
[154] Editorial: High altitude pulmonary hypertension. (Including report on paper, by VOGEL, J. H. K., W. F. WEAVER, R. L. ROSE, S. G. BLOUNT, and R. F. GROVER: at Fifth Annual Conference on Research in Emphysema, Aspen, Colorado, U.S.A. 1962). Lancet 2, 233 (1962).
[155] Union Statistics for Fifty Years, Union of South Africa. Jubilee Issue 1910—1960, Pretoria 1960.
[156] JOUBERT, S. M., C. SLOME, J. H. ABRAMSON, G. GAMPEL, and N. SCOTCH: Plasma cholesterol values of urban Zulu adults. S. Afr. J. Lab. clin. Med. 7, 35 (1961).
[157] CRAIB, W. H.: Heart disease in general practice. Leech (Johannesburg) 23, 5 (1953).
[158] ELLIOTT, G. A.: The Johannesburg Heart. Leech (Johannesburg) 23, 11 (1953).
[159] WAINWRIGHT, J.: Atheroma in the African (Bantu) in Natal. Lancet 1, 366 (1961).
[160] STRONG, J. P., J. WAINWRIGHT, and H. C. McGILL: Atherosclerosis in the Bantu. Circulation 20, 1118 (1959).
[161] LAURIE, W., J. D. WOODS, and G. ROACH: Coronary heart diseases in South African Bantu. Amer. J. Cardiol. 5, 48 (1960).
[162] METZ, J., N. W. LEVIN, and D. HART: Effect of altitude on the body venous haematocrit ratio. Nature 194, 483 (1962).
[163] BARLOW, J. B., L. H. KLUGMAN, and M. M. ZION: Obstructive cardiopathy: Paper presented at 3rd Biennial Congress Southern African Cardiac Society, July, 1962.
[164] GOODWIN, J. F., H. GORDON, A. HOLLMAN, and M. B. BISHOP: Clinical aspects of cardiomyopathy. Brit. med. J. 1, 69 (1961).

Electrocardiographic and Pathologic Features of Myocardial Infarction in Man *

R. S. Wilkinson, Jr., M. D. **, J. A. Schaeffer, M. D. and J. A. Abildskov, M. D.

A correlative study

Myocardial infarction is not always associated with the electrocardiographic features that are considered indicative of this lesion by present standards. Better understanding of the mechanisms of electrocardiographic alteration by infarction may make it possible to improve current diagnostic criteria. Our present observations on man supplement previous theoretic and experimental investigations of the mechanism by which localized myocardial lesions affect the electrocardiogram [1, 2].

Prior theoretic investigation of these lesions was based on the ventricular excitation sequence reported by SCHER [3]. The form of electrocardiographic leads that would result from this sequence was derived and compared with that of leads derived after postulating various areas of localized tissue loss. Results were consistent with clinical and electrocardiographic experience in the recognition and localization of infarcts, but there were several findings of additional interest. Thus, while appropriate lateral wall lesions resulted in "pathologic" Q waves in the derived lead I, other lateral wall lesions of different size, shape or location resulted only in decreased amplitude of R waves in this lead. Further, on the basis of the excitation sequence employed, it appeared that subendocardial and intramural areas of tissue loss were the lesions most likely to result in "pathologic" Q waves. Transmural tissue loss was not necessary to account for such deflections. Lesions confined to the subepicardial myocardium altered only mid or late portions of the QRS complex, while septal lesions in various locations were capable of altering any portion of the QRS, depending on location, size and shape of the lesion.

The aforementioned theoretic study was supplemented by an experimental investigation of localized lesions in the dog heart. Results of this study were

* From the Departments of Medicine and Pathology, State University of New York, Upstate Medical Center and Veterans Administration Hospital, Syracuse, New York. This investigation was supported by Research Grant H-3241 from the National Heart Institute of the National Institutes of Health and by a grant from the Heart Association of Onondaga County. Published in Amer. J. Cardiol.

** Study made during the tenure of a postdoctoral fellowship from the National Heart Institute, U. S. Public Health Service.

consistent with those of the theoretic investigation with respect to the electrocardiographic effects of localized loss of tissue. For example, certain lesions confined to the subendocardial and intramural myocardium resulted in definite "pathologic" Q waves, while lesions in a variety of other locations left the initial portion of the QRS unaltered but changed later portions of the complex. The experimental lesions also resulted in a variety of QRS alterations that could not be accounted for on the basis of localized tissue loss. These changes, which reflected an altered excitation sequence in areas not involved by the lesions, must be attributed to conduction disorders. Such disorders have been reported on the basis of clinical electrocardiographic observations under the title of peri-infarction block [4, 5]. Conduction disorders due to localized myocardial lesions may be the result of either interruption of specialized conduction paths or alteration of the spread of the excitatory process around the lesion itself, or both. In the previous experimental study there was a striking correlation of conduction disorders with lesions located in the interventricular septum where specialized conduction system is most densely concentrated. This finding suggested interruption of elements of this system as the major factor in conduction disorders due to localized lesions. In most instances, electrocardiographic effects of conduction disorders and of tissue loss were oppositely directed.

The observations in this report concern myocardial infarction in the human heart. The number of observations is relatively small since they concern only cases for which electrocardiograms prior to and following infarction were available. They also concern cases in which pathologic demonstration of the lesions with documentation of location, size, and shape was made by the same observer using uniform technics. The correlation of electrocardiographic and pathologic findings was based on the theoretic and experimental studies already summarized.

Materials and Methods

Ten cases were selected for study; myocardial infarcts had been demonstrated at autopsy, and electrocardiograms prior to and following the probable occurrence of infarction were available. In 2 cases the initial electrocardiogram was obtained after the onset of symptoms suggesting myocardial infarction, but further alterations of the QRS complex occurred in subsequent tracings.

The initial postmortem examination of the heart was made before fixation. The ventricles were opened by longitudinal incisions from the A-V valves to the apices. Routine measurements of wall thickness, heart weight and valve circumference were made at this time. The specimens were then formalin-fixed, and with the cut surfaces of the ventricular walls approximated, the specimens were sectioned transversely at 1 to 2 cm. intervals from apex to base. The dimensions of myocardial infarcts were measured and the shape and location of the lesions diagrammed on outlines of horizontal plane sections of the heart. Outlines of four such composite sections were employed to correspond with the ventricular excitation sequence data employed in previous studies of the theoretic effects of localized tissue loss.

Differences between the pre- and postinfarction electrocardiograms were interpreted in terms of the previous theoretic and experimental studies. In each case the electrocardiographic changes that could be attributed to tissue loss were identified. This identification was based on the ventricular excitation sequence reported by Scher [3] and was of necessity made in qualitative terms. For example, Scher's data indicate that activation of the apical one-half of the heart is largely completed during the initial three-quarters of the total ventricular activation time. It was, therefore, considered that the direct effects of tissue loss in this region would be confined to the initial three-quarters of the QRS complex. Alteration of the terminal portion of the QRS complex by an apical lesion was thus attributed to a conduction disorder.

The direction of electrocardiographic changes which could be attributed to tissue loss was also compared to that predicted on the basis of the excitation sequence. This comparison was also of necessity in qualitative terms. Finally the direction of QRS alterations attributed to conduction disorders was compared to that of alterations resulting from localized tissue loss.

Results

The details of lesion location, size, and shape were different in each specimen. The form of the electrocardiograms and the time they were recorded in relation to the occurrence of infarction and to the time of death varied in all cases. For these reasons, results will be presented and illustrated for each case. Cases have been grouped with respect to whether evidence of conduction disorders was or was not identified.

Cases with conduction disorders

Case 1. The control electrocardiogram (Fig. 1) was obtained 14 months before clinical evidence of acute myocardial infarction was noted. The postinfarction tracing was obtained three weeks after the onset of clinical evidence of myocardial infarction. The patient died four days later.

Postmortem examination showed a recent myocardial infarct involving the posterior left and right ventricular walls, the interventricular septum and the anterior and lateral left ventricular walls near the apex. Approximate dimensions of the lesion were 5 by 4.5 by 1.5 cm.

Electrocardiographic changes attributed to loss of excitable tissue in the area of the lesion were decreased amplitude of R waves in lead II, wider Q waves in III and Q waves in aVF. All were attributable to loss of tissue in the inferior wall. There was also a decrease in the amplitude of R waves in V_5 consistent with tissue loss in the lateral wall, and decreased amplitude of R waves and increased amplitude of S waves in leads V_2 through V_4 which were attributable to loss of excitable tissue in the anterior wall. There were no changes attributed to loss of excitable tissue in the posterior wall, and it seems likely that their absence was related to the involvement of the anterior wall by the same lesion.

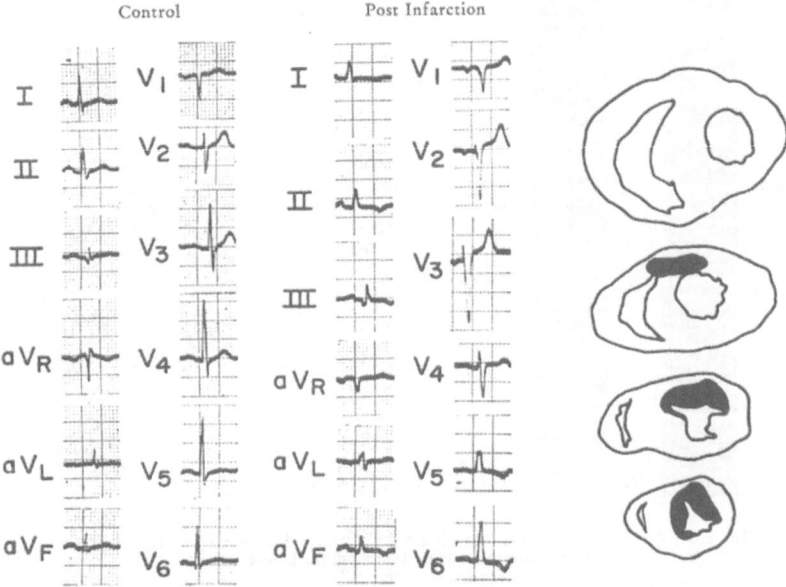

Fig. 1. Case 1. The control electrocardiogram was obtained 14 months prior to and the postinfarction record three weeks after clinical evidence of acute myocardial infarction. In this and subsequent figures, diagrammatic sections of the heart are shown with the acute infarct represented by solid black areas. These sections are arranged with the upper one representing that nearest the base

There were also alterations of the terminal portion of the QRS complex which could not be attributed to tissue loss. S waves in the control tracing in leads I, II, a VF, V_5 and V_6, were absent or of greatly decreased amplitude in the postinfarction tracing. The direction of these changes was opposite those attributed to tissue loss. For example, in lead I the amplitude of the R wave decreased after infarction which could be attributed to lateral wall tissue loss, but the change in the terminal portion of the QRS in that lead was to convert an S wave to an R wave.

Case 2. The control electrocardiogram (Fig. 2) was obtained six and a half years before the patient died. The history did not suggest acute myocardial infarction, but an electrocardiogram one year after the control tracing was made showed evidence of old anterior wall infarction. Subsequent tracings showed a stable pattern, and the postinfarction tracing (Fig. 2) was obtained three months before the patient's death.

Autopsy findings included an old myocardial infarct involving the anterior wall of the left ventricle and the left side of the interventricular septum. This lesion was located in the apical three-fourths of the heart, being transmural in the apical one-half and subendocardial in the remaining portion. The approximate dimensions of the lesion were 6 by 1.5 cm.

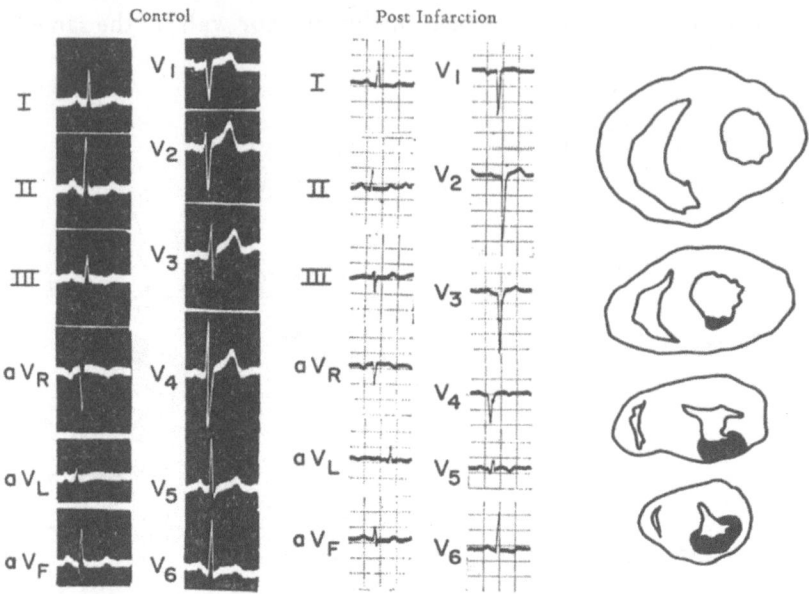

Fig. 2. Case 2. The control electrocardiogram was obtained six and a half years before the patient's death, and the postinfarction tracing three months before death

Electrocardiographic changes attributed to tissue loss were Q waves in leads V_2 through V_5. These changes were consistent with loss of tissue where normal activation proceeded in an anterior direction. *There were also alterations of the terminal portion of the QRS complex* evidenced by large S waves in lead III and aVF. Since the apical anterior wall and anterior portion of the ventricular septum are normally activated before the terminal portion of the QRS complex, alteration of this portion of the complex was considered evidence of a conduction disorder.

Case 3. The "control" electrocardiogram (Fig. 3) was obtained a few hours after onset of the substernal pain suggesting myocardial infarction. There were subsequent changes in the form of the QRS complexes represented in the tracing labeled "post infarction", which was obtained 22 days after onset of symptoms and eight days before the patient died.

Autopsy showed a recent myocardial infarct involving the subendocardial portion of the posteroinferior and lateral walls of the left ventricle and the posterior portion of the interventricular septum on its left side. The approximate dimensions of the lesion, which extended from apex to base, were 8 by 4.5 by 0.5 cm.

Electrocardiographic changes attributed to tissue loss were deeper Q waves in leads I, II, III and aVF, lower peak amplitude of R waves in I, aVL, V_5 and

V_6, and larger R waves in V_1 through V_4. These changes were consistent with the loss of tissue in the lateral and inferoposterior walls, the normal activation of which proceeds toward the left and in a posteroinferior direction, respectively.

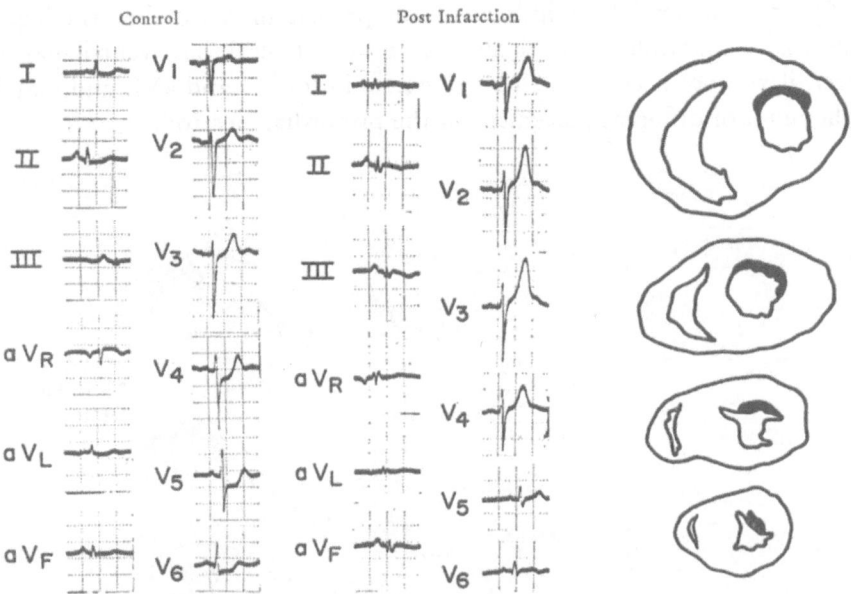

Fig. 3. Case 3. The electrocardiogram titled "control" was obtained a few hours after the onset of substernal pain suggesting myocardial infarction. Later tracings showed changes in the form of QRS complexes. The record labeled "post infarction" was obtained 22 days after the control tracing

Despite the extension of this lesion into basal portions of the heart, its subendocardial localization makes it unlikely that tissue loss effects would extend into terminal portions of the QRS complex. *Alteration of the terminal QRS did occur* as represented by the occurrence of S waves in I, II, III, aVF, V_5 and V_6 and of R′ waves in aVR. These alterations were interpreted as evidence of a conduction disorder. Their direction was the same as that of alterations due to tissue loss.

Case 4. The control electrocardiogram (Fig. 4) was obtained eight months before clinical evidence of acute myocardial infarction. The postinfarction tracing shown was obtained one and a half months after the first evidence of infarction and two days before the patient's death.

Postmortem examination showed a recent infarct of the posteroinferior wall of the left ventricle and of the posterior portion of the left side of the interventricular septum. This lesion was located in the basal three-fourths of the heart, being transmural in the basal one-half and subendocardial in its remaining extent. Its dimensions were 6.5 by 5 by 0.7 cm. There was also an old infarct in the anterior and lateral left ventricular walls in the apical one-half of the heart that measured 5 by 4 by 1 cm. It was almost transmural near the apex and subendocardial above that level.

The presence of an old infarct that could not be dated, complicated the
evaluation of electrocardiographic findings. There were no electrocardiographic
findings suggesting such a lesion either in the tracing six and a half months before
death, or in the record obtained shortly before death. The latter tracing showed
small Q waves in lead V_6 which were not present in the earlier tracing. This
finding was compatible with tissue loss in the lateral left ventricular wall;
however, it was not accompanied by Q waves in leads I and aVL and may have
been the result of different placement of the precordial electrode.

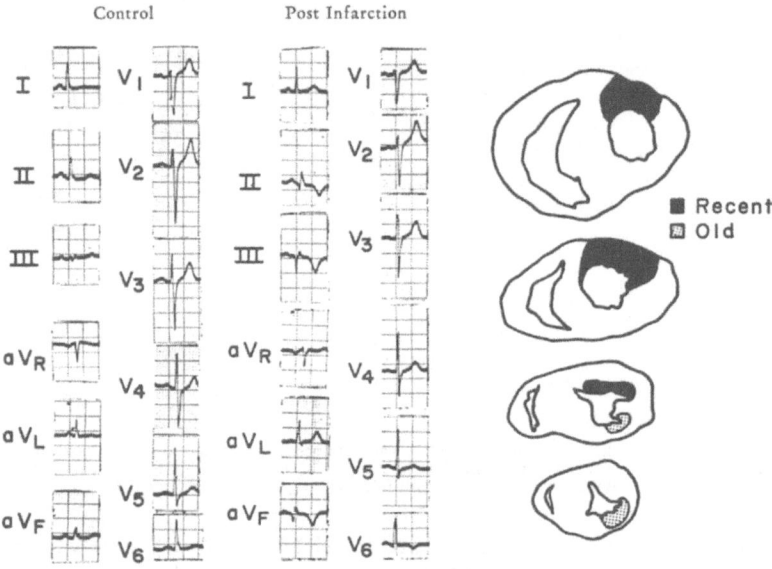

Fig. 4. Case 4. The control record was obtained eight months before and the postinfarction record one and a half
months after clinical evidence of myocardial infarction

The record obtained shortly before death showed findings attributed to tissue
loss at the site of the recent infarct. There were Q waves in leads II, III, and
aVF consistent with loss of tissue in the inferior wall, whose normal mode of
activation is directed downward. The loss of tissue in the posterior wall was not
reflected by a change of the initial portion of the QRS in precordial leads, but
leads V_1 through V_5 showed S waves of decreased amplitude attributable to loss
of tissue, the normal activation of which was directed posteriorly.

There were also definite changes in the terminal portion of the QRS complex.
These alteration included the occurrence of S waves in aVL, slurring of the down-
stroke of the R wave in lead II and a larger terminal R wave in lead III. The
lesion involved the basal subepicardial portion of the left ventricular wall which
is normally activated during the terminal portion of the QRS complex. The
direction of the change in this portion of the complex was, however, roughly
opposite that expected on the basis of tissue loss. This is best evidenced in lead III
where an initial R wave was changed to a Q wave as a result of tissue loss, while

a later small R wave became more prominent after infarction. The direction of the changes in the terminal portion of the QRS suggest they were the result of a conduction disorder.

Case 5. The control tracing (Fig. 5) was obtained 16 months before clinical evidence of the terminal acute infarct. The postinfarction tracing was obtained a few hours after the onset of symptoms suggesting myocardial infarction and 10 weeks before the patient died. Later records did not show further alteration of QRS complexes.

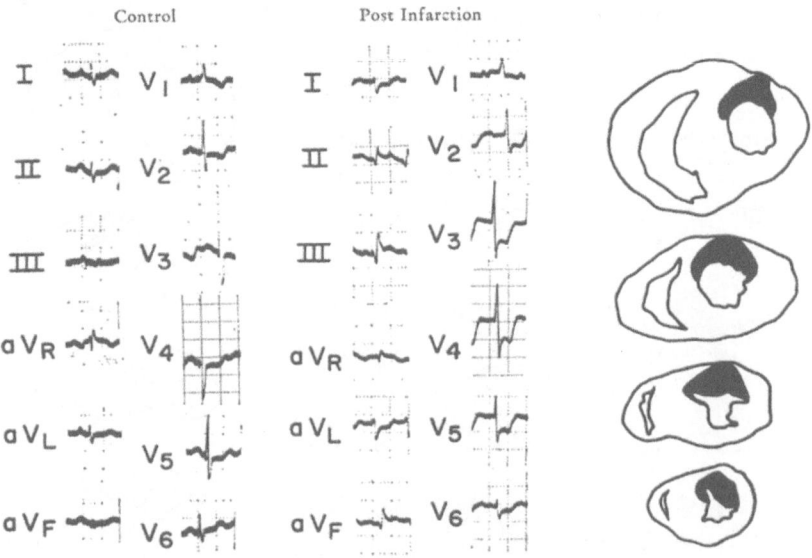

Fig. 5. Case 5. The control tracing was obtained 16 months before and the postinfarction tracing a few hours after clinical evidence of myocardial infarction

Autopsy showed a recent myocardial infarct in the posteroinferior and lateral left ventricular walls and the left side of the posterior portion of the interventricular septum. This lesion extended from base to apex and was subendocardial near the apex and transmural near the base. The infarct measured 8 by 6.5 by 1 cm. There was also an old infarct in the posterior wall in the midportion of base-to-apex dimension of the heart.

The control electrocardiogram showed nonspecific abnormalities of the S-T segments and T waves, and QRS abnormalities including S waves in leads I, II, aVL, V_5 and V_6, R' waves in aVR and prominent R waves in V_1 and V_2. These features were considered secondary to pulmonary emphysema; however, it is possible that they were the result of the old posterior wall infarct demonstrated at autopsy.

The postinfarction record showed QRS alterations attributed to loss of excitable tissue in the posteroinferior and lateral walls and the ventricular septum. There were larger Q waves in leads II, III and aVF, smaller R waves in I, aVL, V_5 and V_6 and loss of the "septal" Q wave in lead I.

In addition, there were alterations of the terminal portion of the QRS in a direction that could not be accounted for on the basis of tissue loss. This was best evidenced in leads II, III and aVF, where the effects of tissue loss resulted in Q waves; but the terminal QRS deflection in the postinfarction record was a large R wave. Because of the direction of alteration of the terminal QRS, this change was attributed to a conduction disorder.

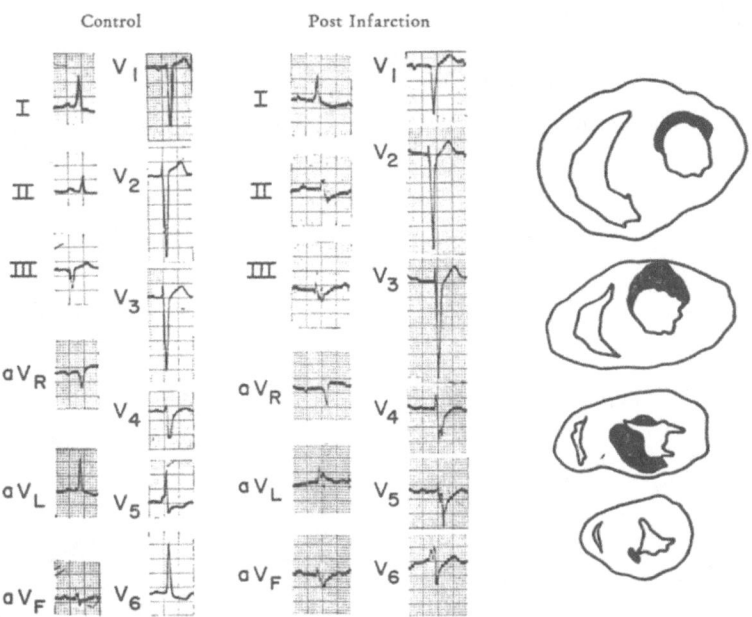

Fig. 6. Case 6. The control record was obtained six and a half months before the occurrence of clinical evidence of myocardial infarction. The postinfarction record was obtained one day before the patient's death

Case 6. The control record (Fig. 6) was obtained six and a half months before clinical evidence of acute myocardial infarction. The postinfarction tracing shown was obtained one day before the patient's death. He had a history of several episodes of severe substernal pain during the four months preceding his death.

Autopsy showed two recent myocardial infarcts, both estimated to have been present less than one month. One lesion was located in the posterior and lateral walls of the left ventricle and in the left posterior portion of the interventricular septum. This infarct was located in the basal three-quarters of the heart, was transmural in its midportions and subendocardial in other portions, and measured 4 by 3 by 1 cm. Another infarct involved the anterior wall of the left ventricle and the left side of the anterior portion of the interventricular septum. This lesion was located in the apical half of the heart and was subendocardial near the apex and transmural in other portions. It measured 8 by 6 by 0.8 cm. Both pathologic and clinical evidence suggested that the two lesions occurred after the available control electrocardiogram. The lesions will, therefore, be considered as a single entity, namely, a large lesion extending from base to apex and involving anterior, posterior and lateral left ventricular walls as well as the interventricular septum.

The widespread extent of this lesion made it difficult to define the expected effects of tissue loss. *Alterations of both initial and terminal portions of the QRS complex occurred.* It did not seem likely that the terminal QRS changes were the direct result of tissue loss. All areas involved by the lesion, including the subendocardial basal myocardium, are normally activated prior to the terminal portion of the QRS complex. Definite alterations of the terminal QRS consisting of the development of S waves in leads II, III, aVF and V_5 and V_6 were, therefore, considered evidence of a conduction disorder.

Alterations of earlier portions of the QRS complex cannot be specifically attributed to loss of excitable tissue in all of the areas occupied by this lesion. Decreased amplitude of R waves in leads aVL, V_5 and V_6 were attributable to tissue loss in the lateral wall. There were no electrocardiographic changes specifically attributable to tissue loss in the anterior and posterior walls and the interventricular septum. These findings illustrate the dependence of QRS changes, usually attributed to localized tissue loss, on a normal sequency of activation in portions of the myocardium not involved by the lesion.

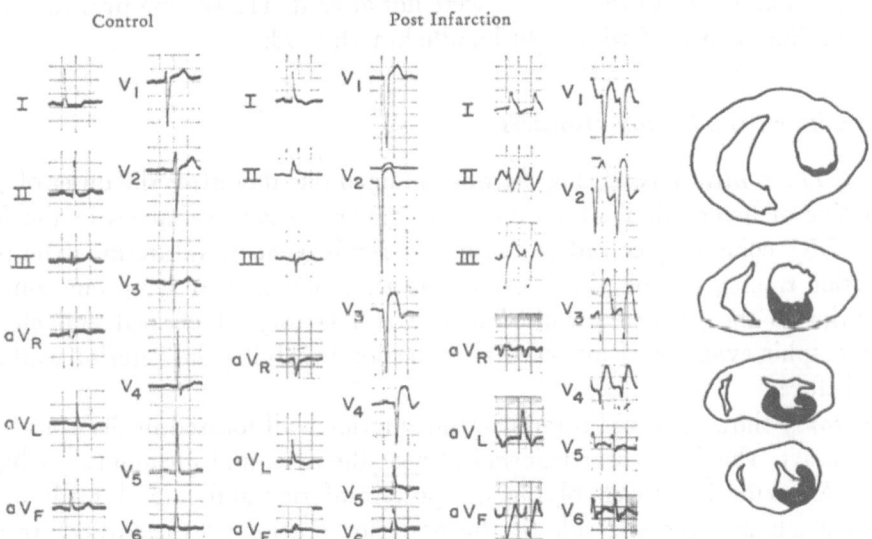

Fig. 7. Case 7. The control tracing was obtained six months before and the postinfarction tracings two and four days after clinical evidence of myocardial infarction

Case 7. The control tracing (Fig. 7) was obtained six months before clinical evidence of acute myocardial infarction. Two postinfarction tracings are shown, these having been obtained two and four days after infarction, and the patient died two days later.

Autopsy showed a recent myocardial infarct in the anterior and lateral left ventricular walls and in the left side of the anterior portion of the interventricular septum. This lesion extended from apex to base; it was transmural in the apical and subendocardial in the basal half of the heart.

The first postinfarction tracing showed only changes attributed to tissue loss. These included Q waves in leads V_2 through V_4 and larger Q waves in V_5. These findings were explicable on the basis of loss of excitable tissue in the anterior wall where activation normally proceeds anteriorly. There was also a decreased amplitude of R waves in V_5 and V_6 attributable to tissue loss in the left lateral wall where activation normally moves toward the left. Decreased amplitude of R waves in leads II, III and aVF are explicable on the basis of loss of tissue in the apical portion of the interventricular septum. In this tracing the polarity of terminal QRS deflections was the same as in the control record; so a conduction disorder could not be identified.

The later postinfarction record showed further alteration of the QRS complex. All of the evidences of tissue loss in the earlier tracing remained; but there was prolongation of the QRS interval and large S waves were present in leads II, III, aVF, V_5 and V_6. These changes were considered evidence of a conduction disorder. This disorder was unlikely to be the result of complete left bundle branch block since the previously described evidences of tissue loss in initial portions of the QRS complex were not altered. The tracing presented none of the findings expected with right bundle branch block.

Cases without conduction disorders

Case 8. The control record (Fig. 8) was obtained one day after the onset of pain suggestive of myocardial infarction. Later tracings showed changes in the form of the QRS complexes considered to be the result of acute infarction. The postinfarction tracing was obtained seven days after the onset of symptoms and one day prior to the patient's death. There was a history of clinical and electrocardiographic evidence of myocardial infarction involving the anterior wall nine years before.

Autopsy showed an old infarct in the anterior wall located in the apical half of the heart. This lesion was transmural near the apex and intramural at higher levels. An acute infarct involving the posteroinferior and lateral walls of the left ventricle and the left side of the posterior portion of the interventricular septum was present. This lesion was located in the basal three-fourths of the heart. In its midportion, in the base to apex dimension, the lesion was transmural and at the other levels was subendocardial. It measured 7 by 6 by 1.2 cm.

The control electrocardiogram showed Q waves in V_1 through V_5 compatible with the old anterior wall infarct demonstrated at autopsy. The later tracing exhibited decreased amplitude of R waves in I, aVL, V_5 and V_6. These changes were consistent with tissue loss in the lateral wall where normal activation is directed to the left. There was also a decreased amplitude of R waves in leads II and aVF consistent with tissue loss in the inferior wall where normal activation is directed downward.

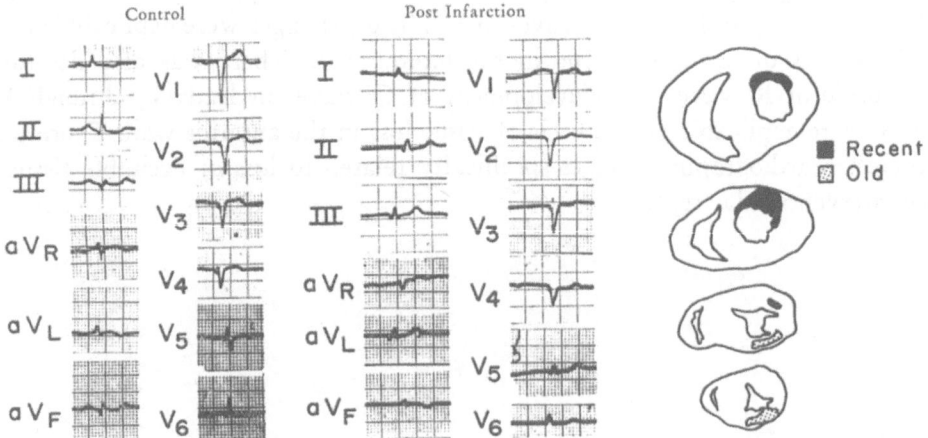

Fig. 8. Case 8. The tracing labeled "control" was obtained one day after the onset of pain suggestive of myocardial infarction. Later tracings showed changes in the form of QRS complexes. The record labeled "post infarction" was obtained seven days after the probable occurrence of infarction

The postinfarction tracing also showed alteration of the terminal portion of the QRS with the development of S waves in leads II, III and aVF. This alteration was in the appropriate direction to be attributed to tissue loss in the posteroinferior wall, and this lesion included the subepicardial basal portions of the left ventricular wall which are normally activated during late portions of the QRS complex. Since the direction of alteration of the terminal QRS was consistent with tissue loss in the area of the lesion, and because the lesion involved areas normally activated during late portions of the QRS, the records were not interpreted as providing evidence of a conduction disorder.

The electrocardiogram did not show the features predictable on the basis of loss of tissue in the posterior wall. The reason for this lack is not certain; however, the presence of the extensive anterior infarct would be expected to modify the manifestations of a posterior lesion.

Case 9. The control electrocardiogram (Fig. 9) was obtained 11 months before clinical evidence of acute myocardial infarction. The postinfarction record shown was obtained four days after the initial evidence of infarction and two days before the patient's death.

Autopsy demonstrated an acute infarct involving the anterior and lateral left ventricular walls and the left side of the interventricular septum. This lesion was located in the apical three-fourths of the heart and measured 9 by 6 by 1 cm. It was transmural in the anterior wall and subendocardial in the lateral wall and septum. There was also an old intramural infarct in the inferoposterior left ventricular wall. This was located midway between apex and base and measured 7 by 5 by 1 cm.

The control tracing showed evidence of the old infarct consisting of Q waves in leads II, III and aVF. These findings were consistent with tissue loss in the inferior wall whose normal activation is in a downward direction. *Electrocardiographic changes after the acute infarct* were decreased amplitude of R waves in I, aVL, V_5 and V_6 and larger Q waves in V_5. These changes were explicable on the basis of loss of excitable tissue in the lateral wall. There was also decreased amplitude of R waves and development of Q waves in leads V_2 through V_4, which were explicable on the basis of tissue loss in the anterior wall. There were no electrocardiographic changes specifically related to loss of excitable tissue in the interventricular septum.

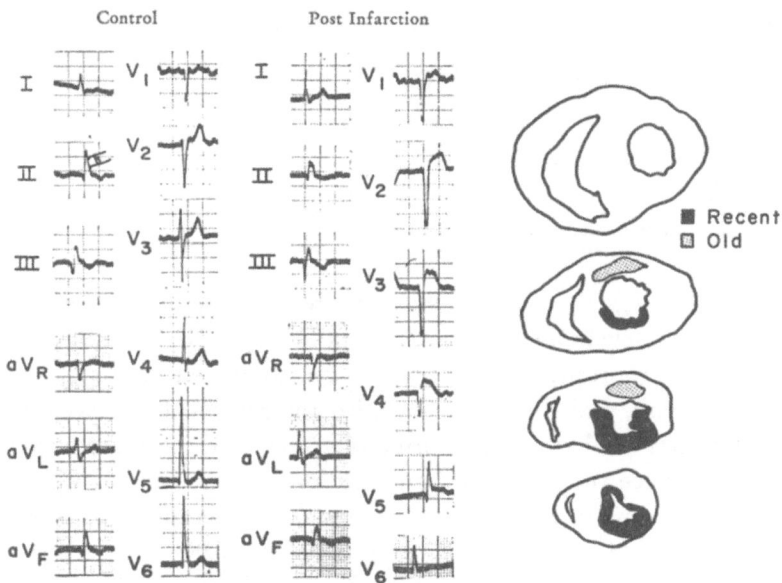

Fig. 9. Case 9. The control record was obtained 11 months prior to and the postinfarction record four days after the occurrence of clinical evidence of infarction

The S-T segment displacement in the postinfarction tracing made it difficult to evaluate the terminal portion of the QRS complex. The polarity of this portion of the complex was the same in control and postinfarction records. Since no definite alterations of the terminal QRS could be identified and since tissue loss in the region of the lesion accounted for the changes in other portions of the QRS, this case was not considered to provide evidence of a conduction disorder.

Case 10. The control electrocardiogram (Fig. 10) was obtained four months before the patient's death. He was admitted to the hospital in a confused state, and the diagnosis of myocardial infarction was not made ante-mortem. The postinfarction record shown was obtained three days before the patient's death.

Autopsy showed a recent infarct confined to the lateral wall of the left ventricle. This lesion was confined to the basal half of the heart and measured

4 by 3 by 0.9 cm. The lesion was intramural nearest the base and transmural at lower levels.

Electrocardiograms were of special interest since the postinfarction record did not show findings considered diagnostic of infarction by present standards. There were, however, changes that are explicable on the basis of tissue loss in the area where the lesion was demonstrated. The changes consisted of decreased amplitude of R waves in I, aVL and V_5 and increased amplitude of Q waves in aVL. These findings were explicable on the basis of tissue loss in the lateral wall where normal activation is directed toward the left. There was also a difference

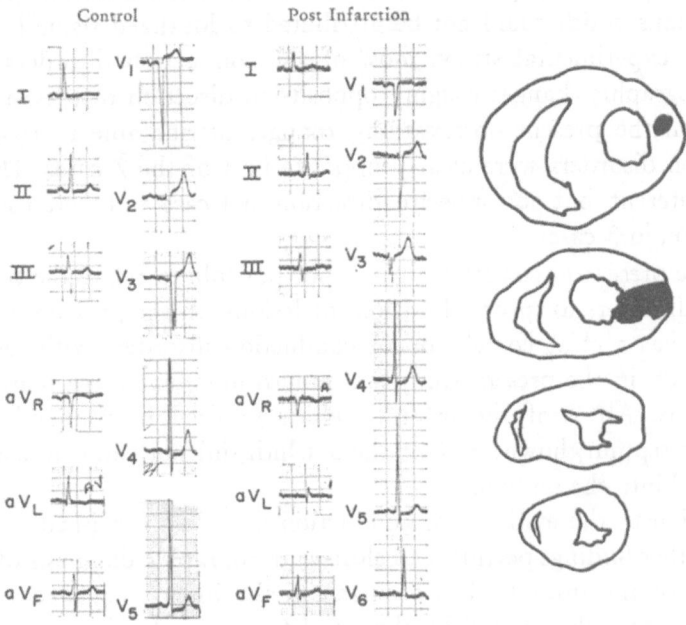

Fig. 10. Case 10. The control record was obtained four months before and the postinfarction record three days before the patient's death

in the form of QRS complexes in lead V_3; however, both the control and postinfarction records showed notching of the S wave. The specific differences are probably the result of different electrode placement. The polarity of terminal QRS deflections is the same in control and postinfarction tracings, and it was not necessary to postulate a conduction disorder to account for QRS changes.

Discussion

There are many shortcomings of the present observations. The control electrocardiograms were obtained at variable intervals before myocardial infarction and may have been modified in the interim by factors other than infarction. The electrocardiograms were recorded by routine technics which included a recording paper speed of 25 mm. per second. This paper speed was not appropriate for detailed evaluation of the QRS complex, and it was necessary to evaluate changes grossly as involving initial or terminal portions of the complex. Most of the infarcts in this series were large lesions; some were multiple, which complicated the correlation of lesion location and electrocardiographic findings. Despite these limitations, the observations provided certain information concerning the mechanism of alteration and the diagnostic merits and limitations of the electrocardiogram in myocardial infarction.

The observations indicated that myocardial infarction in man may produce intraventricular conduction disorders similar to those previously identified with experimental lesions in dogs. In 7 of the 10 cases reported, infarction resulted in QRS alterations which could not be attributed to localized tissue loss alone. In the previous experimental study, most of the conduction disorders resulted in electrocardiographic changes roughly opposite in direction to these produced by tissue loss. In the present observations, changes attributable to tissue loss and to conduction disorders were clearly opposite in 3 of the 7 cases. These changes were in a different, but not opposite, direction in 1 case and were roughly in the same direction in 3 cases.

From the present observations it was not possible to relate the occurrence of conduction disorders to specific locations of lesions. In the previous experimental study there was a clear correlation of conduction disorders with septal lesions. All the infarcts in the present study were much more extensive than the experimental lesions. All 7 of the infarcts which resulted in conduction disorders involved the septum; however, 2 of the 3 which did not result in such disorders also extended into the septum.

In addition to the evidence of conduction disorders furnished by this study, there were other findings pertinent to electrocardiographic diagnosis of infarction. All but one of the infarcts that occurred in the interval between control and postinfarction records resulted in abnormal Q waves. In the case without such deflections (Case 6) the lesion was massive, extending from apex to base and involving anterior, posteroinferior and lateral walls as well as the septum. The occurrence of pathologic Q waves in myocardial infarction is dependent not only upon localized loss of excitable tissue but also upon the activation pattern in uninvolved myocardium. For example, the occurrence of Q waves in precordial leads after anterior wall infarction is the result of activation in the posterior wall no longer opposed to a normal degree by anterior wall excitation. With very extensive tissue loss, as was present in Case 6, such relationships are necessarily modified. In that case the only evidence of loss of excitable tissue was decreased amplitude of R waves in leads aVL, V_5 and V_6 consistent with the lateral wall tissue loss. Electrocardiographic findings specifically attributable to tissue loss in the other areas occupied by this lesion were lacking.

In Case 10 the infarct resulted in increased amplitude of Q waves in lead aVL, but the only evidence of tissue loss in leads I, V_5 and V_6 was decreased amplitude of R waves. The lesion in this case was confined to the basal half of the lateral wall. Activation of a considerable portion of this wall takes place after activation of the septum and right ventricle have been largely completed. There is, therefore, less reason for marked displacement of the excitation direction toward the right by loss of tissue in the basal portion of the left ventricle than by loss of tissue nearer the apex.

The old infarct in Case 4 was not associated with QRS abnormalities which permit recognition of the lesion. The time this infarct occurred was not known, and it may have antedated the first available electrocardiogram; so it was not possible to evaluate the changes which may have resulted. The lesion, however, was located in the anterior and lateral walls near the apex. On the basis of the excitation sequence reported by SCHER characteristic deformities of the QRS complex would be expected. The reason for the absence of these deformities was not apparent.

It is not appropriate to review the voluminous literature concerning myocardial infarction and the electrocardiogram, but certain previous studies are especially pertinent to the present one.

GRANT and MURRAY [5] studied pre- and postinfarction electrocardiograms from 190 patients with clinical and electrocardiographic evidence of myocardial infarction. Findings were suggestive of intraventricular conduction disorders in approximately one third of these. In the present study, the pathologic data available made it possible to assess the contribution of localized tissue loss more exactly, and the incidence of conduction disorders identified was even higher.

COOK and co-workers [6, 7] reviewed the electrocardiograms of 30 patients with subendocardial infarction, including 3 with preinfarction tracings. In the latter cases QRS alterations were decreased amplitude of R waves in precordial leads and, in one of the cases, appearance of Q deflections. In the other cases low amplitude R waves and in some cases Q waves in precordial leads were noted. These authors concluded that small and moderate sized subendocardial lesions produced QRS alterations of limited extent. They also concluded that even large infarcts restricted to the inner half of the myocardial wall produced less marked alterations of the QRS complex than did other nontransmural lesions which included involvement of more than the inner half of the ventricular wall.

In the present study only two of the lesions were not transmural, but both resulted in changes attributed to localized tissue loss, including the occurrence of pathologic Q waves. This is comparable to previous experimental findings where nontransmural lesions also resulted in pathologic Q waves [2]. While these findings demonstrated that at least some nontransmural lesions may result in QRS alterations including pathologic Q waves, they do not prove that the contribution of subendocardial ventricular activation to the QRS complex is comparable to that of subepicardial excitation. The studies of DURRER et al. [8] suggest multidirectional activation of inner layers of the left ventricular wall with less influence on normal QRS form than activation of subepicardial layers. It is also possible that different conductivity of cavity blood and the myocardium itself may modify the contribution of subendocardial and subepicardial activation to the form of the QRS complex. The question of the relative contributions of subendocardial and subepicardial activation to the QRS complex needs further study.

Summary

The electrocardiographic and pathologic findings in 10 cases of myocardial infarction were investigated. In each case, electrocardiograms prior to and following the occurrence of myocardial infarction were available, and the pathologic features were demonstrated by a uniform technic.

The electrocardiographic changes were interpreted in terms of the ventricular excitation sequence reported by Scher. In 7 of the 10 cases, there were QRS alterations which were not explicable on the basis of localized tissue loss applied to that sequence. This finding was considered evidence of intraventricular conduction disorders due to myocardial infarction.

Alteration of the QRS complex which could be attributed to localized tissue loss was associated with all infarcts that occurred in the interim between control and postinfarction electrocardiograms. This evidence of tissue loss did not, however, reflect all of the areas actually occupied by the lesions.

References

[1] Jacobson, E. D., S. Rush, S. Zinberg, and J. A. Abildskov: The effect of infarction on the magnitude and orientation of electrical events in the heart. Amer. Heart J. 58, 863 (1959).

[2] Abildskov, J. A., R. S. Wilkinson, W. A. Vincent, and W. Cohen: An experimental study of the electrocardiographic effects of localized myocardial lesions. Amer. J. Cardiol 8, 485 (1961).

[3] Scher, A. M., and A. C. Young: The pathway of ventricular depolarization in the dog. Circulation Res. 4, 461 (1950).

[4] First, S. R., R. H. Bayley, and D. R. Bedford: Peri-infarction block; electrocardiographic abnormality occasionally resembling bundle branch block and local ventricular block of other types. Circulation 2, 31 (1950).

[5] Grant, R. P., and R. H. Murray: The QRS complex deformity of myocardial infarction in the human subject. Amer. J. Med. 17, 587 (1954).

[6] Cook, R. W., J. E. Edwards, and R. D. Pruitt: Electrocardiographic changes in acute subendocardial infarction. 1. Large subendocardial and large non-transmural infarcts. Circulation 18, 603 (1958).

[7] Cook, R. W., J. E. Edwards, and R. D. Pruitt: Electrocardiographic changes in acute subendocardial infarction. II. Small subendocardial infarcts. Circulation 18, 613 (1958).

[8] Durrer, D., L. H. van der Tweel, and J. R. Blickman: Spread of activation in the left ventricular wall of the dog, III. Amer. Heart J. 48, 13 (1954).

Estudio epidemiologico de la hipertension arterial y de la isquemia miocardica*

L. Méndez, M.C., Sc.D. · R. A. Alva, M.C., M.S.P. · B. R. Ordóñez
de la Mora, M.C., M.S.P. · G. Figueroa, M.C.

En México, como en otros países, la frecuencia de los padecimientos cardiovasculares no reumáticos va siendo cada vez mayor. A ello contribuye, por una parte, la disminución de las enfermedades transmisibles y el consecuente incremento de la esperanza de vida de la población, así como el constante aumento de los factores, conocidos y desconocidos, que están conectados con la vida moderna y que predisponen, coadyuvan o determinan los padecimientos mencionados.

Si bien es imprecisa la información que se tiene sobre la prevalencia de la hipertensión arterial y de la isquemia miocárdica en nuestro medio, es posible apreciar su importancia relevante en determinadas zonas urbanas, al través de algunas observaciones y estudios parciales realizados. Asimismo, las estadísticas de mortalidad, aunque no suelen ser la mejor fuente de información, pueden dar una idea sobre aquellas enfermedades cardiovasculares, sobre todo si se comparan los datos actuales con los de años anteriores.

Es indiscutible la necesidad de realizar investigaciones que ayuden a conocer el problema real que representan en nuestro país los padecimientos señalados; y que además, aporten datos que, comparados con otros similares, permitan establecer la influencia de diversos factores, ofreciendo así bases técnicas para el estudio de medidas preventivas de dichas enfermedades cardiovasculares no reumáticas.

Consciente de estos hechos, el Instituto Mexicano del Seguro Social diseñó un estudio con los siguientes objetivos:

1°. Conocer la prevalencia de la hipertensión arterial y la isquemia miocárdica en algunas áreas del medio urbano de la Ciudad de México.

2°. Establecer la mediana de presión arterial en la población de ese medio, según algunas variables.

3°. Contribuir al conocimiento de la epidemiología de la hipertensión arterial y de la isquemia miocárdica, analizando los factores que pudieran estar interviniendo en la distribución y frecuencia de las enfermedades señaladas.

---

* Trabajo presentado en el IV Congreso Mundial de Cardiología. 1962.

Metodología

Este estudio se llevó al cabo en dos Unidades de Habitación del Instituto Mexicano del Seguro Social (I.M.S.S.), ubicadas en la Ciudad de México y en las que reside población perteneciente a tres diferentes estratos económico-sociales.

Se examinó, en el curso del año de 1961, a toda población de 30 años y más que habita en la Unidad "Legaria" y en el sector "San Ramón" y en las "Torres" de la Unidad Independencia.

Todas la personas fueron visitadas en sus domicilios por pasantes de medicina previamente seleccionados y adiestrados, quienes recabaron, en cuestionarios especiales, datos de identificación; condiciones físicas generales (peso, constitución, etc.); hábitos (tabaquismo, alimentación, actividad física, etc.); ocupación, educación y otras condiciones socio-económicas; antecedentes familiares y personales de posible patología cardiovascular.

Inmediatamente después, a cada una de estas personas se les midió la tensión arterial en ambros brazos tanto en el decúbito como en el ortostatismo y en apnea inspiratoria y espiratoria. A las personas de 40 años o más se les tomó, además, electrocardiograma en las 12 derivaciones.

La crítica de los datos recolectados fué hecha por un médico epidemiólogo, antes de que se estableciera si las personas eran sanas o enfermas. Las personas que no aportaron datos completos, fueron excluídas de este estudio, quedando limitado así a 1,000 personas de 30 años y más que dieron datos utilizables.

Un médico cardiólogo seleccionó y estudió minuciosamente los casos con tensiones arteriales mayores de 140—90, con trazos electrocardiográficos anormales, o con sospecha clínica de patología cardiovascular. A todos estos probables casos se les practicó examen clínico completo incluyendo nuevo electrocardiograma, teleradiografía de tórax y estudio del fondo de ojo, así como química sanguínea con dosificación de electrolitos, análisis general de orina y biometría hemática.

Personal administrativo tabuló los datos, utilizando para ello los aparatos electrónicos del Instituto Mexicano del Seguro Social.

Para la evaluación de los resultados se recurrió a los métodos estadísticos de significancia más comunes.

Antes de señalar los resultados, es conveniente exponer algunas características generales de las 1,000 personas estudiadas y que quedaron distribuídas en tres grupos:

El Grupo B, de clase media superior, reside en las "Torres" de la Unidad de Habitación Independencia; está constituído por personas que en su mayoría son profesionistas, técnicos o están dedicados a labores del hogar, con un promedio de ingreso anual per cápita de 618.6 Dls. Un alto porcentaje de esta población ha realizado estudios superiores.

El Grupo C, de clase media inferior, habita en el sector de "San Ramón" de la misma Unidad. Una proporción elevada de este grupo la forman oficinistas o personas dedicadas a labores del hogar, con un promedio anual de ingresos per cápita de 246.1 Dls.

El Grupo D, de clase baja superior, lo integran personas que viven en la Unidad Habitación "Legaria" y que trabajan como obreros o se ocupan de labores domésticas. El promedio anual de ingresos per cápita es de 106.0 Dls. El 55% de esta población adulta no completó su educación primaria y otro 20% eran analfabetos.

Resultados

Los resultados obtenidos corresponden a cada uno de los objetivos que se fijaron para este trabajo. Ellos son: los relativos a las medianas de tensiones arteriales, a la prevalencia de los padecimientos investigados según algunas variables, y al análisis de otros factores que pudieran estar influyendo.

Medianas de presión arterial

Por lo que se refiere a las presiones arteriales, la mediana hallada en las 1,000 personas incluidas en este estudio es de 128—84, para una edad promedio de 41.3 años. Las curvas de distribución normal de tensiones tomadas en el decúbito y en el ortostatismo, no variaron significativamente entre sí. (Anexo # 1).

Como era de esperarse, la mediana de tensión arterial es progresivamente más elevada conforme mayor es la edad de la población. Así, de los 30 a los 39 años, la mediana es de

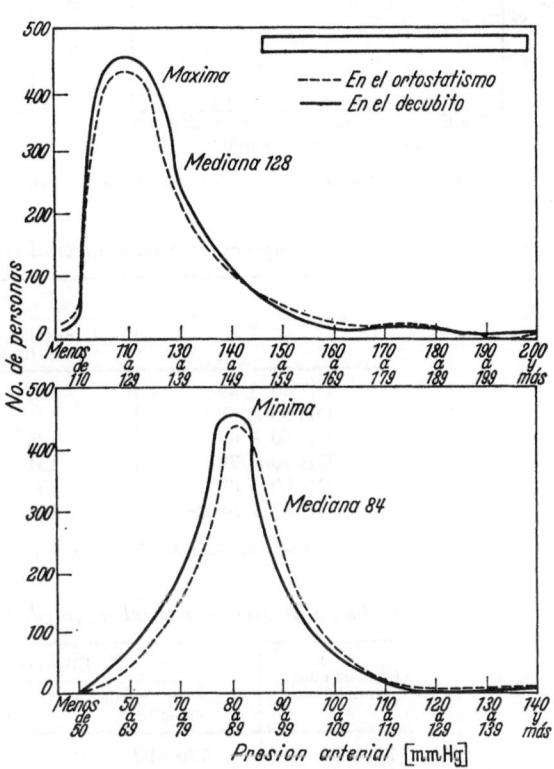

Anexo 1. Presion arterial de la poblacion estudiada

123—82; de los 40 a los 49 años, de 132—86; de los 50 a 59 años, de 141—89; y de los 60 y más años, de 148—89 (Anexo # 2).

En relación con el sexo, se observa que en personas menores de 50 años, la mediana de presión arterial es más alta entre hombres que mujeres; pero en edades más avanzadas es mayor en mujeres, lo que probablemente se debe, entre otros factores, a que es más frecuente la obesidad en personas del sexo femenino de 50 años y más (Anexo # 3).

Se obtuvieron las medianas según el peso corporal de las personas estudiadas, observándose que a cifras mayores de peso corporal, corresponden medianas de presión arterial más elevadas, tanto sistólicas como diastólicas, lo que coincide con otras observaciones hechas en México y en el extranjero (Anexo # 4).

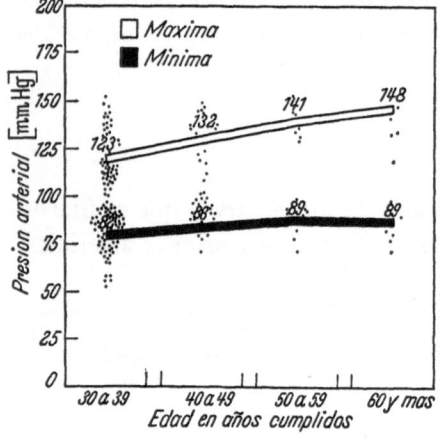

Anexo 2. Presion arterial de la poblacion segun edades   Anexo 3. Medianas de presion arterial por edad y sexo

Medianas de presion arterial segun peso corporal

Peso corporal en Kg.	Presion arterial	
	Sistolica (mm.Hg.)	Diastolica (mm.Hg.)
DE 40 A 49	126	80
DE 50 A 59	126	82
DE 60 A 69	128	84
DE 70 A 79	131	86
DE 80 A 89	136	88
DE 90 Y MAS	139	89

Anexo 4. Medianas de presion arterial segun peso corporal

Medianas de presion arterial segun edad y estrato economico-social

Edad en años cumplidos	Estrato economico-social		
	Clase "B" media superior	Clase "C" media inferior	Clase "D" baja superior
30 A 39	126—82	125—83	123—82
40 A 49	130—85	133—86	131—85
50 A 59	140—89	140—89	140—89
60 Y MAS	155—88	144—89	144—89
Total	132—85	130—84	127—83

Anexo 5. Medianas de presion arterial segun edad y estrato economico-social

Según los estratos económico-sociales, cuyas características se mencionaron en párrafos anteriores, se tienen tensiones arteriales significativamente mayores en estratos con mejores condiciones de vida; pero esta diferencia no es significativa si las medianas se establecen por edades dentro de cada estrato. La variación de presiones arteriales de un estrato en relación con otro se debe, principalmente, a que en clases altas existen personas de mayor edad (Anexo # 5).

En relación con todas estas cifras de normalidad de tensiones arteriales, es pertinente aclarar que no se consideran definitivas, ya que es necesario el estudio de un mayor número de personas, especialmente de determinados grupos de edad y peso. Estos estudios se continúan realizando en población amparada por el I.M.S.S., fuera de las Unidades de Habitación.

Prevalencia de hipertensión arterial e isquemia miocárdica

Ahora bien, en relación con la patología encontrada en todo el grupo estudiado, que como se dijo, lo integraron 1,000 personas de 30 años y más, se señala lo siguiente:

El 11.2% de todo este grupo se halló con hipertensión arterial, siendo las más de las veces asintomática. Así, siguiendo la clasificación de Méndez, tenemos que el 68.8% de los casos son grado I; el 16.9% grado II; el 12.6% grado III y el 1.7% grado IV.

Se encontró isquemia miocárdica en el 5.6% de las personas de 40 años y más, predominando la insuficiencia coronaria. Unicamente en 4 casos coincidieron ambos padecimientos: isquemia miocárdica e hipertensión arterial, lo que resulta un poco sorprendente ya que, como es bien sabido, este último padecimiento predispone a la isquemia del miocardio.

La arterioesclerosis generalizada coincidió, como se esperaba, con la hipertensión arterial o la isquemia miocárdica, excepto en 2 casos. Su prevalencia fué de 6.2 en el grupo estudiado. Accidentes vasculares cerebrales se hallaron en el 0.3%.

Aunque no era objetivo de este trabajo estudiar otros padecimientos cardiovasculares o nó cardiovasculares, puede ser importante señalar que en el 4.6% de la población, se descubrió otro tipo de cardiopatía, siendo de naturaleza reumática en el 95%. Otras enfermedades no cardiovasculares se encontraron en el 7.5% de las 1,000 personas examinadas (Anexo # 6).

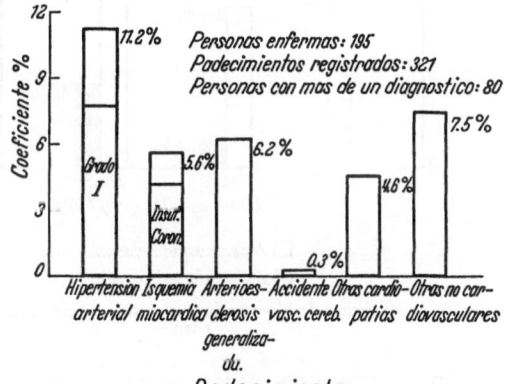

Anexo 6. Padecimientos descubiertos en la poblacion estudia

Un hecho importante debe de resaltarse: un alto porcentaje de los casos descubiertos a través de este estudio desconocían su padecimiento. Como se aprecia en el anexo # 7, este fenómeno se observa en todos los grupos de enfermedades, pero es particularmente ostensible entre los casos de isquemia miocárdica: el 91.3% de estos pacientes ignoraban su enfermedad, en tanto que el 76.0% del grupo de hipertensión arterial, el 82.6% del de otras enfermedades cardiovasculares y el 81.3% de enfermedades no cardiovasculares, desconocían su padecimiento antes del presente estudio.

Todos estos porcentajes creemos son elevados, y hacen evidente la utilidad de este tipo de estudios que, además de revelar el problema actual que representan la hipertensión arterial y la isquemia miocárdica, permiten aplicar medidas preventivas y curativas en fases tempranas de la enfermedad.

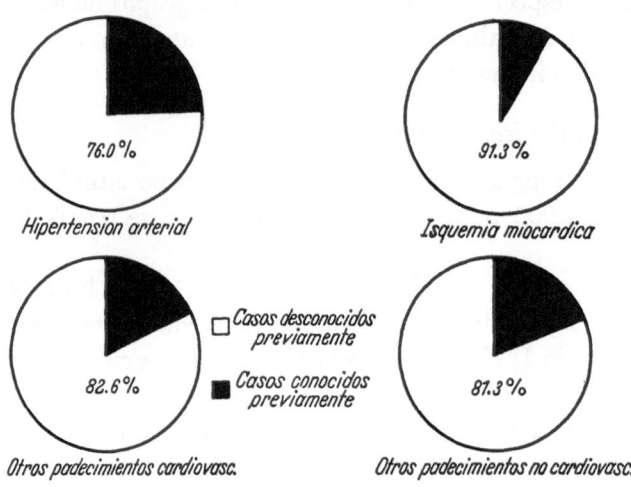

Anexo 7. Conocimiento previo de las enfermedades diagnosticadas

La prevalencia de los padecimientos cardiovasculares investigados varía según las edades de la población en estudio.

En relación con hipertensión arterial, se tienen coeficientes de 6.9% en personas de 30 a 39 años de edad; de 13.7% en las de 40 a 49 años; y de 23.0% y de 19.0%, en las de 50 a 59 años y de 60 y más años, respectivamente. El descenso observado en el último grupo no es significativo.

Los índices de morbilidad por isquemia miocárdica son de 2.5%, 7.0% y 13.6% para las edades de 40 a 49 años, de 50 a 59 años, y de 60 y más años (Anexo # 8).

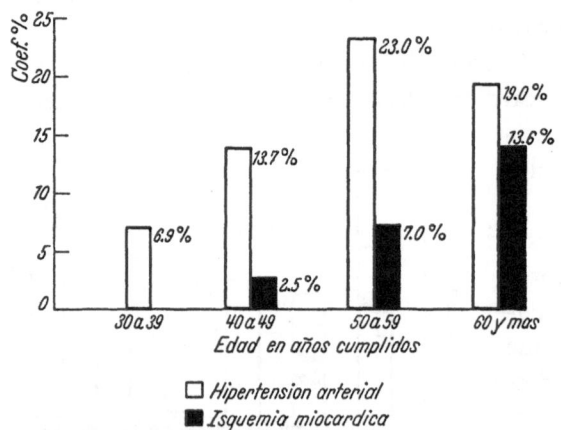

Anexo 8. Coefficientes de hipertension arterial e isquemia miocardica segun edad

Concuerda con otras observaciones y estudios, el hecho de que existen coeficientes más elevados en los dos padecimientos, conforme mayor es la edad de la población.

Por sexo, fué necesario establecer los coeficients dentro de cada grupo de edad, ya que en personas del sexo femenino la edad promedio es mayor. Analizando dichas tasas se aprecia que, en términos generales, son más elevadas las de hipertensión arterial en mujeres y las de isquemia miocárdica en hombres; sin embargo, sólo es estadísticamente significativo el predominio señalado en los grupos de edad de 50 a 59 y de 60 y más años (Anexo # 9).

Se calcularon los índices por ambos grupos de enferemedades según los ingresos de población examinada (Anexo # 10).

A mayores ingresos, se encuentran coeficientes más altos, tanto de hipertensión arterial como de padecimientos isquémicos del corazón; la diferencia más significativa se halló entre personas con ingresos anuales per cápita de menos de 200 dólares, que exhibieron coeficientes de 4.1% para hipertensión arterial y de 0.9% para isquemia del miocardio, en relación con las de más de 200 dólares, cuyos índices fueron de 17.1% en hipertensión arterial y el 13.7% en isquemia miocárdica.

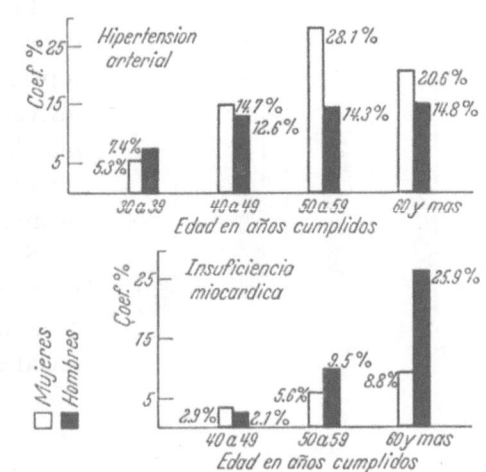

Anexo 9. Coeficientes de hipertension arterial e isquemia miocardica segun edad y sexo

Cabe pensar que las personas de mayores ingresos son las que tienen más edad y que es precisamente el factor edad el que origina que este grupo de personas presenten altos coeficientes para ambos tipos de padecimientos; pero ajustando los índices por edades e ingresos, se mantienen significativamente más elevados en el grupo de ingresos mayores de 200 Dls. por año y por persona.

Según la ocupación de las personas examinadas, los índices de hipertensión arterial e isquemia miocárdica fueron, respectivamente, de 15.9% y 5.6% en profesionistas y técnicos; de 12.7% y 8.0% en oficinistas; de 11.4% y 6.2% en personas dedicadas a las labores del hogar; y de 6.7% y 2.3% entre obreros.

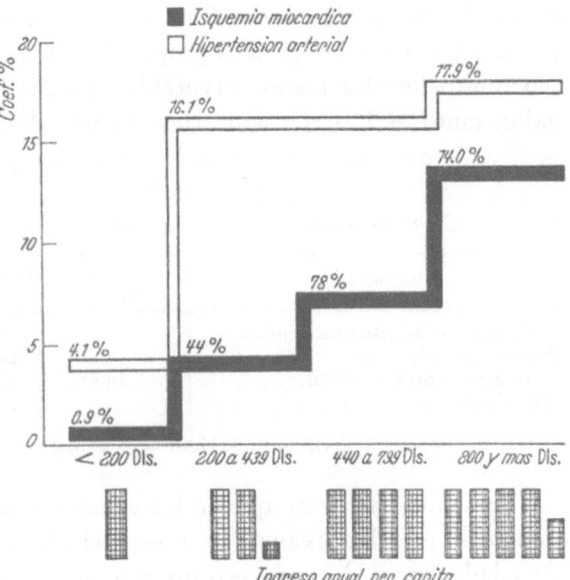

Anexo 10. Coeficientes de hipertension arterial e isquemia miocardica segun ingreso anual per capita

Ambos coeficientes son significativamente inferiores entre obreros. Nótese cómo incluso en personas dedicadas a las labores del hogar (mujeres), las tasas de isquemia del corazón son más elevadas que en obreros, no obstante que, en el total, las mujeres tienen coeficientes más bajos que los hombres (Anexo # 11).

Para evaluar este hecho, debe resaltarse que las personas incluídas en este estudio, que están dedicadas a las labores domésticas, tienen una posición económico-social promedio más elevada que la de los obreros.

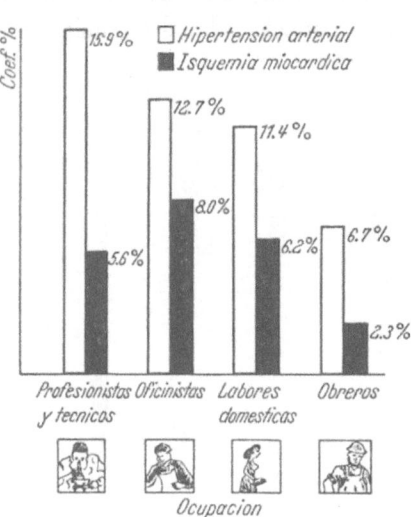

Anexo 11. Coefficientes de hipertension arterial e isquemia miocardica segun ocupacion

Entre personas analfabetas y con educacion primaria incompleta, las tasas de hipertensión arterial (8.1%) e isquemia miocárdica (2.7%) son significativamente más bajas, que entre personas con mayor instrucción (14.4% y 7.1%, respectivamente) (Anexo # 12).

Se establecieron asimismo, los coeficientes por los dos grupos de padecimientos, en cada uno de los tres estratos económico-sociales que se estudiaron. Los de hipertensión arterial son: de 16% en el grupo B, de clase media superior; de 17.2% en el grupo C, de clase media inferior; y de 5.2% en el grupo D, de clase baja superior.

Por lo que se refiere a isquemia del miocardio, las tasas alcanzadas fueron de 9.5% para el grupo B; de 7.7% para el grupo C; y del 1.6% para el grupo D. Como se ve, en el estrato de condiciones económico-sociales menos favorables, grupo D, se encuentran los índices más bajos, tanto de hipertensión arterial como de isquemia miocárdica. No es significativa la diferencia de coeficientes entre los grupos B y C (Anexo # 13).

Coeficientes de hipertension arterial e isquemia miocardica segun instruccion

Instruccion	Coeficiente de hipertension arterial		Coeficiente de isquemia miocardica	
Analfabetos o primaria incompleta		8.1%		2.7%
Primaria completa		10.6%		9.5%
Secundaria o prevocacional. . . .	14.4%	15.5%	7.1%	3.5%
Profesional		14.3%		9.0%

Anexo 12. Coefficientes de hipertension arterial e isquemia miocardica segun instruccion

Tomando en cuenta que en los estratos económicamente débiles existe menos población en edad avanzada, se hizo el ajuste de dichos coeficientes por grupos de edad dentro de cada estrato económico-social, conservándose significativamente más bajas ambas tasas en el grupo D, excepto en edades de 60 a más años, en hipertensión arterial y de 40 a 49 años, en isquemia del miocardio (Anexo # 14).

Análisis de algunos factores

Para cumplir con el tercer objetivo de este estudio, se analizaron algunos otros factores que pudieran intervenir en la frecuencia y distribución de los padecimientos mencionados, cotejando la incidencia de dichos factores en grupos comparables de enfermos y de sanos de la población examinada.

Para la valoración de los datos que a continuación se presentan, como de los que fueron señalados anteriormente, debe tenerse en cuenta, como ya se dijo, que todos los factores fueron investigados antes de saber si las personas eran sanas o

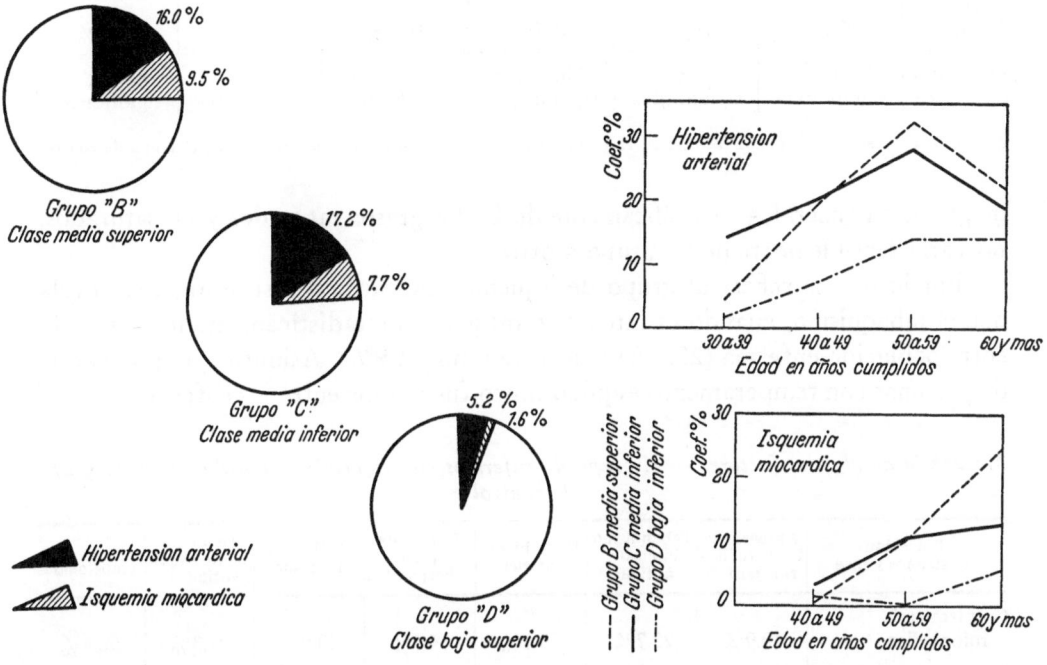

Anexo 13. Coefficientes de hipertension arterial e isquemia miocardica segun estrato economico-social

Anexo 14. Coefficientes de hipertension arterial e isquemia miocardica segun edad y estrato economico social

enfermas; por tanto, hay la misma probabilidad de error en la recolección e interpretación de datos en ambos grupos. Recuérdese, además, que la gran mayoría de los casos, más del 80%, desconocían su padecimiento antes del presente estudio.

De todos los factores investigados, los más importantes aparecen en los Anexos 15 y 16, comparándose su frecuencia en los grupos de enfermos y sanos.

Dos factores mostraron ser significativamente diferentes en el grupo de hipertensos y en el grupo testigo. Uno de ellos es el antecedente de cardiopatía en familiares consanguíneos de primer grado, que se encuentra más frecuentemente en enfermos de hipertensión arterial (42.2%) que en sanos (26.4%); esta diferencia fué altamente significativa.

El otro factor está en relación con la alimentación. En el grupo de hipertensos se encuentran porcentajes significativamente más elevados de personas con dieta hipercalórica (63.3%) y consecuentemente, con exceso de peso (61.5%), en comparación con el grupo testigo (35.7% y 39.8%, respectivamente). La ingestión

Frecuencia de algunos factores en el grupo de enfermos hipertensos y en el grupo de control

Poblacion de 30 años y mas	Antecedentes hereditarios positivos	Tabaquismo intenso y antiguo	Dieta hiper-calorica	Exceso de peso y corporal	Actividad limitada	Problemas emocionales
Con hiper-tension arterial	42.2%	5.5%	63.3%	61.5%	39.4%	30.9%
Sana (control)	26.4%	37%	35.7%	39.8%	31.1%	32.0%
Diferencia estadistica	Altamente significativa	No. significativa	Altamente significativa	Altamente significativa	No. significativa	No. significativa

Anexo 15. Frecuencia de algunos factores en el grupo de enfermos con isquemia miocardica y en el grupo de control

de grasas en general, y específicamente de ácidos grasos saturados y no saturados, no varía sensiblemente de un grupo a otro.

Por lo que se refiere al grupo de isquemia miocárdica y su testigo, se revela que el tabaquismo, cuando es intenso y antiguo, es estadísticamente más elevado entre población enferma (22.7%) que entre sanos (4.9%). Asimismo, el porcentaje de personas con temperamento esquizotímico fué mayor entre los enfermos.

Frecuencia de algunos factores en el grupo de enfermos con isquemia miocardica y en el grupo de control

Poblacion de 40 años y mas	Anteceden-tes heredita-rios post. *	Tabaquismo intenso y antiguo	Dieta hiper-calorica	Exceso de peso corporal	Actividad limitada	Tempera-mento esqui-zotimico.	Problemas emocionales
Con isquemia miocardica . .	40.9%	22.7%	50.1%	54.5%	40.9%	27.3%	52.4%
Sana (control) .	27.0%	4.9%	41.5%	47.3%	38.7%	7.4%	32.6%
Diferencia estadistica . . .	No. signifi-cativa	Altamente signifi-cativa	No. signifi-cativa	No. signifi-cativa	No. signifi-cativa	Signifi-cativa	No. signifi-cativa

* Familiares cosanguineos de 1er. Grado.

Anexo 16. Frecuencia de algunos factores en el grupo de enfermos hipertensos y en el grupo de control

Contrariamente a lo observado en el grupo de hipertensos, la alimentación en personas con padecimientos isquémicos del corazón no es significativamente diferente de la de personas sanas de la misma edad. La actividad física que desarrolla el grupo de enfermos fué también muy similar a la que realiza el grupo testigo.

De todos los factores estudiados, los que mostraron ser significativamente diferentes en los grupos de enfermos y sanos, se correlacionaron con los tres estratos económico-sociales con objeto de investigar si influyen para que estratos con mejor nivel de vida tengan coeficientes más altos, tanto de hipertensión arterial como de isquemia miocárdica. Los datos obtenidos aparecen en el anexo # 17.

Frecuencia de algunos factores en los distintos estratos economicos sociales

Estrato	Dieta hipercalorica	Exceso de peso	Tabaquismo intenso y antiguo	
B-Clase media super.	23.6%	24.5%	5.0%	3.6%
C-Clase media inferior	40.6%	42.9%		5.6%
D-Clase baja super.	35.8%	41.3%		2.9%
Diferencia estadistica	Significativa de B en relacion con C y D	Significativa de B en relacion con C y D	No. significativa	

Anexo 17. Frecuencia de algunos factores en los distintos estratos economicos sociales

Se observa que en relación con la alimentación, el estrato B, teniendo índices de hipertensión arterial sensiblemente más altos que el estrato D después de ajustar edades, tiene un porcentaje significativamente menor de personas con dieta hipercalórica y con exceso de peso.

Por otra parte, el tabaquismo intenso y antiguo, que ostensiblemente fué mayor entre enfermos con isquemia miocárdica que entre sanos, no difiere sensiblemente en los tres estratos.

Estos hechos pudieran indicar que algún otro factor o factores están influyendo en el estrato B y nó en el D; dichos factores están probablemente en relación con la ocupación. No es posible precisarlo a través de este estudio; sin embargo, basándose en estudios semejantes del extranjero, podríamos pensar que posiblemente intervengan la vida sedentaria a la que obligan ciertas ocupaciones y la tensión que origina la responsabilidad.

Síntesis

1. Se presenta un estudio de 1,000 personas de 30 años y más, tendiente a conocer la mediana de presión arterial, la prevalencia de la hipertensión arterial y de la isquemia miocárdica, y a contribuir al conocimiento de la epidemiología de ambos padecimientos.

2. Se establece la mediana de tensión arterial de 128—84 y se analiza según algunas variables.

3. El coeficiente de hipertensión arterial fué de 11.2% y el de isquemia miocárdica de 5.6%.

4. Más del 80% de todos casos hallados desconocían su padecimiento antes del presente estudio.

5. Los índices por las enfermedades señaladas, fueron significativamente más altos en personas de mayor edad y en población de estratos socio-económicos superiores. Fueron particularmente bajos entre obreros.

6. Por sexo, se obtuvieron tasas más elevadas de hipertensión arterial en mujeres y de isquemia miocárdica en hombres, siendo significativos ambos predominios en personas de 50 y más años.

7. Los antecedentes hereditarios de cardiopatía, así como la dieta hipercalórica y el exceso de peso, fueron estadísticamente más frecuentes en el grupo de hipertensión que en el grupo testigo.

8. El tabaquismo intenso y antiguo se halló en mayor proporción entre enfermos con isquemia miocárdica que entre sanos.

9. Los tres últimos factores señalados en los puntos anteriores, no mostraron ser los responsables de la mayor frecuencia de ambos padecimientos en el estrato económico-social más elevado.

Conclusiones

1. El estudio que se presenta contribuye al conocimiento de la situación actual de la hipertensión arterial e isquemia miocárdica en ciertas áreas en el medio urbano de México.

2. Aporta datos que, con los obtenidos en el extranjero, permiten conocer mejor los factores causales, predisponentes o simplemente coincidentes de dichos padecimientos.

3. Además, demuestra la utilidad de estas investigaciones para llegar a descubrir casos incipientes, lo que permite aplicar oportunamente medidas preventivas y curativas.

4. La edad, la alimentación y el tabaquismo, indudablemente intervienen en la frecuencia de las enfermedades estudiadas; pero posiblemente hay un cuarto factor o grupo de factores que está influyendo para que personas de estratos en mejores condiciones económico-sociales tengan más altos coeficientes.

5. Dicho factor o factores pudieran estar conectados con la ocupación, en la que probablemente intervienen la vida sedentaria y la tensión originada por la responsabilidad.

6. Todos los datos obtenidos a través de este estudio no son definitivos; deben ser comparados con los que se recaben en otras investigaciones epidemiológicas que se vayan realizando dentro de este campo.

An Epidemiological Study of Hypertension and Myocardial Ischaemia

In view of the importance of cardiovascular ailments, the Mexican Institute of Social Insurance arranged in 1961 a statistical survey aimed at:

1) ascertaining the extent of hypertension and myocardial ischaemia in an urban area such as Mexico City.

2) Determining the average blood pressure of the population under survey.

3) Contributing to a better knowledge of the epidemiology of these two anomalies by analysing the factors which affect their distribution and frequency.

To this end a study was made of all persons aged 30 or over living in certain housing units owned by the Institute. These persons, at various social levels, were each visited by an investigator (an advanced medical student with appropriate instructions) who noted the necessary information (weight, build, way of life, profession, educational background, personal and family history of cardiovascular disease, etc.). Then the blood pressure was taken on both arms, in the standing and the lying position, and on both inspiration and expiration. An epidemiologist sorted through the questionnaires without drawing a distinction between persons in good health and those who were ill. The incomplete questionnaires were eliminated and at the final count the survey covered 1,000 persons aged 30 or over. Then a cardiologist selected each case showing a tension in excess of 140/90 mm., with an abnormal ECG or with any clinical suggestion of cardiovascular pathology. Each of these selected cases was subjected to a complete examination, with a new ECG, teleradiography of the thorax and examination of the fundus of the eye, chemical analysis of the blood and examination of the blood electrolytes, and general analysis of the urine.

The population surveyed was divided into three groups:

Group B: Upper middle class (those in the skilled or learned professions, technicians, housewives) with an average annual income of 618.6 dollars per capita.

Group C: Lower middle class (largely comprising office employees or housewives) with an average annual income of 246.1 dollars per capita.

Group D: Working class (Labourers, domestic staff) with an average annual income of 106 dollars per capita.

Results

1. Average blood pressure

The 1,000 persons showed an average blood pressure of 128/84 mm. and had an average age of 41.3 years (see graph 1). By age categories, the average pressures were 123/82 mm. (30 to 39 years), 132/86 mm. (40 to 49 years), 141/89 mm. (50 to 59 years) and 148/89 mm. (60 years and over), as will be seen from graph 2.

In persons under 50 years of age, the average blood pressure was higher in men than in women; at later ages the converse was true, with a more significant difference in the systolic pressure; however, it must be noted that obesity was also more marked in the case of women aged 50 and over (graph 3).

In both the systolic and diastolic processes, average blood pressure increased with weight (graph 4). On the whole the blood pressure appeared to be higher with a higher standard of living but it was found that this was not significant if one considered the age categories, the differences being due primarily to the fact that the higher income groups contained more older persons (graph 5).

2. Hypertension and myocardial ischaemia

Of the persons under survey, 11.2% showed hypertension and 5.6% had myocardial ischaemia. The incidence of other diseases is indicated in graph 6.

That a high proportion of the cases had no knowledge of their ailment (76%) for hypertension, 82.6% for cardiovascular diseases in general, and as much as 91.3% for ischaemia) is illustrated by graph 7.

Graph 8 provides a percentage breakdown by age of the cases of hypertension and ischaemia. It will be seen that no case of ischaemia was recorded for the ages 30—39.

For all age categories apart from ages 30—39 the percentage of women with hypertension was higher than that of men but the contrary applied (apart from ages 40—49) with regard to ischaemia (graph 9).

Graph 10 gives the hypertension and ischaemia percentages with reference to annual income. As the financial situation improved, so the percentages rose for these two ailments. The relationship between age and income played its part and the annual income had a pronounced effect when it exceeded 200 dollars.

Depending upon the individual occupation, the incidence of hypertension corresponded to the socio-economic standard, whilst the highest rate of ischaemia occurred in office employees (graph 11).

With regard to the educational standard (graph 12) the highest incidence of hypertensives was found in persons who had had the benefit of a "secondary" education, whilst ischaemia occurred principally in persons with a "primary" education and, to almost the same degree, in persons in the learned or skilled professions.

Graph 13 provides a classification according to the socio-economic standard: for hypertension, Group C (lower middle class) is the one worst affected at 17.2%, as against 16% for Group B and the relatively low rate of 5.2% for Group D; for ischaemia the percentages decreased with the standard of living (9.5%, 7.7% and 1.6% for Groups B, C and D respectively). The percentage difference between Groups B and C is not significant.

Bearing in mind that the weaker financial groups comprised the younger population, the percentages have been related to age categories. Group D is affected considerably less than the others, except at age 60 and over by hypertension and at 40—49 years of age by ischaemia (graph 14).

3. Analysis of certain other factors

What other factors can influence the frequency and distribution of the two diseases in question? The answer is given in graphs 15 and 16, which quote comparative figures for sick persons and for those in good health (control group). It is apparent from graph 15 that heredity, high caloric diet and excess weight are highly significant as regards hypertension. In the case of ischaemia (graph 16) contributory factors are nicotinism and, to a lesser extent, a cyclothymic temperament.

Graph 17 clearly shows that Group B (the upper middle class) has an appreciably lower percentage of persons who are on a diet and overweight, whereas there is hardly any difference in nicotinism between the three socio-economic groups mentioned. Thus there must be other contributory factors, possibly of an occupational nature and arising from a sedentary life and the nervous tension of responsibility.

Recapitulation

1. This study covers 1,000 persons aged 30 or over and is aimed at determining the average blood pressure, and the extent of hypertension and myocardial ischaemia, as well as increasing knowledge of the epidemiology of these two diseases.
2. The average blood pressure was 128/84 mm. Hg.
3. The coefficient of hypertension was 11.2%; for ischaemia 5.6%.
4. Over 80% of all the cases studied had no knowledge of their ailment at the time of the survey.
5. The coefficients of the diseases studied were perceptibly higher for older persons and those in the upper social scale. They were particularly low for labourers.
6. In the case of hypertension, the percentages were higher for women whilst for myocardial ischaemia the incidence was higher in men, the preponderance being in both instances especially marked in persons aged 50 and over.
7. The hereditary antecedents of cardiopathy, was well as high caloric diet and excess of weight, were more frequent in the group with hypertension than in the control group.
8. Intense and long lasting nicotinism was found in greater proportions among sufferers from myocardial ischaemia (22.7%) than among persons in good health (4.9%).
9. The four factors mentioned in points 7 and 8 do not appear to be responsible for the greater frequency of the two diseases in persons in the upper social scale.

Anti Hypertensive Therapy and its Effect on Risk Evaluation

H. E. UNGERLEIDER, M.D.

IRVING PAGE in a recent editorial of the magazine "Circulation" states, "Even though it is often not so thought of, the problem of the *control* of arterial hypertension is, next to atherosclerosis, civilized man's greatest cardiovascular problem". It is, then of more than passing importance to decide whether the use of the new formidable array of hypertensive drugs is of real value and as underwriters, it becomes our function to assess their impact on the selective process.

With the profusion of agents which have been advocated for hypertension in the past few years, there has been a tendency to overlook the simple fact that high blood pressure is a disorder involving the patient and not the mercury manometer. This is unfortunate because blood pressure is only one and often a minor aspect of hypertensive disease, and it has not been sufficiently recognized that various remedies may *improve the blood pressure* and *hurt the patient*.

Viewing hypertension from the aspect of the applicant the underwriter's order of business is approximately the following:

1. Is hypertension present and what is its degree? It is pertinent to remark that hypertension and the evaluation of measures used in its control can never be decided on the basis of casual blood pressure readings. It is important to know the range of blood pressure through which the particular patient lives. This can be determined in a variety of ways, most simply perhaps at the time of initial examination, by the combination of the breath holding pressor test and combined hyperventilation and carotid sinus depressor test which we described sometime ago. Unfortunately, we as underwriters must assess the risk only on casual readings. This is a handicap, but due to the urgency of our business we have no other alternative.

We do have some factors that operate somewhat in our favor. We should ask our examiners to record all the blood pressures they take and not to report only the lowest. When increased blood pressure is present, at least three (3) readings should be made. We should not be misled by such statements that the applicant has a rise in blood pressure when he is examined by a physician or a strange examiner and finally, basal blood pressures, or those taken after a period of rest, should be looked upon with some suspicion. Basal blood pressures are helpful in determining the floor of the blood pressure but as underwriters, our concern is the blood pressure that is present during the applicant's working day — or what

I like to call his "carrying blood pressure". The latter, if abnormal, is significant from a selection viewpoint.

2. The next problem is to determine whether hypertension is due to a curable cause. Time does not permit a consideration of all of these, such as coarctation of the aorta, phaeochromocytoma and others, but among recent developments the most interesting perhaps from a point of view of curability is the demonstration at the Cleveland Clinic that almost one-quarter, 16 of 67 patients to be exact, of hypertensive patients investigated by trans lumbar aortography exhibited gross abnormalities in renal arterial flow. Cures were affected by arterial grafts in younger persons, by nephrectomy in older persons.

Blackman, describing the post-mortem findings in fifty (50) cases of essential hypertension reported finding sclerotic placques in 86% of the renal vessels, and I. M. PAGE showed that in 427 patients studied at the Cleveland Clinic, 131 occlusive renal lesions were discovered.

These studies are important because arterial lesions of the type found may not be disclosed by conventional renal function tests and pyelograms. Hypertension can result from renal involvement even when there is no gross abnormality in function or structure.

A vast majority of cases of hypertension cannot be related to surgically curable causes, but there has been considerable progress in understanding factors which may produce hypertension. Thus, VON EULER has shown that some 10 % of hypertensive patients excrete increased amounts of catechol amines indicating increased norepinephrine output which may be playing a casual role in hypertension in such persons. Another endocrine factor which has recently been clarified is the syndrome of aldosteronism, an increased secretion of the sodium retaining hormone of the adrenal cortex. Increased knowledge has developed also concerning the commoner types of hypertension seen in the young and in the old, which are two quite different diseases in their effects. WIDIMSKY of Prague reported at the European Congress of Cardiology that 70% of hypertensives under the age of 30 exhibited a high cardiac output as revealed by the HAMILTON dye method. This revives an old and almost abandoned concept of hypertension as due to increased cardiac output. Another European investigator, HEYMANS, of Belgium has presented fairly substantial evidence that hypertension, at least in older persons, is often due to arterial inelasticity causing an increased pressor reactivity of the baro receptors in the carotid sinus. These receptors are sensitive to stretch in the arterial wall, and when the artery is inelastic and unstretched, pressor activity is increased. In support of this concept is the known frequency of hypersensitivity to carotid sinus pressure in older persons.

3. After the physician has determined if hypertension is present, what its degree is, and whether it is due to a recognizable and curable cause, the next aspect of the diagnostic work-up is to decide whether the elevated blood pressure is giving the patient any trouble. Observation and note must be made of the patient's symptoms, particularly headache, involvement of the heart (which is

evaluated more sensitively by electrocardiography than by X-ray methods), the state of the kidneys, cerebral involvement including observation of the retinal vessels, and observation of the major arteries. It may seem trite to mention these points, but this type of investigation is imperative if one is to make proper use of the newer developments in therapy.

4. Beyond the question of whether hypertension is giving the patient trouble, the physician must also assess whether it is *likely* to give trouble. In this question aspects of importance include not only the degree of hypertension, but questions of sex, race, age, family history, and the presence of associated conditions such as diabetes. Again mention of these points appears trite, but the outlook in two patients with uncomplicated hypertension of 180/100 is entirely different where one is an obese female of 55 with good family history, and the other is a negro male of 30 of slender build and a strong family history of hypertensive disease.

With this as a preface, we may turn to questions of treatment. If treatment appears to be indicated, this must be approached with the recognition that this is apt to be a lifelong affair, and consideration must be given to the cooperation and economic circumstances of the patient. Parenthetically, I might remark that when drugs of the many types now being used are employed, few patients find themselves spending less than $5.00 weekly for medication alone, and sometimes considerably more.

It is a seeming paradox that the treatment of hypertension with the methods that have become available in the past decade have been most spectacularly successful in the worst cases i.e., malignant hypertension, and have been relatively disappointing in the milder cases of hypertension. In some respects the situation is analogous to the situation with steroids in rheumatoid arthritis i.e., dramatic results in short term treatment of the severe case and less decisive benefit compounded by iatrogenic problems in long term management of patients with less severe disease. It is interesting to note that fully 50% of patients with malignant hypertension now survive five years, whereas formerly few survived more than one to two years.

Unquestionably, the antihypertensive drugs are improving the outlook for a proportion of hypertensive patients. However, there are many patients receiving drug therapy who are either slightly benefited or not at all, and a few are actually harmed by the drugs. Patients most likely to be benefited are men below fifty (50) years of age whose diastolic pressures are fixed at 110 or above who have eye ground changes such as papilledema, impaired cardiac reserve and renal function, enlarged hearts, and electrocardiographic evidence of left ventricular hypertrophy. Women over fifty (50) with diastolic pressure around one hundred (100), and particularly those patients who are uncooperative in that they remain overweight or even gain weight, smoke heavily, discontinue or take their drugs irregularly, continue activities which induce severse physical or mental stress, or are psychologically incapable of prolonged periods of supervision and careful attention to the treatment program are least likely to benefit from these drugs.

Let us consider the new developments and the present status of various therapeutic measures in hypertension. The treatment of hypertension properly begins with diet. There are at least three aspects; weight, fat intake, and salt consumption. Personally, I doubt that obesity has any direct connection with hypertension, despite their frequent association, beyond the fact that the high calorie eater is usually a high salt eater. It has been shown neatly in a study conducted at the Brookhaven, Long Island National Laboratory that when people are divided into three groups, salt abstainers, salt sprinklers, and an intermediate group, hypertension is found preponderantly in the salt sprinklers, and is notably absent in the salt abstainers. Dietary fat intake is also an important consideration from the long range point of view in hypertension because the most common complications of hypertensive diseases are arteriosclerotic in nature. There is good evidence that reducing fat intake to a palatable minimum is a simple and very useful procedure in reducing the risk of arteriosclerotic complications such as coronary artery disease. Although vigorous salt restriction, confining sodium intake to less than 200 milligrams daily has unquestionably been successful as a sole measure in controlling hypertension, the studies of KEMPNER and others must be viewed as a laboratory experiment, unsuitable for the long term management of patients who wish to live as well as to exist. This was shown clearly in the study conducted by GUTMAN and others at the Goldwater Memorial Hospital on Welfare Island in New York. The patients fared very well during prolonged periods of drastic sodium restriction while leading a monastic life in an institution, but only a negligibly small percentage were able to maintain an adequate sodium restriction voluntarily after leaving the hospital and returning to their environment.

Nevertheless, salt restriction should be encouraged in hypertensive patients and salt depletion may be aided by the use of diuretics, sodium depleting resins, and thiocyanate which increases urinary salt loss. Evidence has accumulated recently that extreme sodium depletion may have adverse effects, notably in the presence of renal insufficiency. In addition, salt loss leads to a compensatory increased secretion of the sodium retaining hormone aldosterone by the adrenal gland. For all these reasons diet alone has not provided an answer to the problem of hypertension.

Of the various drugs used in treating hypertension, rauwolfia preparations enjoy by far the widest use. These include the whole root (raudixin), the alseroxylon fraction (rauwiloid) and syrosingopine. All of these have similar hypotensive effects and it should be emphasized, undesirable and even dangerous effects. The alkaloids may be used orally. The rauwolfia preparations produce a modest hypotensive effect when used orally. The situation is analogous to the use of PAS in tuberculosis which has some mild utility of its own, but which is valuable primarily to enhance the effectiveness of additional and more potent therapy. When patients with high blood pressure are treated with drugs, it is generally desirable to begin with one of the rauwolfia preparations. In some degree the untoward effects of the ganglion blocking agents, and also of apresoline, two of the major antihypertensive drugs employed today, are mitigated by the previous and concurrent employment of rauwolfia. The untoward effects of reserpine are by no means confined to a stuffy nose, bradycardia, loose bowels, and an increased appetite as the pharmaceutical manufacturers would like us to believe. These drugs may cause a variety of serious complications. Among them, and we have seen them all, are severe mental depression with suicidal tendencies which do not disappear on discontinuing the drug, but may require a full course of shock therapy. Another serious complication is peptic ulcer and hemorrhage which may result from the increased acid secretion provoked by reserpine. We have seen a fatal gastric hemorrhage probably attributable to this cause. An additional complication is sodium retention produced by reserpine in certain persons, which may actually cause heart failure and pulmonary edema. We have seen this as well, and currently, therefore, do not employ reserpine in patients with hypertensive heart disease without giving an accompanying diuretic. Another complication which may be very distressing to the patient is the production of basal ganglia tremors and in patients with Parkinsonism, tremor may be greatly aggravated. For these reasons, reserpine is by no means a harmless drug and patients using it must be kept under observation. These untoward effects are perhaps somewhat less evident with the alseroxylon fraction (rawiloid).

The past decade has witnessed the successive introduction of a variety of ganglion blocking agents beginning with tetra ethyl ammonium salts which were active only very briefly when injected intravenously. The object of the newer derivatives has been to provide longer acting compounds which are effectively absorbed orally. The first and most extensively employed, hexamethonium, while effective in small dosage parenterally is absorbed very poorly and erratically so that oral doses must be one hundred times or more than that of the injected dose. Categorically, it may be stated that this drug has no place in the oral management of hypertension because it may be ineffective on the one hand and dangerous on the other. Parenterally it has enjoyed wide use, particularly in England and Australia, and in several centers patients have been taught to administer hexamethonium by injection much as a diabetic takes insulin. In this country interest has centered on the oral employment of ganglion blocking agents. Ansolysen (i.e., pentolinium) has attained a fair measure of use, but its absorption likewise, is erratic and doses up to several milligrams daily are usually required. Another, which has not become very popular is Ecolid. A drug which seems destined to be used increasingly as a ganglion blocking agent is mecamylamine (inversine) which differs somewhat in structure from the others, and which has the virtue of being very well absorbed orally. It is administered as 2.5 mg. tablets twice daily initially, the dosage being gradually increased according to the patient's tolerance until a dosage of approximately 20 milligrams daily is attained, which may be administered as two 10 milligram tablets daily. Ostensin, another drug in this category has recently been introduced.

There are serious problems attending the administration of the ganglion blocking agents, whichever one is employed, and they are all similar in their adverse effects. Among the important adverse effects in this group of drugs are postural hypotension of severe degree, bladder and bowel paralysis which may lead to urinary retention, severe constipation, and even ileus. Other adverse effects are disturbances in vision which increase the hazard in driving automobiles, constipation, difficulty in urination, tremors, augmentation of glaucoma and orthostatic hypertension. Some of these blocking agents produce excitement and confusion leading to erratic conduct. In addition, renal blood flow is decreased by these drugs. Consequently, they should not be employed in the treatment of hypertension in the presence of coronary disease, cerebral vascular disease, renal involvement and prostatic disorders. In significant measure, the untoward effects of the ganglion blocking agents are prevented by rauwolfia preparations, which should therefore always be used as a preliminary measure prior to starting the ganglion blocker and should be continued with them. It should be noted that some tolerance usually develops to the ganglion blocking agents so that their dosage has to be increased.

Another agent which has come to be widely employed in the drug therapy of hypertension is apresoline, or hydrazino phthalazine. This drug has effects quite unlike those of the ganglion blocking agents and untoward effects as well, differing from those of a ganglion blocker. The precise mechanism of action of apresoline is not entirely clear, but it inhibits a variety of amine oxidase enzymes. This action, which is probably responsible for its blood pressure lowering effect, is also responsible for some of the toxic effects of apresoline. It is a potent inhibitor of the histamine detroying enzyme, histaminase. Consequently, its use is commonly attended by symptoms resembling those produced by histamine. The most disturbing of which to the patient although not the most serious effects of apresoline are headache and palpitation with accompanying tachycardia. These are minimized somewhat by prior administration of rauwolfia preparations, and can also be helped by use of one of the common antihistamines. It is important to begin dosage with apresoline in small amounts on the order of 20 to 40 milligrams twice a day initially, increasing as the patient's tolerance permits. Ultimately, a dosage of about 400 milligrams total daily given in divided doses is desirable. If doses much above this are employed or even in this dose over protracted periods, in certain instances a polyarthritis or a full blown picture of collagen disease can develop. This is a small but important risk of apresoline therapy. In addition, a variety of blood disorders and skin lesions have been described in rare instances. Apresoline has the effect of increasing cardiac output and consequently, in patients with heart failure or coronary disease, its use may be undesirable. Many patients taking apresoline experience anginal pain. Apresoline has the virtue of increasing renal blood flow and is therefore a lot safer to employ than ganglion blocking agents if hypertension is accompanied by renal disease.

A combined use of one of the rauwolfia preparations, one of the ganglion blockers and apresoline judiciously employed enable us to exert a beneficial effect on the blood pressure, and less regularly on the patient, in the greater number of instances. There are many other agents which have been extolled and damned in the treatment of hypertension. One of these is thiocyanate which is not too dramatic in its blood pressure lowering effect, but which is unexcelled in relieving hypertensive headaches, and which is quite safe if properly employed with controlled blood levels maintaining the blood level below 12 milligrams per cent. Veratrum alkaloids have enjoyed a recent flurry of interest, but I believe they belong with the snows of yesteryear. Their unpleasant gastro intestinal effects can make a patient far prefer his hypertension to a cure. Peripherally acting agents such as hydergine and dibenzyline are quite useless in treating hypertension.

Recently a host of new compounds has found widely accepted usage in the treatment of hypertension. The first of these, chlorothiazide or diuril, is gradually being replaced by newer members of the series. Among these are:

hydrochlorthiazide (hydro-diuril, esedrix & oretic)

flumethiazide (ademol)

hydroflumethazide (saluron)

benzydroflumethazide (natureton)

dichlorhydroflumethazide (naqua)

chlorthalidone (hygraton)

polythiazide (renese).

The exact mode of action of these agents in hypertension has not yet been entirely understood. Their ability to mobilize and cause a loss of body sodium is an important factor. Their site of action is thought by some to be on the arterial wall. Doses vary from 1 gram to 1 milligram daily.

These drugs do not seem to produce the toxic effects of those previously described, but they too produce serious effects at times, among these are increase in the blood uric acid, with gouty attacks, blood disorders, lowering of potassium levels, hyperglycemia, and even acute pancreatitis. In patients who are taking digitalis, it has produced toxicity, arrhythmias, and even death.

There are still two other agents which are of recent vintage and are sure to be joined by others. These belong to the class of "Sympathetic Inhibitors". The two are designated guanethidine sulfate (Ismelin) and brethylium tosylate (Darentin). Their virtue lies in their ability to selectively block peripheral adrenergic activity. Evidence indicates that they inhibit the release of norepinephrine usually freed by adrenergic activity. Darentin does not deplete the tissues of catecholamines, but Ismelin does, which also has the advantage in that it is longer acting. These drugs to date are not widely used, but when they are, we should be alerted to the possibility of their producing toxic effects.

Selection

The rating of this class of applicants will test the acumen of any underwriter, no matter what his sophistication. The complexities attending hypertension under treatment are of such an order that they cannot be dismissed by merely the application of some digits or numbers derived from an underwriting manual. Underwriting considerations such as age, sex, overweight, albuminuria with or without microscopic findings, cardiac enlargement, electrocardiograph changes, eye ground changes, and family history all enter the picture with varying degrees of importance. Some of these may be favorable at times; others may blacken the picture so that no underwriting offer can be made. The useful addition to our medical examination forms when elevation of blood pressure is recorded would be the question, "Have you, or are you now taking any treatment for your blood pressure?" Until this is part of the form, the examiner should be requested to supply this information whenever he finds the blood pressure elevated.

Some years ago, we made a study of some 450 applicants who were homogeneous as to age, sex, body build, and blood pressure. They were all 40 years of age, of the male sex, with build −5 to +5% of the average, and with blood pressure 160/100. We tested this group with the electrocardiogram, which is more sensitive than the X-ray in eliciting cardiac hypertrophy, and by doing so we hoped to establish an index of the duration of the hypertension and the subsequent mortality. Using the criteria for hypertrophy by the electrocardiogram, previously published, we found that those with a normal electrocardiogram gave a mortality of 180%; those exhibiting a so-called "borderline" type of 230%; those with the pattern of left ventricular hypertrophy of 350%, or twice that of the normal group. This is good evidence to show the need of procuring an electrocardiogram where the amount of the application is sufficient to bear the expense. This amount, to my mind, should be in excess of $10,000. The presence of hypertrophy, or cardiac enlargement, in the applicants who are hypertensive, is always an unfavorable situation from the standpoint of selection. For the most part, it signifies the presence of hypertensive heart disease.

The influence of overweight, albuminuria, family history, etc. has been described so frequently by other authors, it need not be discussed here.

In considering the actual underwriting decision, what are the factors to be considered, or in other words, "What are the criteria for selection?".

(1) The applicant must be under treatment at least one year — with at least one visit every three months to his physician.

(2) Type of treatment:
   (a) Class of drug
   (b) Doses of drug
   (c) Duration of treatment
   (d) Side effects — if any
   (e) Response to treatment

(3) Sex — age — body build — family history.

(4) Range of the blood pressure:
   (a) Highest
   (b) Lowest
   (c) Present

(5) Electrocardiogram

(6) X-ray of heart and lungs

(7) Urinary findings

(8) Eye ground changes

The actual process of determining the final rating as practiced by the North American Reassurance Company is as follows:

I. Average the current blood pressure readings as outlined below:

(A) Average all blood pressure recordings taken on the same day whether reported in the Medical Examination, a Medical Recheck Heart Chart, an Attending Physician's Statement or the Impairment Records dated within three (3) months of the current examination. Example:

Medical Examination: June 20, 1960			Medical Recheck: June 27, 1960		
156	/	94	142	/	90
152	/	94	146	/	92
148	/	92			
3)456		)280	)288		)182
(a) 152	/	93	(b) 144	/	91

Attending Physicians's Statement of June 29 re a May 15, 1960 exam:			Impairment Record:				
160	/	98	May 15, 1960	(d) 170	/	100	
150	/	90	Apr. 3, 1960	(e) 180	/	98	
3)310		)188					
(c) 155	/	94					

(B) Average these results to secure a final current average:

Medical Examination	(a)	152	/	93
Medical Recheck	(b)	144	/	91
Attending Physician's Statement	(c)	155	/	94
Impairment Records	(d)	170	/	100
	(e)	180	/	98
		5)801		476
		160	/	95

II. Record as a single reading the highest Pre-treatment systolic blood pressure and diastolic blood pressure from among prior Medical Examinations, Impairment Records or Attending Physician's Statements. That is, a series of blood pressures including: 178/98, 166/104, 176/102, and 170/100 would be recorded as a Pre-treatment Blood Pressure of: 178/104.

III. If the Pre-treatment Blood Pressure is ratable, i.e., it falls within the limits of the Blood Pressure Table, record the Table rating and then reduce it by the following percentages based on the level of the Current Blood Pressure Average:

Current blood pressure average

Systolic Blood Pressure	Diastolic Blood Pressure		
	Under 90	90 to 96	Over 96
Under 140 . . .	50%	40%	0
140 to 155 . . .	30%	20%	0
Over 155 . . .	0	0	0

IV. If the Pre-treatment Blood Pressure is not ratable, i.e., it does not fall within the limits of the Blood Pressure Table and the Current Blood Pressure Average is higher than 140 systolic and/or 90 diastolic, the application should usually be declined.

V. If the Pre-treatment Blood Pressure is not ratable, i.e., it does not fall within the limits of the Blood Pressure Table, and the Current Blood Pressure Average is 140/90 or lower: Assess a minimal rate of +250.

This rate will be increased in relation to the known height of the Pre-treatment Blood Pressure and the length of time since it existed, i.e., the higher the Pre-treatment Blood Pressure is above the Blood Pressure Table limits and the shorter the period of time since it was present, the more the rate of +250 should be increased. The several methods of averaging blood pressures should be used in an effort to establish a reasonably accurate rate. Any Pre-treatment Blood Pressure over 200 systolic and/or 114 diastolic should usually call for declination.

It would be well to keep in mind, particularly in considering the older age groups, that while the lowered level of blood pressure may signify good response to treatment, it may also indicate serious heart impairment. More than simple blood pressure readings are needed to evaluate the over-all picture in these cases.

These suggested methods of underwriting blood pressure cases under treatment are to be combined with medical judgment. In any case having other cardiovascular — renal impairments, e.g., albuminuria, hypertrophy, suspicious electro-cardiographic changes, arrhythmia, eye ground changes, history of cardiac symptoms, or an unfavorable family history, etc., these procedures are no longer practical guides since they deal only with the single element of blood pressure elevation and the case should usually be declined.

Aglycosuric Diabetes *

W. B. Spaulding, M.D., F.R.C.P.(C), F.A.C.P. · W. O. Spitzer, M.D. ·
P. W. Truscott, M.D.

A number of surveys to detect diabetes mellitus have demonstrated that tests for
glycosuria may fail to reveal mild diabetes [1—9]. In most of the reported
studies those investigated were either members of one community such as a town,
or workers in an industrial organization. This report concerns patients attending
a medical out-patients clinic in a teaching hospital. By means of random determinations of the blood sugar, it has been possible to detect a group of diabetic
patients with hyperglycemia but without glycosuria at the time of initial visit
to the clinic. The term "aglycosuric diabetes" has been used to designate the
disease in this group. By using the term it is hoped to draw attention to a sizeable
but occult segment of the population of diabetic patients. The segment is
important because it consists of patients whose diabetes may be unrecognized for
a long time. The routine use of blood sugar tests may reveal the disease in some
of these patients before they suffer from complications such as retinopathy or
neuropathy.

Method

Urine and blood specimens were obtained from 2,000 patients attending the
Medical Out-patients Clinic at the Toronto General Hospital. Most of the
patients had eaten breakfast before coming to the clinic, which is held in the
morning. While the urine specimens were obtained shortly after the patients
arrived, the blood specimens were usually drawn within the next two hours.
The interval was occasionally greater than two, or even three hours.

The method employed for the measurement of the blood sugar is a modification of the procedure proposed by W. S. Hoffman [10]. An Auto-Analyzer
was used to make the determinations. The normal range for fasting levels of
glucose in the blood is 60 to 100 mg. per 100 ml. at this hospital. The figures
analyzed in this study represent a very close approximation to the true levels of
glucose in the blood. In our hospital, specimens analyzed after treatment with
glucose oxidase were found to contain not more than 1.0 mg. per 100 ml. of

* From the Department of Medicine, University of Toronto and the Medical Out-Patients
Department, Toronto General Hospital. — Presented at the Annual Meeting of the Royal College
of Physicians and Surgeons of Canada, January 19, 1963.
Published in Canad. med. Ass. J. **89**, 329—333, August 24, 1963.

reducing substances, indicating that the method practically excludes reducing substances other than glucose.

The presence and approximate concentration of sugar in the urine were determined using commercially prepared reagent strips (Combistix) and tablets (Clinitest). The tablets were employed to confirm all positive results obtained with the reagent strips.

Criteria for diagnosis

Of the 2,000 patients only those found to have either glycosuria or levels of glucose in the blood of at least 140 mg. per 100 ml. were studied further. They were divided into two groups:

Aglycosuric — Patients with negative urine tests but with levels of glucose in the blood of 140 mg. per 100 ml. or higher.

Glycosuric — Patients with glycosuria, regardless of the blood sugar level.

The clinical records of all patients falling into the aglycosuric and the glycosuric groups were examined. Patients already known to be diabetic were not investigated further. The remainder were tested subsequently to determine whether or not they were diabetic.

Although no perfectly satisfactory definition of diabetes can be formulated, some arbitrary definition is necessary to avoid confusion. A patient was considered to be "diabetic" who had a fasting or two-hour postprandial hyperglycemia (140 mg. per 100 ml. or higher) on at least two occasions, or had an abnormal glucose tolerance curve following the ingestion of 100 g. of glucose. The glucose tolerance test was judged to be abnormal if the peak blood sugar value exceeded 160 mg. and the level at two hours was above 120 mg. per 100 ml.

No attempt was made to control the diet during the days before the glucose tolerance tests were carried out. Marked restriction of the intake of carbohydrate may produce a diabetic type of response in glucose tolerance tests of normal subjects [12]. However, the patients tested were attending the clinic because of inability to afford private medical care, and most clinic patients eat large amounts of carbohydrate because it is cheaper to do so. Furthermore, the study of WILKERSON et al. [13] has shown that it is unnecessary to modify the diet before doing glucose tolerance tests on adequately nourished patients.

Results

The survey was conducted in two steps: screening, and investigation. Tables and graphs were prepared to compare the results of this survey with one which might have been conducted with the same population but without determinations of the level of glucose in the blood.

Table I shows that 80 patients had glycosuria but an additional 46 patients with a normal urine test had a random blood sugar level of 140 mg. per 100 ml.

Table I. *Results of screening stage of survey*

Designation of patients	1st thousand patients	2nd thousand patients	Total
Aglycosuric group	26	20	46
Glycosuric group	42	38	80
Total	68	58	126

or higher. The figures in Table II demonstrate further the advantage of including measures of glucose in the blood at the screening stage. Firstly, the blood tests resulted in a higher number of total diabetics detected (85 compared to 52). Secondly, one half of the *new* diabetics in this survey (15 out of 30) exhibited no glycosuria at the screening stage. Finally, a considerable number of the known diabetics were aglycosuric with hyperglycemia at the time of initial testing. Such a patient might lie about his past health in an attempt to obtain insurance at standard rates. The likelihood of detecting his disease would be greater if the blood sugar were measured in addition to testing for glycosuria.

Table II. *Results of investigation for diabetes, second stage of survey*

Designation of patients	Diabetics detected		Diabetes excluded by		Untraced or deceased	Total
	New	Known	Normal G.T.T'S	Subsequent blood, urine tests normal		
Aglycosuric group	15	18	6	—	7	46
Glycosuric group	15	37	—	23	5	80
Total	30	55	6	23	12	126

The characteristics of the disease in what shall be termed the "aglycosuric diabetics" were compared with the characteristics of the disease in the remainder of the diabetics detected. The sex incidence, age incidence, levels of glucose in the blood, and treatment necessary for the control of new diabetics in both groups, were compared.

Table III. *Sex incidence of diabetics*

	Aglycosuric diabetes	Glycosuric diabetes	Total
Males	17	26	43
Females	16	26	42
Total	33	52	85

The sex incidence is similar in the two groups (Table III). As shown in Table IV and Fig. 1 the aglycosuric diabetics tend to be older than the glycosuric diabetics.

Table IV. *Age of diabetics*

Age group	Number of patients	Aglycosuric diabetics	Glycosuric diabetics
10—19	135	1—0.7%	1—0.7%
20—29	290	0—0	1—0.3
30—39	381	0—0	8—2.3
40—49	271	7—2.6	6—2.3
50—59	342	9—2.6	12—3.5
60—69	316	6—1.9	12—3.8
70—79	211	7—3.3	9—4.3
80—89	53	3—5.7	3—5.7
90—99	1	0—0	0—0
Total	2000	33—1.6	52—2.6

The group of aglycosuric diabetics for the most part had levels of glucose in the blood below 220 mg. per 100 ml. at the screening stage (Fig. 2). On the other hand most of the glycosuric diabetics had levels above 220 mg. per 100 ml.

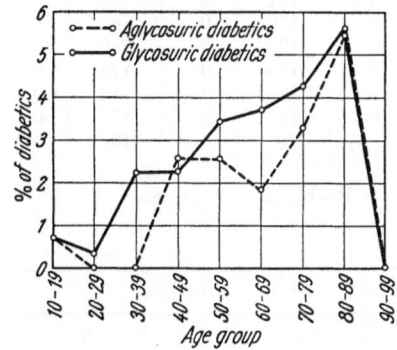

Fig. 1. Percentage of diabetics within each age group

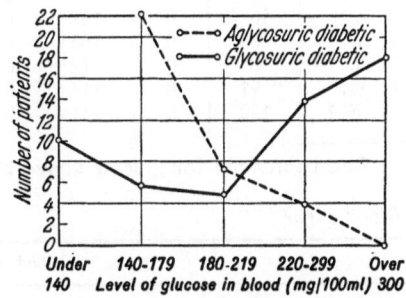

Fig. 2. Comparison of levels of glucose in blood in aglycosuric and glycosuric diabetics

Almost all the newly discovered aglycosuric diabetics (14 out of 15) were controlled with regulation of diet only, indicating the mildness of their disease. The glycosuric diabetics required insulin in 5 cases, oral hypoglycemic drugs in

Table V. *Treatment of new diabetics discovered*

Type	Aglycosuric diabetics	Glycosuric diabetics
Insulin	1	5
Oral drugs.	0	4
Diet only	14	6
Total	15	15

4 instances and 6 patients were controlled with dietary regulation only (Table V). The incidence of more severe disease was higher in this group. Twelve of the newly discovered aglycosuric diabetics were diagnosed as a result of glucose tolerance tests. Two patients were diagnosed on the basis of repeated fasting levels of sugar in the blood over 140 mg. per 100 ml. A third was

considered to be diabetic as a result of finding the fasting level to be 155 and the level three and one-half hours after a meal to be 303 mg. per 100 ml. (Table VI). One of the newly discovered aglycosuric diabetics had a diabetic retinopathy with hemorrhages and exudates. An ophthalmologist had noted this finding two years before and had advised him to be tested for diabetes. He had ignored the advice.

Table VI. *Newly discovered aglycosuric diabetics*

A. *Glucose tolerance test*

Patient	Fasting		Half hour		One hour		Two hours		Three hours	
	B	U	B	U	B	U	B	U	B	U
1. B. S.	134	0	160	0	237	tr	231	3 +	204	4 +
2. W. M.*	117	0	180	0	243	0	258	3 +	177	1 +
3. K. P.*	115	0	202	0	243	3 +	204	3 +	171	tr
4. F. M.	152	0	192	0	204	tr	288	tr	195	tr
5. G. V.*	107	0	207	0	255	4 +	231	4 +	132	4 +
6. F. Z.	110	0	200	2 +	197	4 +	191	0	99	4 +
7. M. V.	85	0	153	0	172	0	188	0	68	0
9. R. Z.	102	0	132	0	158	0	192	0	169	0
9. A. S.*	85	0	163	0	200	0	153	0	174	0
10. T. C.	83	0	172	0	204	tr	186	3 +	116	0
11. O. W.	91	0	114	0	174	0	162	0	174	0
12. A. W.*	120	0	231	0	315	4 +	240	4 +	180	4 +

* Renal threshold for glucose above 200 mg./100 ml. — B=blood, U=urine.

B. *Blood sugar*

		Blood sugar		Urine sugar	
1. E. S.	1st value	193	Fasting	0
	2nd value	164	Fasting	0
2. M. K.	1st value	142	Fasting	0
	2nd value	148	Fasting	0
3. G. C.	1st value	155	Fasting	0
	2nd value	303	3½ hrs p. c.	2 +

Discussion

The results of this survey indicate that considerably more diabetics are discovered when screening methods include determinations of the level of glucose in the blood. The need to include these tests arises, in part, from the fact that high renal thresholds for glucose are probably more common than is realized [8, 14]. An examination of the 12 glucose tolerance curves (Table VI) lends support to such a supposition. It is interesting to note that in 5 patients (indicated with *) the threshold value would appear to be at least 200 mg. per 100 ml.

4.2 per cent of 2,000 medical out-patients at the Toronto General Hospital were diabetics. Significantly, the diabetic patients who showed no sugar in their urine at the screening stage represented 1.6 per cent of this out-patient group (Table IV). Such out-patients represent as close an approximation to the type of patients seen by a general practitioner as a teaching hospital can provide, although it does not include children under 15, obstetrical patients and non-indigent patients.

Conducting a continuing programme of routine testing for diabetes in the offices of medical practitioners or in hospitals, has a number of advantages over community surveys. No mobile public health team is required to advertise the diagnostic survey and obtain the cooperation of members of the community. Patients attending a doctor's office or an outpatient department expect to have laboratory tests and usually cooperate well. They are easier to follow and often remain under supervision for a long time. Routine blood sugar tests can be the basis of a continuing survey, in the same way that serological tests for syphilis and miniature radiographs of the chest are employed in many hospitals. The introduction of automation into laboratory work has markedly reduced the cost per test. The cost, in terms of money and technician time, is low enough to make routine measurements of glucose in the blood feasible. Since many patients have at least one venepuncture during their investigation, the additional work involved in drawing blood for a determination of the blood sugar level is minimal.

We have chosen to use the term "aglycosuric diabetes" because it directs attention to a group of diabetic patients who warrant special consideration, but the term has its semantic drawbacks. Diabetes mellitus means the running through of honey-tasting liquid and is a picturesque allusion to glycosuria. Some authorities still consider glycosuria necessary for the diagnosis of diabetes mellitus [15] but many now define the disease in terms of hyperglycemia and abnormal glucose tolerance as revealed in glucose tolerance tests. As this study demonstrates, there exists a group of diabetic patients who have elevated blood sugar levels without glycosuria, or who have glycosuria only intermittently when the blood sugar level is high. Strictly speaking, to call this condition "aglycosuric diabetes" means saying a running through of no sugar in the urine! Despite this semantic absurdity the terminology appears understandable and medically reasonable in view of current criteria for the diagnosis of diabetes mellitus. Table VII sets out a number of differences between aglycosuric and glycosuric diabetes in accordance with the experience in this study.

Was it desirable to detect the aglycosuric diabetics? They suffered from a mild form of the disease; some were elderly; none had the usual symptoms of diabetes. A few may have suffered psychological trauma unnecessarily on discovering their new disorder. Nevertheless it was considered worthwhile to detect and treat the disease in these patients for the following reasons. Firstly, half of these individuals were under 60 years of age and had years of life ahead and one already had retinopathy. Secondly, of the new diabetics all but one were controlled by diet alone, which means that their living habits were altered little as a result of the diagnosis. Thirdly, the older diabetic patient with poor circulation is the one who is prone to develop gangrene if left untreated and unaware of the need for good care of the feet.

Table VII. *Differences between aglycosuric and glycosuric diabetes*

Aglycosuric	Glycosuric
1. Lacks symptoms dependent on glycosuria, e. g. polydipsia, polyuria, weight loss, pruritus vulvae.	Often presents with these symptoms.
2. Symptoms of complications (e. g. retinopathy, neuropathy) may occur before diabetes diagnosed.	If symptoms of complications occur, patient usually known to be diabetic.
3. Initial random urine test normal.	Initial random urine test abnormal.
4. Blood sugar test necessary for diagnosis.	Blood sugar test necessary to confirm diagnosis.
5. Urine tests of limited value in control.	Urine test useful in control.
6. Mild diabetes.	Diabetes tends to be more severe.
7. Renal threshold for glucose often elevated.	Renal threshold for glucose usually not elevated.

Of all the diabetics detected in this survey 33 out of 85 would not have been suspected on the basis of laboratory tests had the screening been restricted to urinary sugars. Exactly half (15 out of 30) of the new diabetics discovered would have been missed. These figures are significant in insurance medicine. There is a strong probability that many supposedly healthy individuals receiving life insurance policies at standard rates are actually diabetic. The implication these figures have in public health are important with regard to diabetes surveys. Finally, the findings are relevant to medical practice. In many private practitioner's offices testing for glucose in the urine is a routine procedure. It is felt that the private practitioner would increase considerably the efficiency of his detection of diabetes by having the blood tested in addition to carrying out tests of urinary sugar.

Summary

A survey of 2,000 patients was conducted to compare the relative reliabilities of urinary sugar tests and determinations of the level of the glucose in the blood in the detection of diabetes mellitus. Of 85 diabetics detected by screening all patients with tests of urinary sugar *and* determinations of the level of glucose in the blood, 33 would not have been suspected by performing only urinary tests. Exactly one half of the new diabetics discovered would have been missed (15 out of 30). The diabetics who did not exhibit glycosuria at the screening stage of the survey had a mild form of the disease, were predominantly elderly and were controlled, in nearly every case, by diet only. An elevated renal threshold for glucose was common in these patients. These results have significance in practice, hospital routines, insurance medicine and population surveys to detect diabetes.

Acknowledgements

Mrs. Eva Braun has given valuable technical assistance. A grant for the investigation of diabetes from the Faculty of Medicine, University of Toronto helped to support the project.

References

[1] KENNY, A. J., A. L. CHUTE, and C. H. BEST: Canad. med. Ass. J. **65**, 233 (1951).

[2] KURLANDER, A. B., A. P. ISKRANT, and M. E. KENT: Diabetes **3**, 213 (1954).

[3] WILKERSON, H. L. C., A. S. COHEN, and B. G. KENADJIAN: J. chron. Dis. **2**, 464 (1955).

[4] JOSLIN, E. P., H. F. ROOT, P. WHITE, and A. MARBLE: The Treatment of Diabetes Mellitus. 10th ed. Philadelphia: Lea and Febiger 1959, pp. 37—38.

[5] REMEIN, Q. R., and H. L. C. WILKERSON: J. chron. Dis. **13**, 6 (1961).

[6] PACKER, H., J. M. HAWKES, and R. F. ACKERMAN: Diabetes **10**, 280 (1961).

[7] JORDE, R.: The Diabetes Survey in Bergen, Norway, 1956. Bergen-Oslo: Norwegian Universities Press 1962.

[8] GROTT, J. W., L. MARZEC, W. GINTOWT-DZIWILL, J. KORZON, R. PITEROWA, W. POSKUTA, and J. W. ZURKOWSKI: Pol. Tyg. Lek. **16**, 1569 (1961).

[9] College of General Practitioners Working Party. Brit. med. J. **1**, 1497 (1962).

[10] HOFFMAN, W. S.: J. biol. Chem. **120**, 51 (1937).

[11] PORTER, J. S.: Head of Division of Biochemistry, Toronto General Hospital: Personal Communication.

[12] CONN, J. W.: Amer. J. med. Sci. **199**, 555 (1940).

[13] WILKERSON, H. L. C., H. HYMAN, M. KAUFMAN, A. C. McCUISTON, and J. O'S. FRANCIS: New Engl. J. Med. **262**, 1047 (1960).

[14] PEDERSEN, J., and N. I. NISSEN: Acta med. Scand. **163**, 477 (1959).

[15] JOSLIN, E. P., H. F. ROOT, P. WHITE, and A. MARBLE: The Treatment of Diabetes Mellitus. 10th ed. Philadelphia: Lea and Febiger 1959, p. 212.

Changing Concepts in Vascular Surgery *

Michael E. De Bakey, M.D.

My first thought at this time is to express my sincere and grateful appreciation
for the signal honor that you have accorded me in electing me President of
the International Cardiovascular Society. In observing the distinguished group
with which I am surrounded, my pleasure in receiving this honor is exceeded
only by my sense of humility. My next thought is to express my deep gratitude to
the other officers of the Society who have performed their duties with the utmost
diligence and efficiency. It has been a pleasure to work with such a group of
dedicated men.

In selecting an appropriate topic for this occasion I wished to choose a subject sufficiently challenging to merit your attention and also one in which I have
had intense interest for a number of years. My topic is, of course, peculiarly
appropriate to this organization in that the contributions toward the changes and
improvements in vascular surgery have come from widely divergent geographical locations and schools of surgical thought. In surgery there is a universality
that is perhaps not found so clearly demonstrated in other fields of endeavor.

During the past decade my associates and I have devoted our main efforts to
surgical approaches to certain cardiovascular problems, among which I have been
especially concerned with diseases of the aorta and its major branches. Accordingly, I should like to discuss some of the more significant observations derived
from our surgical experience during this period with over 3,000 cases, as they per-
tain particularly to changing conceptual and technical developments (Table I).

One of the major factors, if not the most important, in the rapid advancement
of this field of surgery in recent years has been the principle of arterial graft replacement. To be sure, this principle was well developed by experimental workers
and even applied sporadically by a few surgeons more than half a century ago,
but for a number of reasons its widespread clinical application was delayed
until recent years. For one thing, certain ancillary measures in surgery, including
particularly anesthesia, blood transfusion, and chemotherapy, had not developed
adequately to support extensive surgery of this type, and the precise diagnostic

* Published in J. Cardiovasc. Surg. (Torino) 1, 3 (1960).

Presidential address, International Cardiovascular Society, Munich, Germany. — Supported
in Part by Grants from the United States Public Health Service and the Houston Heart
Association.

Table I. *Tabulation of data on surgery of the aorta and major arteries*

Location	No. cases	per cent
Thoracic aorta		
Aneurysms of aortic arch	56	2
Aneurysms of descending aorta . .	111	4
Dissecting aneurysms	48	2
Thoraco-abdominal aneurysms . .	25	1
Coarctation	150	5
Injuries.	4	0.1
Abdominal aorta		
Aneurysms	806	26
Occlusive disease	769	25
Injuries.	10	0.3
Major peripheral arteries		
Injuries.	151	5
Aneurysms	132	4
Occlusive disease	829	27
Femoro-popliteal	*634*	*21*
Innominate, carotid, vertebral,		
subclavian	*195*	*6*
Total	3091	100

procedure of angiography was not available to delineate its proper application. For another, the general status of surgical endeavor had not matured sufficiently to accept this more vigorous and aggressive approach to these difficult and complex surgical problems. The first successful form of arterial graft replacement was

Table II. *Comparison of results following use of dacron grafts with other forms of grafts in various vascular diseases*

Dacron grafts	No. cases	Deaths	Graft failures	Successful
Thoracic aorta				
Aneurysms	113	26 (23 %)	0	87 (77 %)
Occlusions.	34	2 (6 %)	0	32 (94 %)
Abdominal aorta				
Aneurysms	436	19 (4 %)	1 (0.2 %)	416 (95 %)
Occlusions.	407	4 (1 %)	5 (1 %)	398 (98 %)
Peripheral arteries				
Aneurysms	56	2 (4 %)	1 (2 %)	53 (95 %)
Occlusions.	552	10 (2 %)	26 (5 %)	516 (94 %)
Total dacron grafts . .	1598	63 (4 %)	33 (2 %)	1502 (94 %)
Total other synthetic grafts	341	29 (9 %)	27 (8 %)	285 (84 %)
Total homografts . . .	593	62 (10 %)	24 (4 %)	507 (85 %)
Total all grafts	2532	154 (6 %)	84 (3 %)	2294 (91 %)

the arterial homograft, but it had certain disadvantages such as inconvenience associated with its procurement and preparation and inadequate availability. For these reasons we, like others, have directed our efforts toward development of a

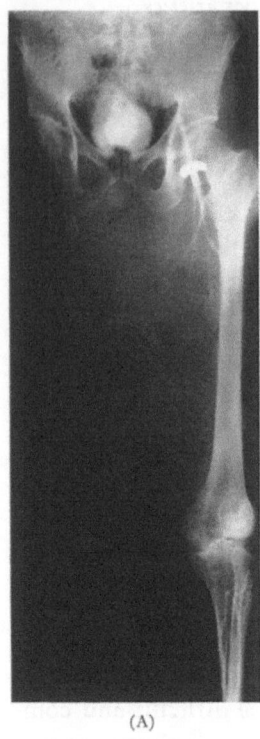 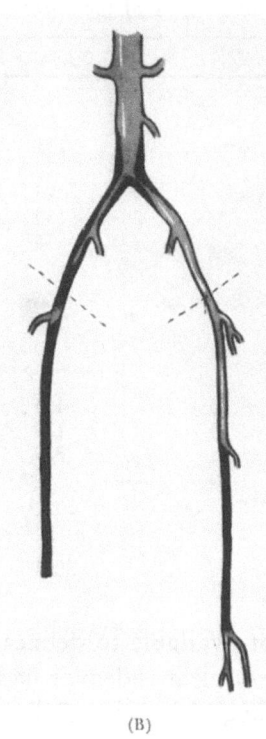

Fig. 1 (A) Aortogram and left femoral arteriogram in 36-year-old white male patient with typical manifestations of thromboangiitis obliterans showing extensive occlusive disease of both iliac arteries and left superficial femoral and popliteal arteries. Patient had above knee amputation of right lower extremity twelve years previously for gangrene. (B) Diagrammatic representation of extent and location of occlusive disease

(A)   (B)

Fig. 1. (C) Drawing illustrating method of treatment employing bypass graft from abdominal aorta to left common femoral artery and to popliteal artery with patch graft angioplasty to restore normal lumen to popliteal artery. (D) Postoperative aortogram and left femoral arteriogram showing restoration of normal circulation by means of bypass graft

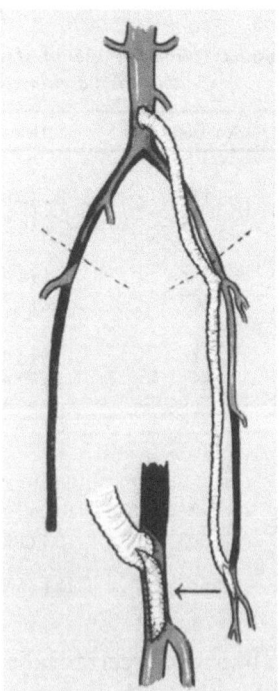 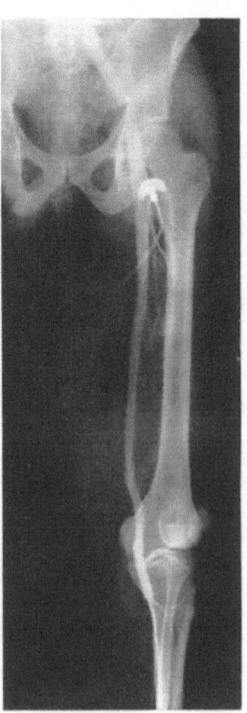

(C)   (D)

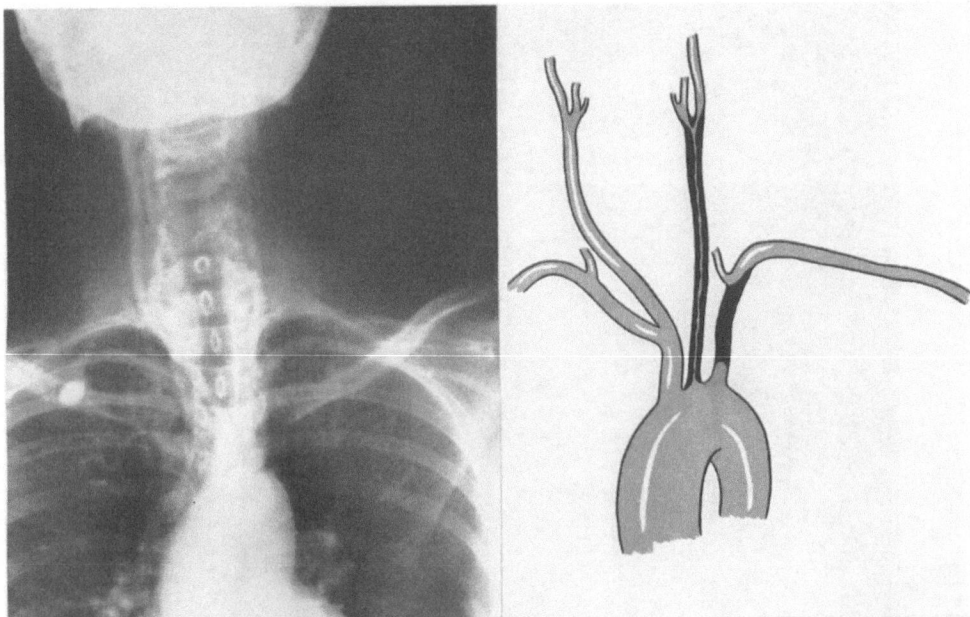

Fig. 2 (A)

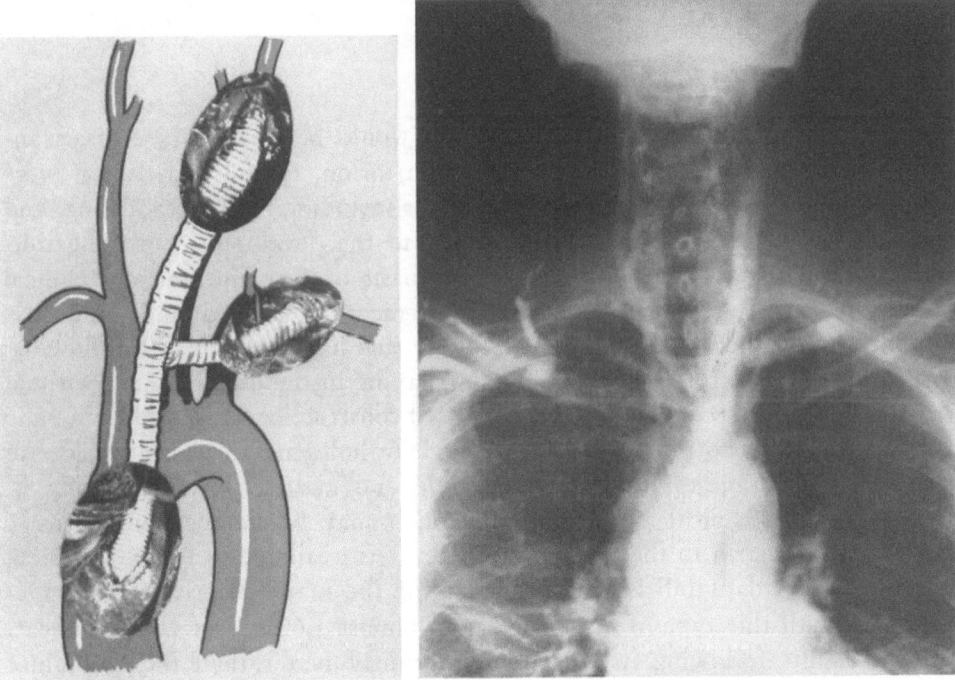

Fig. 2 (B)   Fig. 2 (C)

Fig. 2. (A) Angioaortogram in patient with atherosclerotic occlusive disease of major branches of aortic arch showing incomplete occlusion of left common carotid artery and complete occlusion of left subclavian artery as depicted in drawing on right. (B) Photograph in same patient made at operation with drawing illustrating application of bypass principle from ascending aorta to left common carotid artery opposite bifurcation with side-arm from this graft to left subclavian artery. (C) Postoperative angioaortogram showing restoration of normal circulation through bypass graft

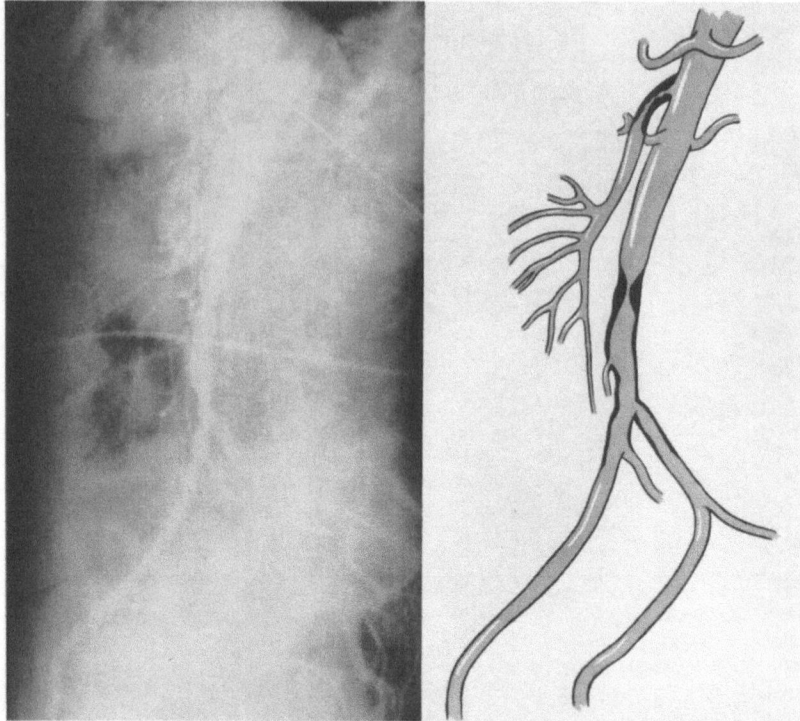

Fig. 3 (A)

satisfactory substitute for homografts, which would be free of these disadvantages. Various materials such as ivalon, nylon, orlon, teflon, and dacron were tried, fashioned into tubes by different methods including braiding, knitting, and weaving. Our own efforts in this regard led to the development of a flexible, knitted, seamless dacron tube, which on the basis of experimental and clinical studies was found to meet the essential requirements of strength and durability, flexibility, and function. Among its desirable characteristics are the following: first, it may be repeatedly sterilized by autoclaving in the usual manner without harm to the fabric; second, owing to its knitted construction, it is nonfraying and may be cut with scissors or scalpel at any angle or holes may be cut in its side for anastomosis of branches; third, it is flexible and elastic, thus facilitating its anatomical and technical application; fourth, it may be clamped with arterial clamps without harm to the fabric; and fifth, it is available in tubes of various sizes for ready adaptability to all segments of the major arterial system. Our experience with this type of dacron graft in almost 1,600 cases would indicate that the results following its use are significantly better than those obtained in our previous experience with homografts and other types of synthetic grafts (Table II).

Diseases of the aorta and its major branches, with which we are mainly concerned, may be broadly classified into two categories, namely, aneurysms and

Fig. 3. (A) Lumbar aortogram showing incomplete segmental occlusive lesions involving superior mesenteric artery near its origin and abdominal aorta near bifurcation as depicted in drawing on right in patient with manifestations of "intestinal angina" and intermittent claudication of lower extremities

Fig. 3. (B) Photograph made at operation with drawing illustrating application of bypass principle. The bifurcation dacron graft has been attached by end-to-side anastomosis to abdominal aorta above occlusive lesion and in similar manner both limbs of graft have been attached to external iliac arteries below occlusive lesion. Using similar end-to-side anastomoses a segment of tubular dacron graft is attached to trunk of abdominal aortic graft and to superior mesenteric artery distal to occlusive leson

Fig. 3. (C) Aortogram made after operation in same patient showing restoration of normal circulation through bypass graft as indicated in drawing on right

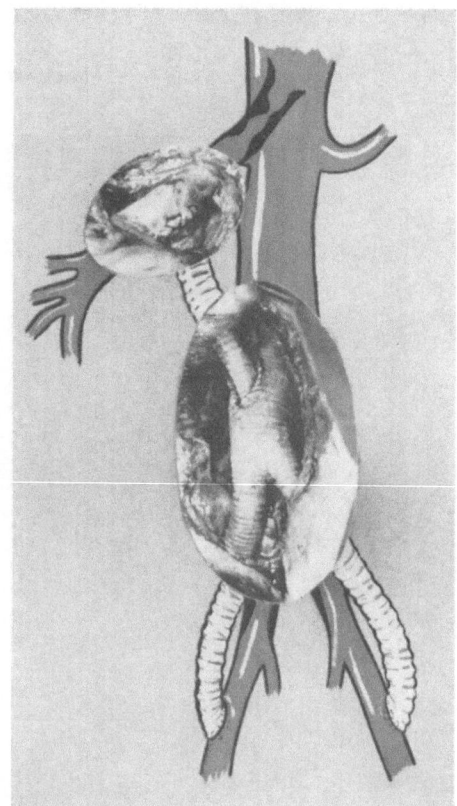

Fig. 3 (B)

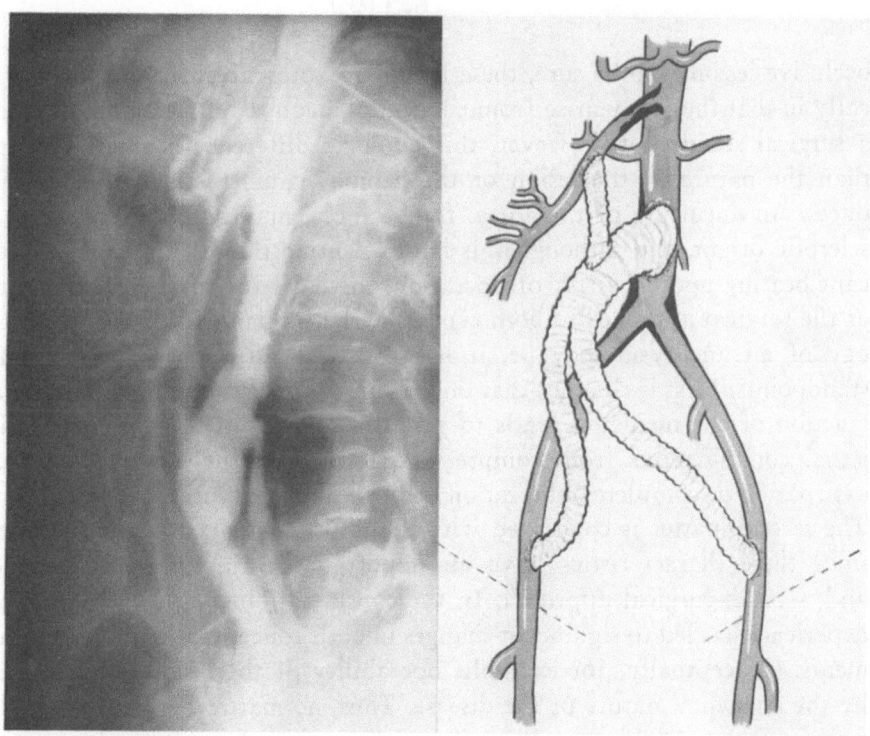

Fig. 3 (C)

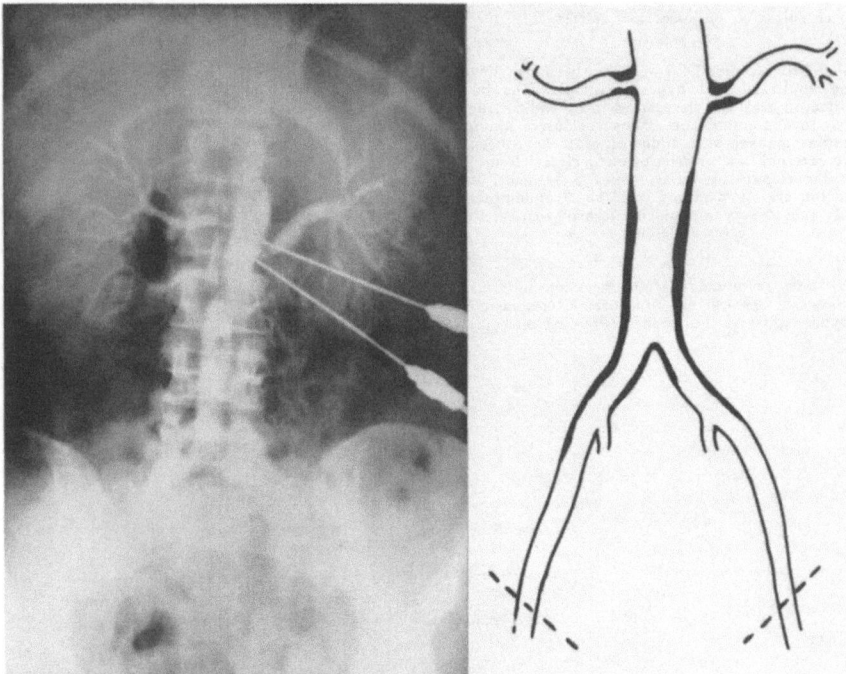

Fig. 4 (A)

occlusive lesions. To be sure, these lesions in both categories may differ etiologi-
cally in that they may arise from congenital, acquired, or traumatic origin. From
a surgical standpoint, however, this etiologic difference is much less significant
than the nature of the lesion or the hemodynamic disturbances which it produces. An aneurysm of the aorta, for example, may be of traumatic or arteriosclerotic origin, and although this is of scientific interest and may have significant bearing upon the risk of operation, the basis for surgical treatment as well
as the surgical approach to both types may be similar. No matter what the etiology of an aneurysm may be, it has practical surgical meaning from several
standpoints. First is the fact that once it has formed through weakening and des-
truction of the media, it tends to progress and ultimately produce serious and
lethal complications from compression of surrounding tissues. For this reason
extirpation or complete obliteration of the lesion is essential for effective therapy.
The second matter is concerned with its nature, extent, and site of involvement
since these characteristics have an important bearing upon, first, operability
and, second, surgical approach. In the consideration of these factors, increasing
experience has led to significant changes in both conceptual and technical developments. Conceptually, for example, operability of the lesion itself is determined
by the segmental nature of the disease. Thus, no matter how extensive the lesion
may be, it is operable providing it is delimited with a relatively normal proximal and distal vascular segment. So far as site of involvement is concerned, all

Fig. 4. (A) Lumbar aortogram showing segmental occlusive lesion involving both renal arteries near their origin and aorto-iliac segment as depicted in diagram on right in patient with severe hypertension and intermittent claudication

Fig. 4. (B) Photograph made at operation with drawings illustrating application of bypass principle employing dacron bifurcation graft attached by end-to-side anastomoses to abdominal aorta above and to both external iliac arteries below occlusive lesion with side-arms from trunk of bifurcation graft to both renal arteries

Fig. 4. (C) Postoperative aortogram showing restoration of circulation to both renal arteries and to both external iliac arteries through bypass graft as depicted in diagram on right. Patient was completely relieved of intermittent claudication and hypertension

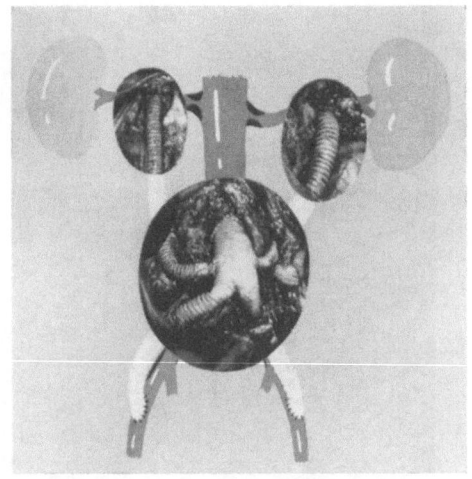

Fig. 4 (B)

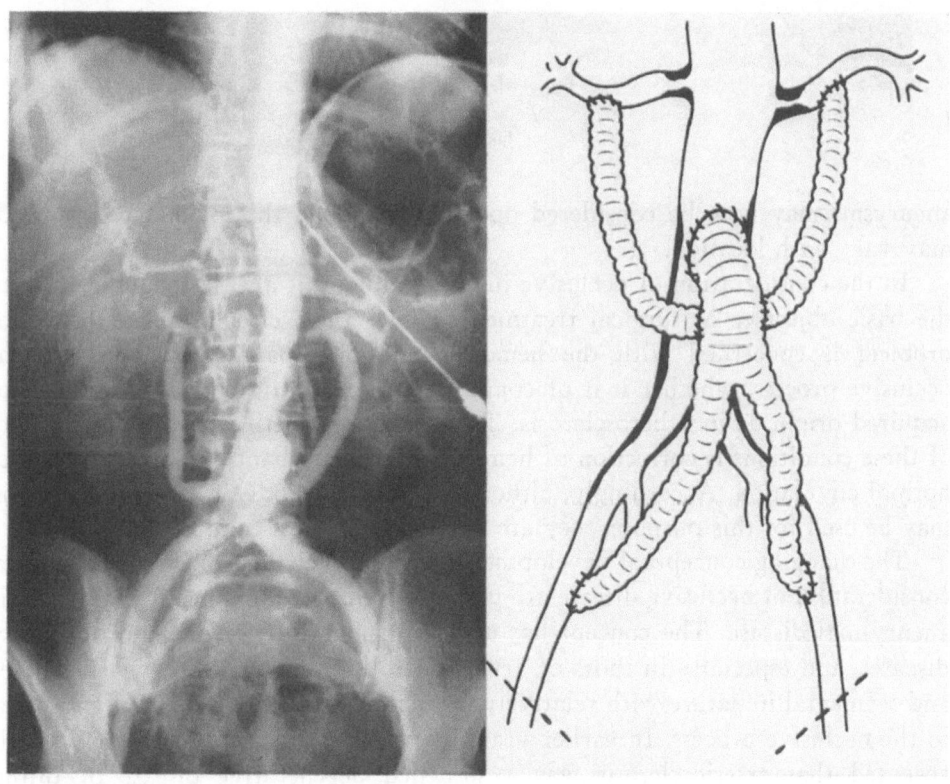

Fig. 4 (C)

10*

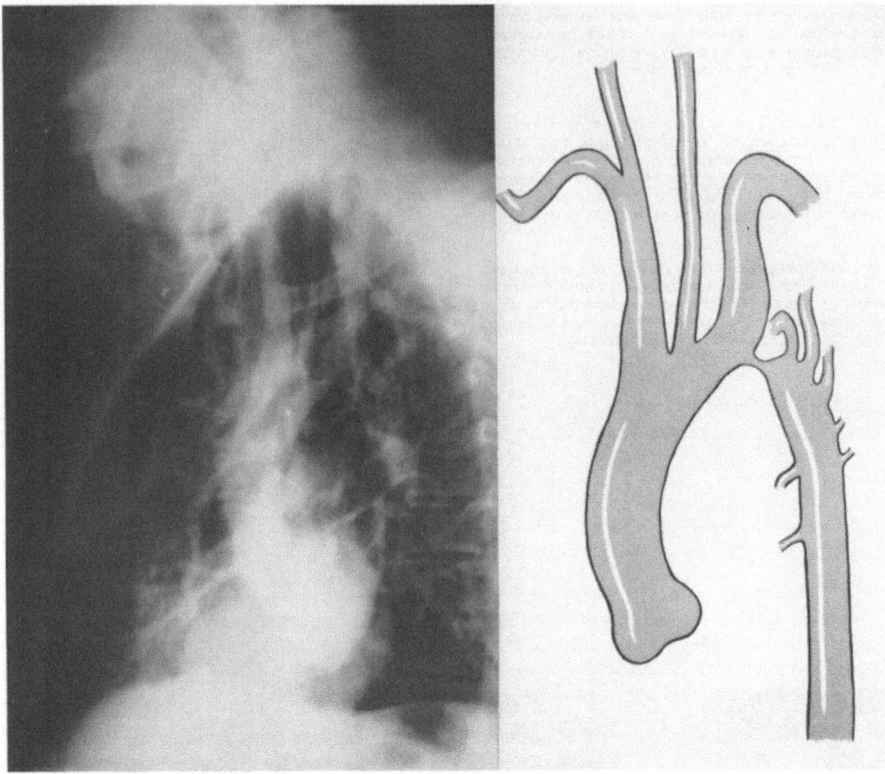

Fig. 5 (A)

aneurysms may now be considered operable, although the method of approach
may vary with location.

In the consideration of occlusive diseases etiology is also less significant than
the basic objective of surgical treatment. Under these circumstances the major
problem is concerned with the hemodynamic disturbances produced by the
occlusive process, whether it is of congenital origin such as in coarctation or of
acquired origin as in atherosclerosis. The primary objective of therapy in both
of these conditions is correction of hemodynamic disturbances and restoration of
normal circulation. Accordingly, although several methods of surgical treatment
may be used for this purpose, they are applicable to both conditions.

The changing conceptual developments which have taken place in the surgical
consideration of occlusive disease are perhaps even more significant than those in
aneurysmal disease. The concept has evolved that the lesion in many occlusive
diseases, and especially in those of arteriosclerotic origin, may be well localized
and segmental in nature with relatively normal arteries both proximal and distal
to the occlusive process. In earlier years it was generally considered and widely
accepted that arteriosclerosis was a so-called degenerative disease of diffuse
nature. More recently, however, and through investigations derived largely

Fig. 5. (A) Preoperative angioaortogram in 50-year-old patient with coarctation showing coarcted segment as depicted in diagram on right

Fig. 5. (B) Photograph made at operation with drawing showing application of bypass principle employing dacron graft attached by end-to-side anastomosis to left subclavian artery above and to descending thoracic aorta below coarcted segment

Fig. 5. (C) Postoperative angioaortogram showing restoration of normal aortic circulation through bypass graft as depicted in drawing on right

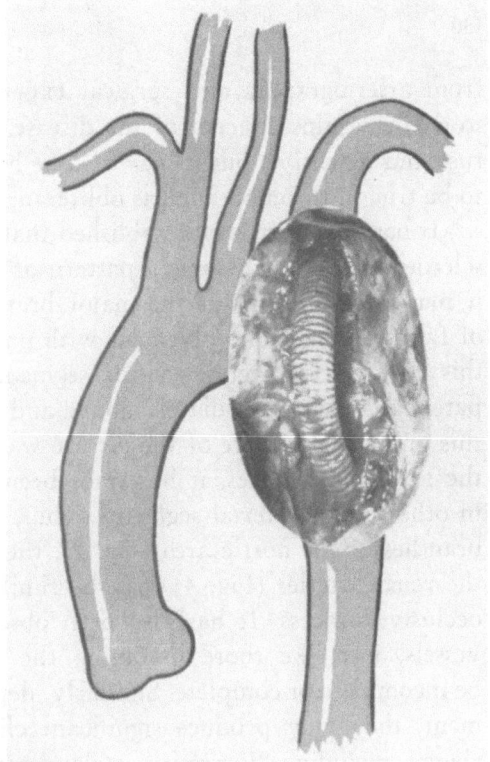

Fig. 5 (B)

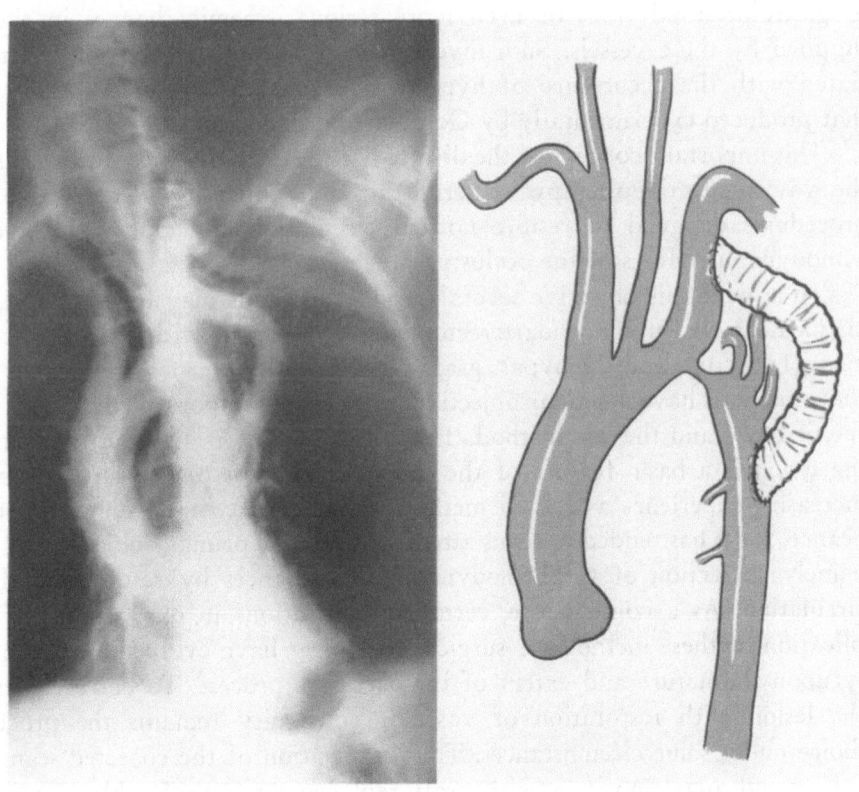

Fig. 5 (C)

from arteriographic and surgical experiences, much evidence has accumulated to challenge this concept of the disease. To be sure, arteriosclerosis may be diffuse and extensive, but it may also be highly localized. This has also been found to be true in thrombo-angiitis obliterans (Fig. 1).

It has now been well established that there is a great tendency for the atherosclerotic process to assume a pattern of localized or segmental involvement, and it may occur in any of the major branches of the aorta. Even in the presence of fairly extensive involvement with multiple sites of occurrence, it may assume this characteristic tendency for segmental involvement with relatively normal patent channels immediately above and below the limits of the lesion. Although this important feature of the disease was earlier recognized in the arterial bed of the lower extremities, it has since been found to occur in much the same way in other major arterial segments. Thus, it has been demonstrated that the major branches of the aortic arch (Fig. 2), the superior mesenteric artery (Fig. 3), and the renal arteries (Fig. 4) may be similarly involved in this type of segmental occlusive process. It has also been observed that the occlusive lesions in these vessels, just like those involving the arteries of the lower extremities, may be incomplete or complete. Similarly, depending on the site and extent of involvement, they may produce significant clinical manifestations of arterial insufficiency, including "intermittent claudication" of the brain and upper extremities or gastrointestinal tract or even more serious ischemic changes in the organs supplied by these vessels. Such involvement of the renal arteries is often associated with the occurrence of hypertension presumably on the same basis as that produced experimentally by Goldblatt and his associates (Fig. 4).

This important concept of the disease has great significance since it has opened the way to effective therapy by permitting the application of corrective surgical procedures designed to restore normal circulation and thus to overcome the hemodynamic effects of the occlusive process.

To achieve this objective several surgical methods may be employed, including particularly thromboendarterectomy (DOS SANTOS), excision with graft replacement (LERICHE), and the bypass graft procedure (KUNLIN). Although all three of these methods have a similar objective, there is one important difference between the first two and the last method. This difference lies in the fact that removal of the lesion is a basic feature of the first two but not of the last method. With increasing experience with these methods this difference has assumed greater significance, for it has tended to focus attention upon the primary objective of therapy, namely correction of the hemodynamic disturbances by restoration of normal circulation. As a consequence, certain modifications in our concept of the application of these methods of surgical treatment have evolved, depending largely upon the nature and extent of the occlusive process. To be sure, removal of the lesion with restoration of vascular continuity remains the procedure of choice under some circumstances. Thus extirpation of the coarcted segment with end-to-end anastomosis or with graft replacement is preferable in most of the usual forms of coarctation and should always be done in those associated with aneurysmal formation. In some of the more unusual types, however, particularly in those associated with relatively long coarcted segments extending in some instances into the abdominal aorta, the use of the bypass graft principle has been found to be an equally effective but much simpler technical procedure (Fig. 5).

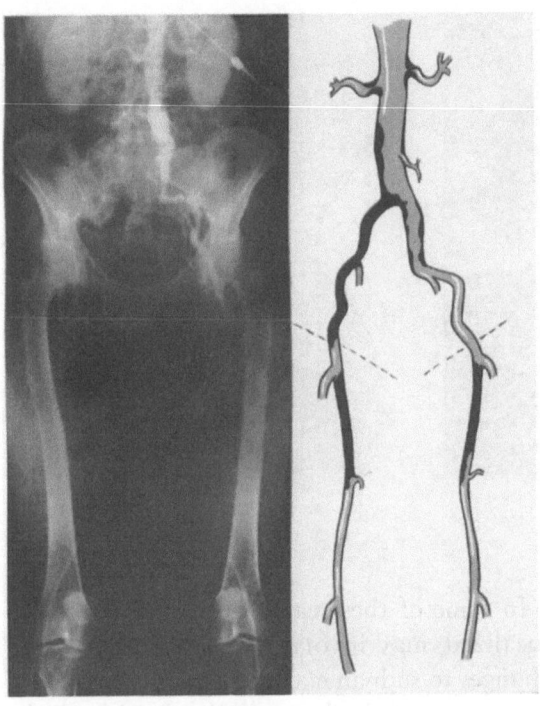 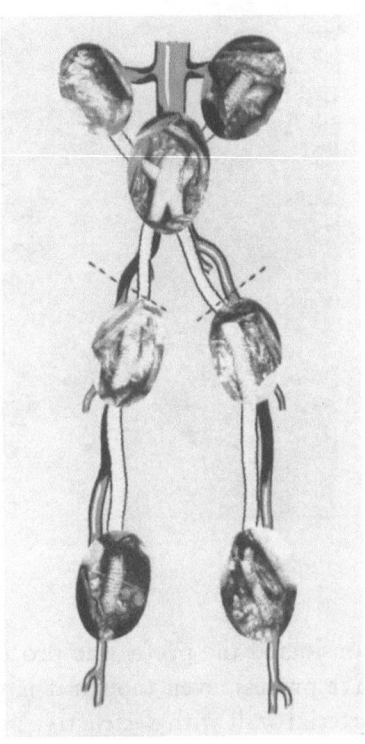

Fig. 6. (A) Preoperative aortogram showing multiple segmental occlusive lesions involving renal, iliac, and femoral arteries bilaterally as depicted in diagram on right in 62-year-old white female patient with severe hypertension and intermittent claudication

Fig. 6. (B) Photograph made at operation with drawings illustrating application of bypass graft to restore normal circulation distal to multiple segmental occlusive lesions

Similarly, in occlusive lesions involving the major branches of the aortic arch, most of which are of atherosclerotic origin, the bypass graft principle has proved to be the most satisfactory procedure in most cases (Fig. 2). This bypass graft procedure is particularly desirable in patients with multiple segmental occlusive lesions since it permits restoration of normal circulation with minimal operative trauma (Fig. 6).

It has also been found to be the preferable procedure in certain forms of occlusive disease of the superior mesenteric and renal arteries (Figs. 3 and 4). In other forms of the disease, in which, for example, the occlusive lesion is fairly discrete and well localized with relatively normal outer layers which permit the development of a well defined cleavage plane between the involved intimal and uninvolved medial layers of the artery, thromboendarterectomy is still

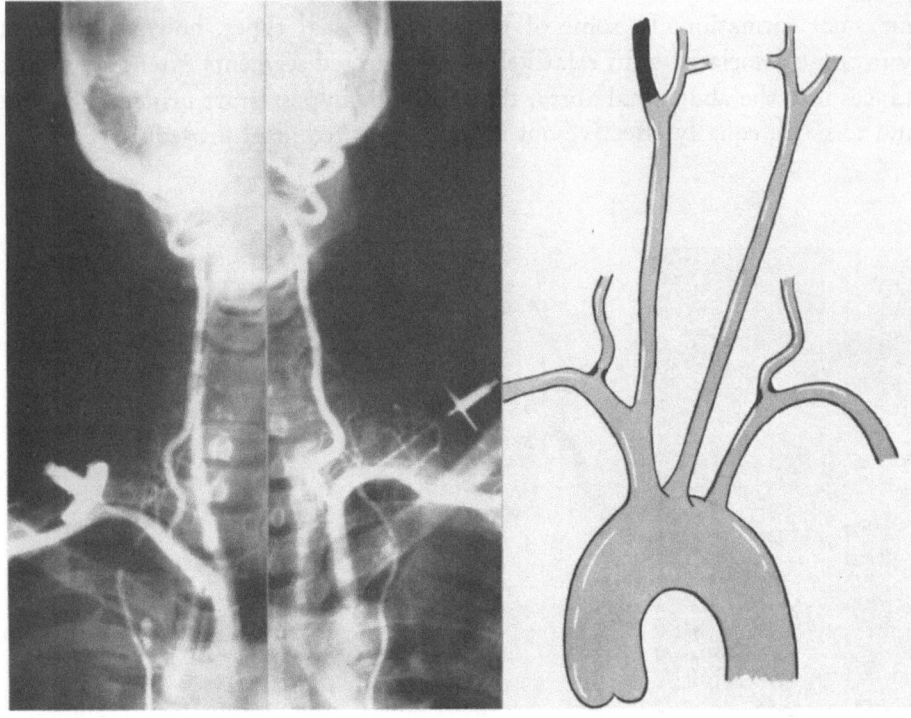

Fig. 7 (A)

considered the preferable procedure. In some of these cases, however, the occlusive process, even though it is well localized, may involve the outer layer of the arterial wall with destructive mural changes to such an extent that endarterectomy either is not feasible or results in compromise of the lumen following its repair.

In some cases of this type it is possible to employ the patch graft angioplasty principle of repair (Figs. 7—9). This method has proved to be particularly valuable in extending application of these methods of restorative vascular surgery to occlusive disease of the smaller, more peripheral arteries and in converting some of these cases from inoperable to operable lesions (Fig. 1).

In still other cases in which the mural atherosclerotic process, although segmental, is extensive and involves multiple sites of the arterial channels or is associated with aneurysmal formation, the combined use of two or more of these methods may be required (Figs. 10 and 11). It is thus apparent that several methods are available which may be employed individually or in combination depending upon the type and extent of the occlusive process as well as certain systemic factors. Growing experience and the shift of emphasis from excisional therapy to the primary objective of restoration of normal circulation have permitted more effective application of these different methods in accordance with their proper indications with increasingly gratifying results (Tables III—V).

Fig. 7. (A) Preoperative arteriograms showing incomplete occlusive lesions near origin
of vertebral arteries as depicted in diagram
on right in patient with manifestations of
basilar artery insufficiency. Patient also
had complete occlusion of right internal
carotid artery of long duration

Fig. 7. (B) Photograph made at operation
showing application of dacron patch graft
angioplasty to restore normal lumen size
of vertebral arteries at their origin from
subclavian arteries

Fig. 7. (C) Postoperative arteriogram showing restoration of normal circulation in
vertebral arteries by means of patch graft
angioplasty as depicted in drawing on right

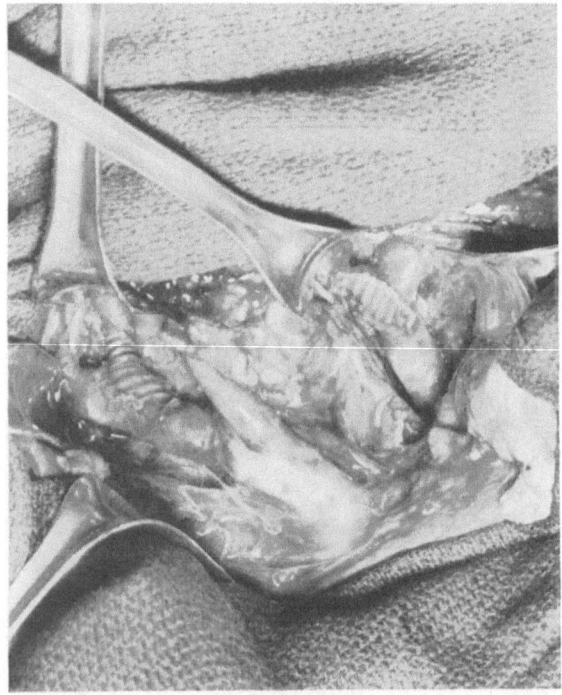

Fig. 7 (B)

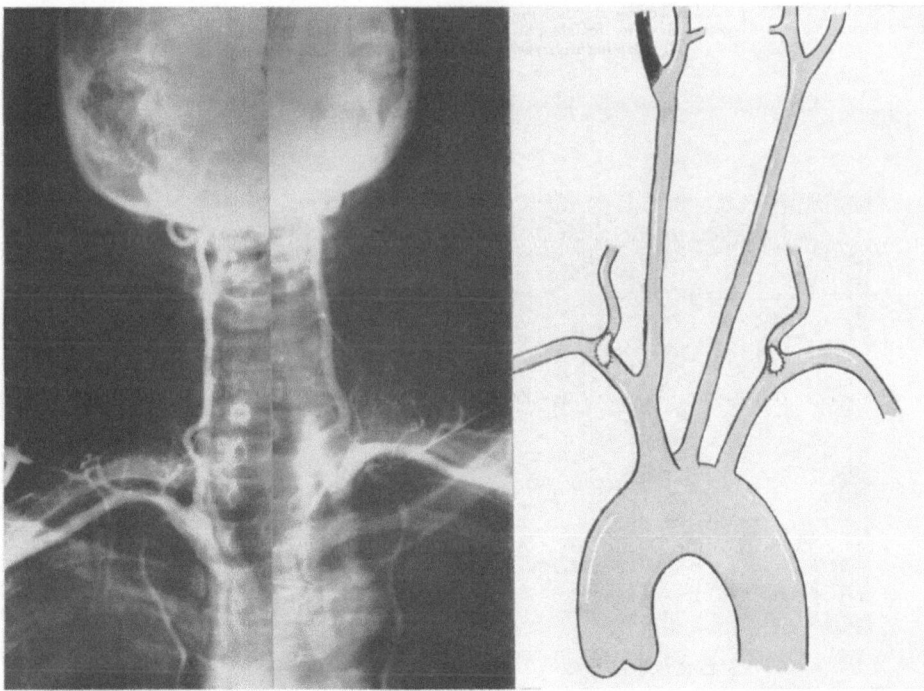

Fig. 7 (C)

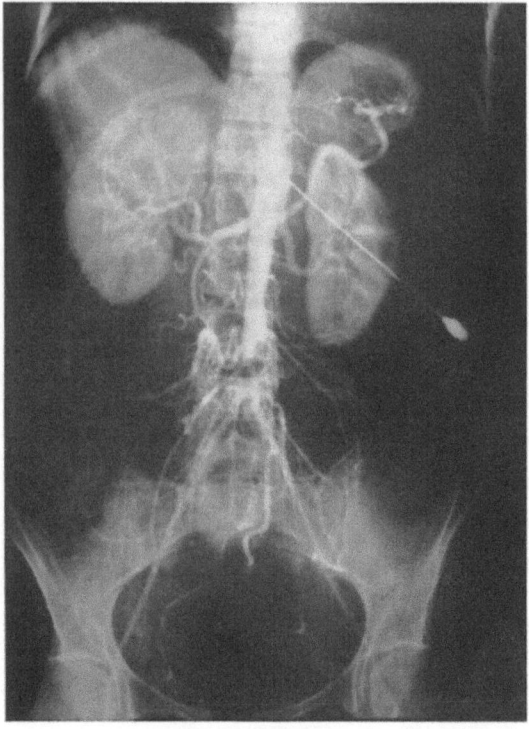
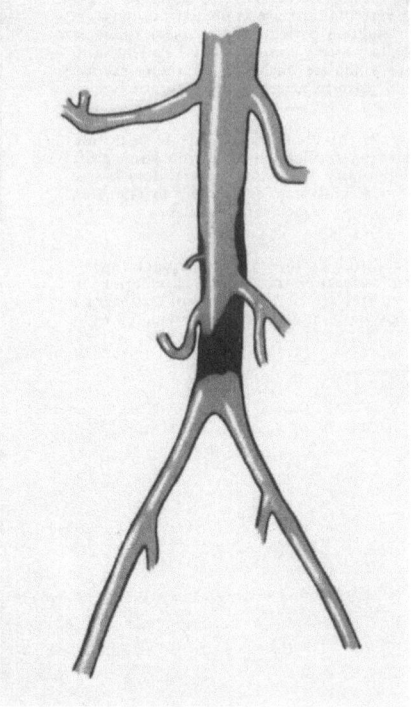

Fig. 8. (A)   Fig. 8. (B)

Fig. 8. (A) Preoperative lumbar aortogram showing well localized segmental occlusive lesion in abdominal aorta just above bifurcation in 44-year-old white female patient suffering with intermittent claudication of lower extremities. (B) Drawing illustrating site and extent of occlusive lesion

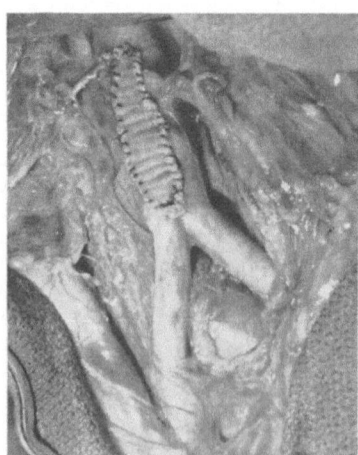
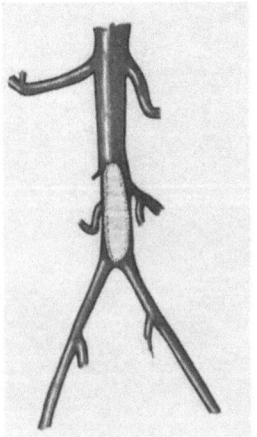

Fig. 8. (C)   Fig. 8. (D)

Fig. 8. (C) Photograph made at operation showing dacron patch graft angioplasty employed to restore normal aortic lumen after removal of occlusive lesion by endarterectomy as depicted in drawing (D)

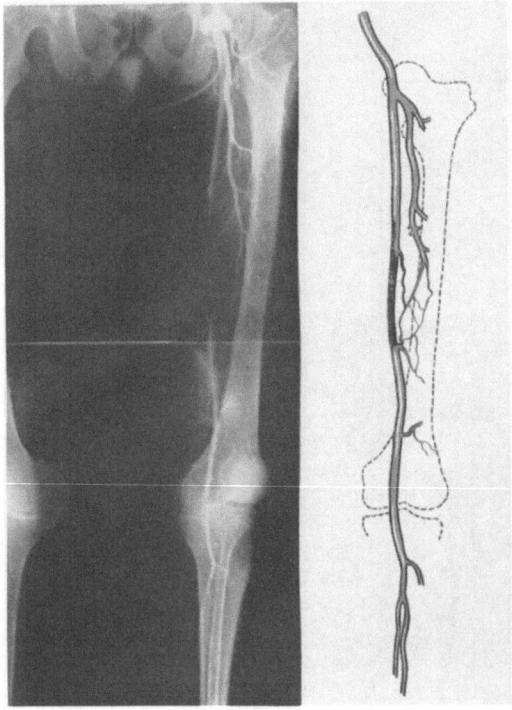

Fig. 9 (A)

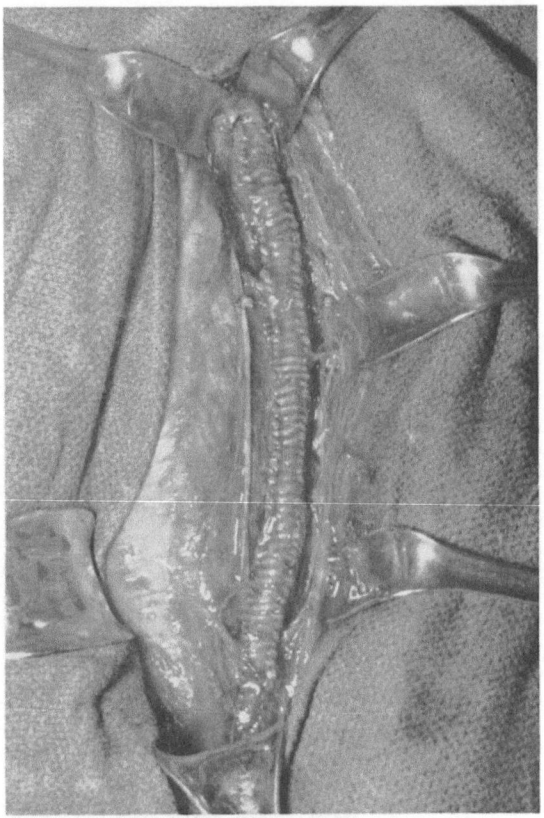

Fig. 9 (B)

Fig. 9. (C)

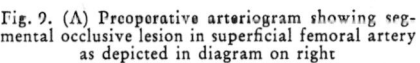

Fig. 9. (A) Preoperative arteriogram showing segmental occlusive lesion in superficial femoral artery as depicted in diagram on right

Fig. 9. (B) Photograph made at operation showing application of dacron patch graft angioplasty to restore normal lumen after removal of occlusive lesion by endarterectomy

Fig. 9. (C) Postoperative arteriogram showing restoration of normal circulation following endarterectomy and patch graft angioplasty as depicted in drawing on right

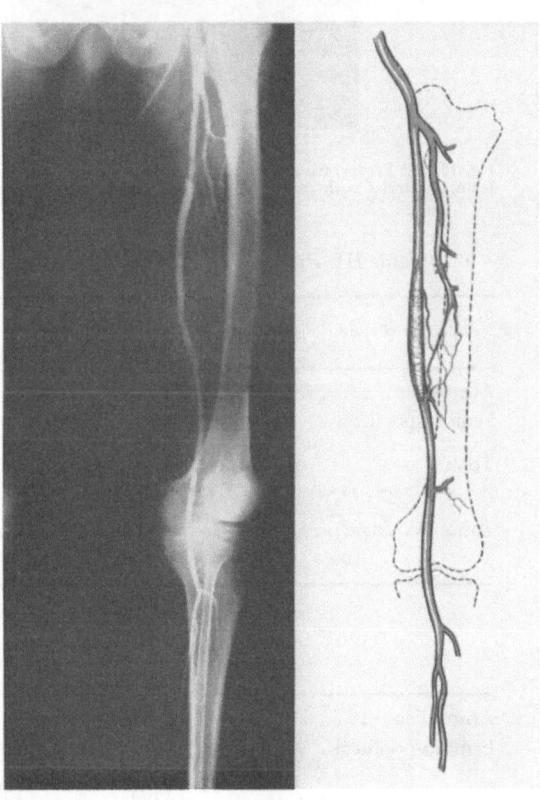

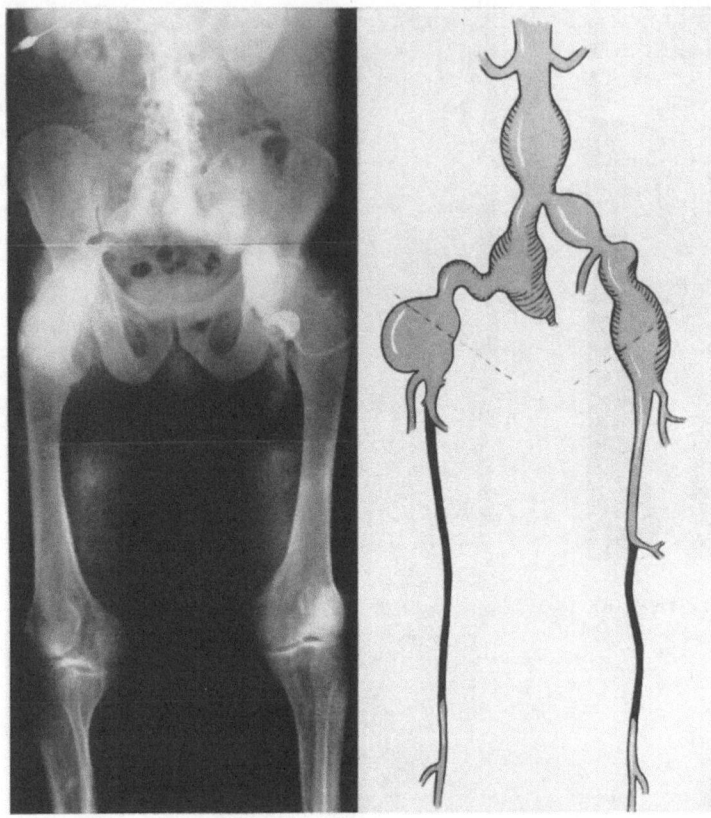

Fig. 10. (A) Preoperative aortogram showing extensive aneurysmal lesions involving abdominal aorta and both iliac and femoral arteries with segmental occlusive lesions in both superficial femoral arteries as depicted in drawing on right

Table III. *Results of treatment in aorto-iliac and femoro-popliteal occlusive disease*

Type	No. cases	Successful		Mortality	
		No. cases	Per cent	No. cases	per cent
Aorto-iliac	769	738	96	17	2.2
Femoro-popliteal . . .	634	558	88	3	0.5
Total	1403	1296	92	20	1.4

Table IV. *Incidence of recurrent occlusions in cases of aorto-iliac and femoro-popliteal occlusive disease*

Type	No. cases	Recurrent occlusion		
		No. cases	Reoperation	
			No. cases	No. successful
Aorto-iliac	769	37 (5 %)	36	36
Femoro-popliteal . . .	634	121 (19 %)	86	77
Total	1403	158 (11 %)	122	113

Fig. 10. (B) Drawing illustrating method of treatment
consisting in resection and dacron graft replacement
of aneurysms of abdominal aorta, iliac and femoral
arteries with bypass grafts to both popliteal arteries

Fig. 10. (C) Postoperative aortogram showing restoration of normal circulation to both lower extremities

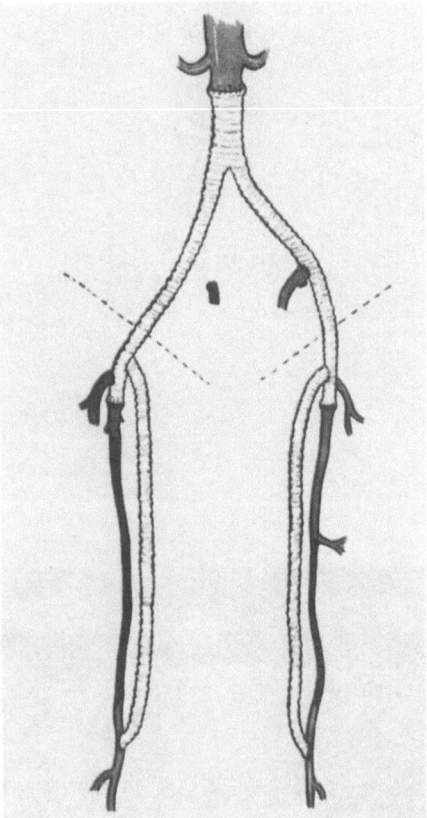

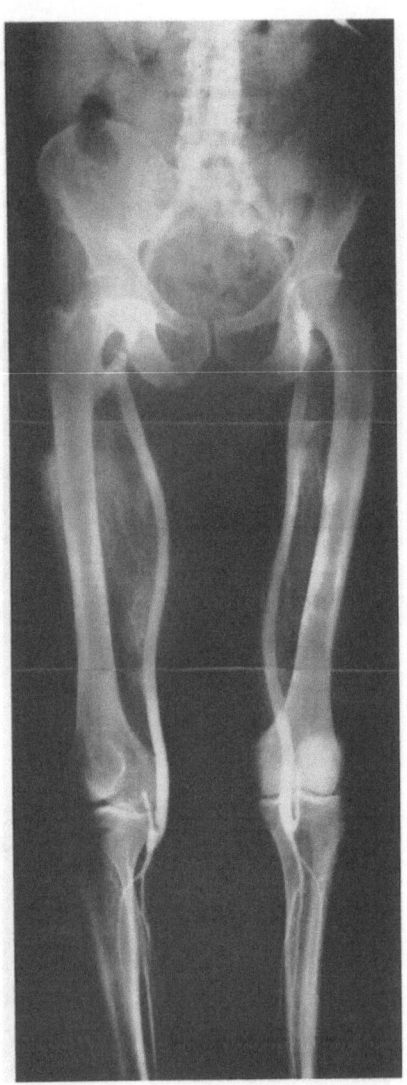

Fig. 10. (B)   Fig. 10. (C)

Table V. *Incidence of operability and results of operation in patients with occlusive disease of innominate, carotid, subclavian, and vertebral arteries*

Location	No. cases	No. explored	No. circulation restored
Internal carotid	128	117 (91 %)	100 (85 %)
Common carotid	14	14 (100 %)	14 (100 %)
Innominate	15	14 (93 %)	14 (100 %)
Subclavian	23	21 (91 %)	21 (100 %)
Vertebral	28	19 (68 %)	16 (84 %)
Total	208	185 (89 %)	165 (89 %)

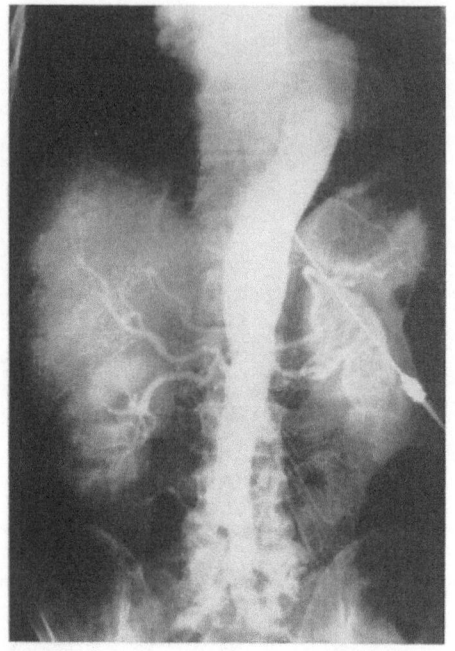

Fig. 11. (A)

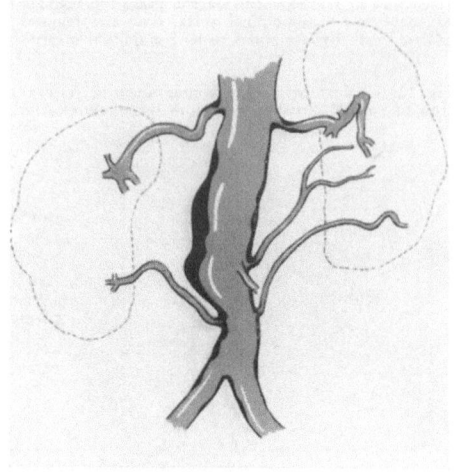

Fig. 11. (B)

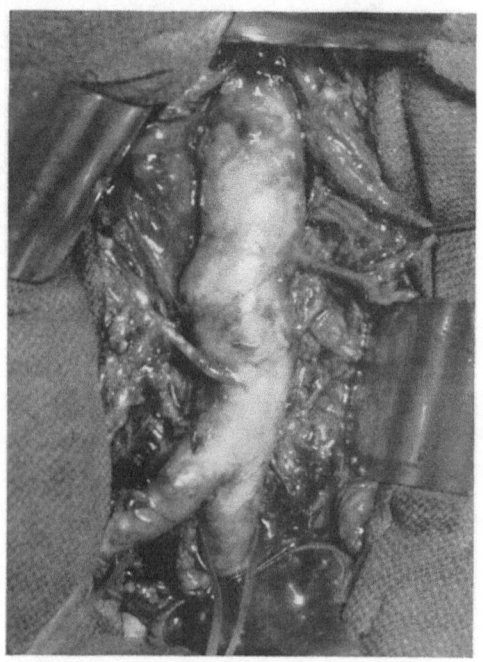

Fig. 11. (C)

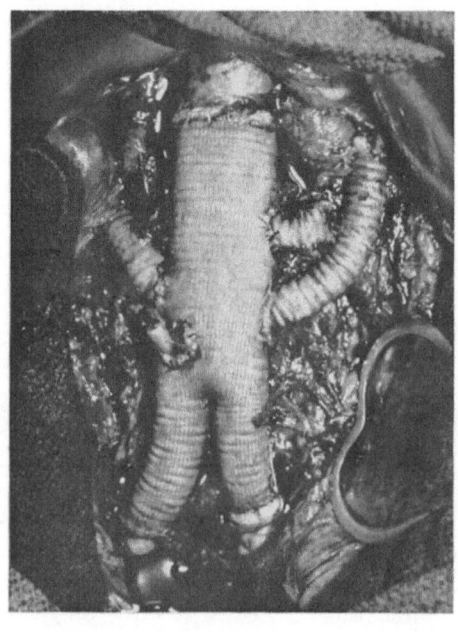

Fig. 11. (D)

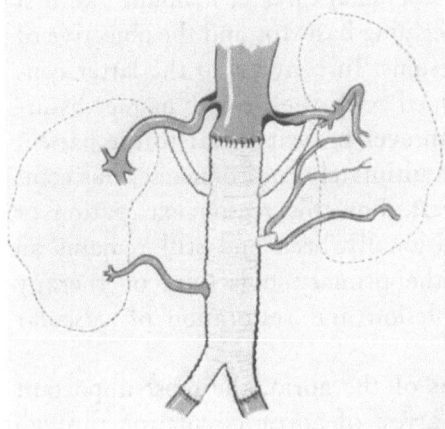

Fig. 11. (E)

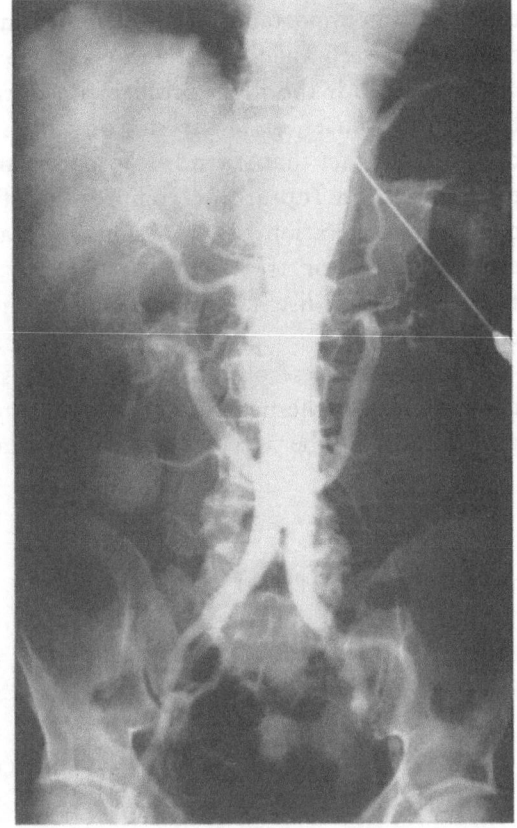

Fig. 11. (F)

Fig. 11. (A) Preoperative aortogram showing small aneurysm of abdominal aorta with segmental occlusive lesions involving both renal arteries near their origin and several accessory renal arteries in patient with severe hypertension

Fig. 11. (B) Drawing illustrating nature and location of lesion

Fig. 11. (C) Photograph made at operation showing small aneurysm of abdominal aorta and accessory renal arteries

Fig. 11. (D) Photograph made at operation showing method of treatment by resection and dacron graft replacement of abdominal aorta with bypass grafts to both renal arteries and attachment of accessory renal arteries to graft as depicted in drawing (E)

Fig. 11. (F) Postoperative aortogram showing restoration of normal circulation through dacron graft to both renal arteries, accessory renal arteries, and iliac arteries

In returning now to a consideration of aneurysmal disease, I should like first to indicate an important difference in the underlying basis for and the objective of therapy between aneurysmal and occlusive lesions. In contrast to the latter condition, in which the main problem is concerned with the hemodynamic disturbances it produces, an aneurysm constitutes an ever-present threat to the patient owing to the fact that it tends to progress and ultimately to produce serious complications from rupture or compressive effects. For this reason extirpation or complete obliteration of the lesion has traditionally been and still remains an essential basis for treatment. Accordingly, the primary objectives of therapy for aneurysmal disease are removal of the lesion and restoration of vascular continuity.

To achieve these objectives for aneurysms of the aorta, the most important consideration is the necessity for temporary arrest of aortic circulation through the segment to be resected. The potentially hazardous consequences of this procedure are concerned first with the resultant sudden increased vascular resistance upon the heart with left ventricular strain and second with ischemic damage to the tissues distal to the occlusion. In this connection it should be stated that this problem assumes significance only for aneurysms arising above the origin of the renal arteries, but from this point upward it assumes increasing significance. Accordingly, for aneurysms of the abdominal aorta, most of which fortunately arise below this level,

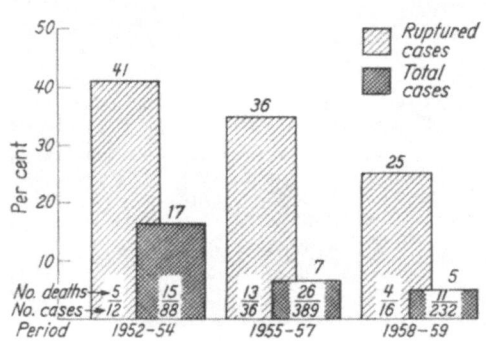

Graph 1. Graph showing decreasing mortality with chronologic periods in surgical treatment of aneurysm of abdominal aorta

there are few surgical problems worthy of consideration, and these are concerned mostly with rupture and certain systemic factors such as advanced age, hypertension, and heart disease which have important bearing upon the risk of operation. To be sure, some variations in technic may be required in accordance with the different pathologic circumstances encountered, but the essential technical principles are now fairly well standardized, and with increasing experience in their application the results have been progressively more gratifying (Graph 1).

For aneurysms arising above the level of the renal arteries, control of the problems emanating from temporary arrest of aortic circulation is of vital importance. Several methods have been devised and used for this purpose, and their application depends largely upon the nature, extent, and location of the lesion. For this reason and in accordance with our experience, these aneurysms may be classified into the following categories:

(1) Those located in the aortic arch proximal to the left subclavian artery;

(2) Those arising distal to the left common carotid artery and involving the descending thoracic aorta; and

(3) Those involving the thoraco-abdominal segment of aorta.

Aneurysms involving the aortic arch may be further subdivided into two groups, depending upon whether or not the lesion involves the proximal 3 or 4 cm. of the ascending aorta. The reason for this distinction lies in the fact that different methods of excisional therapy are necessary for each of these lesions. Thus in cases in which the aneurysm does not involve the proximal segment of the ascending aorta, the temporary bypass principle is the procedure of choice since by this means relatively normal aortic circulation can be maintained during the entire procedure (Fig. 12). In this connection it is worthy of note that with the development of the dacron tube as a vascular replacement it is possible and sometimes desirable to convert the temporary dacron shunt into the permanent graft (Fig. 13).

For fusiform aneurysms involving the proximal segment of the ascending aorta, it is necessary to employ cardiopulmonary bypass with the artificial heart-lung apparatus (Fig. 14). Unfortunately, this method imposes additional hazards to the operative procedure derived largely from possible interference with coronary circulation and the necessity for heparinization, which may lead to difficulties in control of hemorrhage in the grafted segment despite measures to counteract heparinization. The former factor is particularly important since many of these patients are in an older age group and are likely to have varying degrees of associated heart disease. In such cases it may be desirable to maintain coronary circulation by direct cannulization and perfusion of the coronary arteries. While some gratifying success has been achieved in this form of the disease, further investigative efforts are indicated in providing a more effective solution to some of these problems.

Aneurysms of the second category, i.e., those arising in the descending thoracic aorta distal to the left common carotid artery, are associated with fewer difficulties and hazards than the former group. Moreover, several methods are available for overcoming some of the problems resulting from the necessity for temporary cross-clamping of the aorta. These include hypothermia and temporary shunts. The former method was used in our early experience, but because of certain disadvantages associated with its application in recent years, we have preferred some form of temporary bypass depending upon the type and location of the lesion. Thus for aneurysms that involve the left subclavian artery or extend distally along the descending thoracic aorta, the most satisfactory method consists in the use of a pump-bypass in which oxygenated blood is removed from the left auricle and pumped through a plastic cannula inserted upward into the left femoral artery into the aorta distal to the lower occluding clamp (Fig. 15). The major advantage of this method lies in the fact that it provides adequate circulation distal to the level of the aortic occlusion to permit

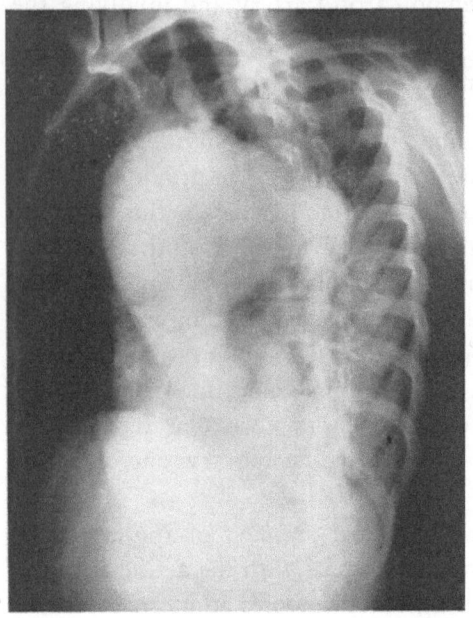

Fig. 12. (A)

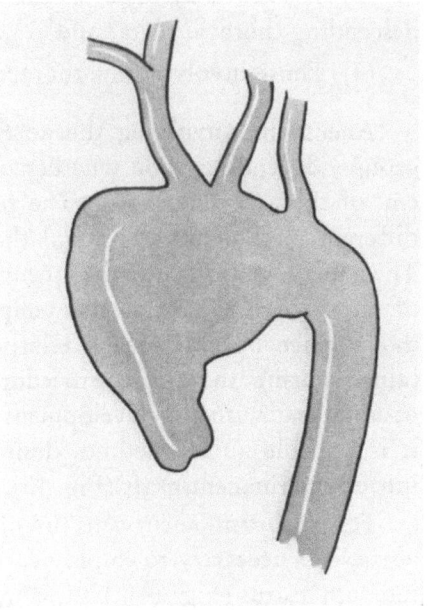

Fig. 12. (B)

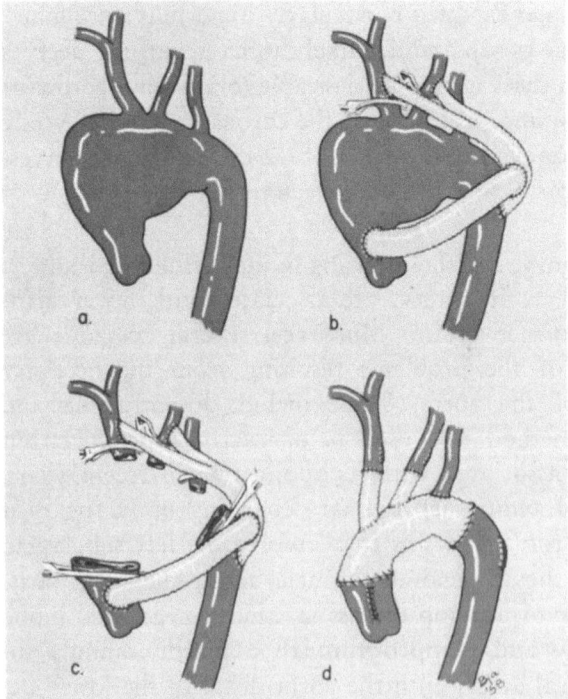

Fig. 12. (C)

Fig. 12. (A) Preoperative aortogram showing fusiform aneurysm involving ascending aorta and transverse arch

Fig. 12. (B) Drawing illustrating location and extent of aneurysm

Fig. 12. (C) Drawings illustrating method of treatment utilizing temporary bypass grafts to maintain normal aortic circulation during excision and graft replacement of aneurysm

Fig. 12 (D) Photograph made at operation showing completed procedure as depicted in drawing on right

Fig. 12. (E) Aortogram made approximately one and one half years after operation showing normal aortic circulation

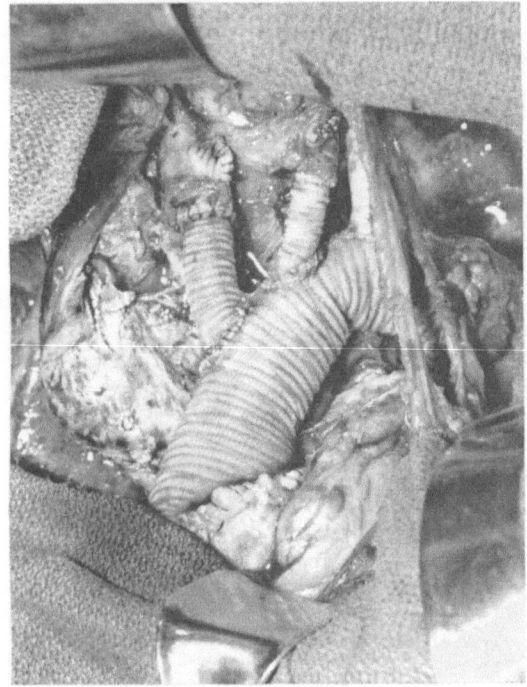

Fig. 12 (D)

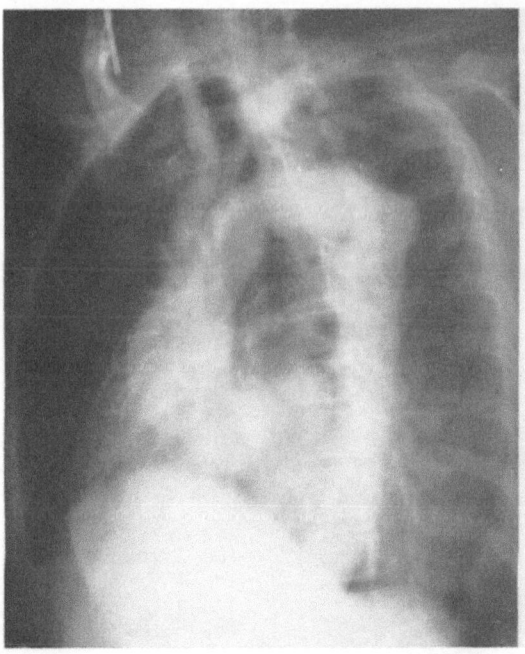
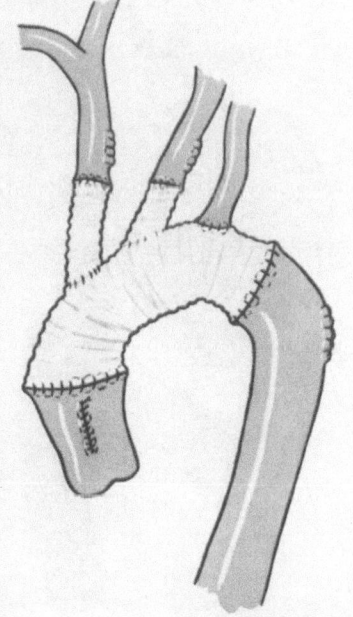

Fig. 12. (E)

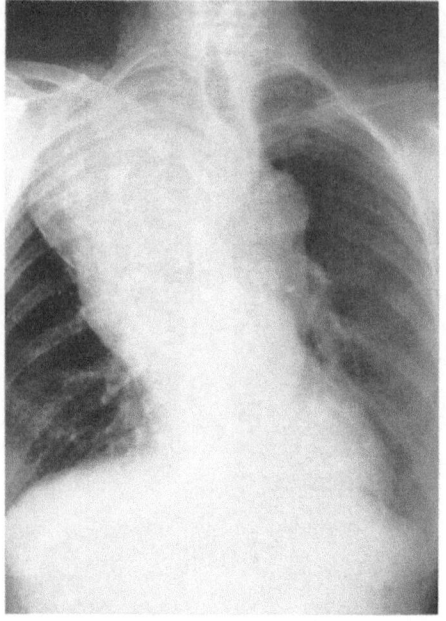

Fig. 13. (A)

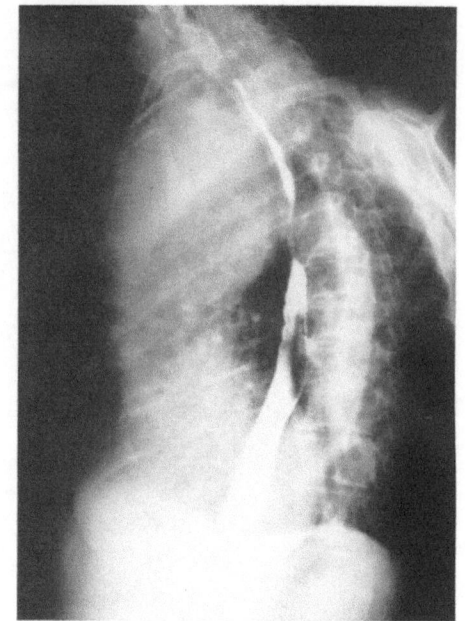

Fig. 13. (B)

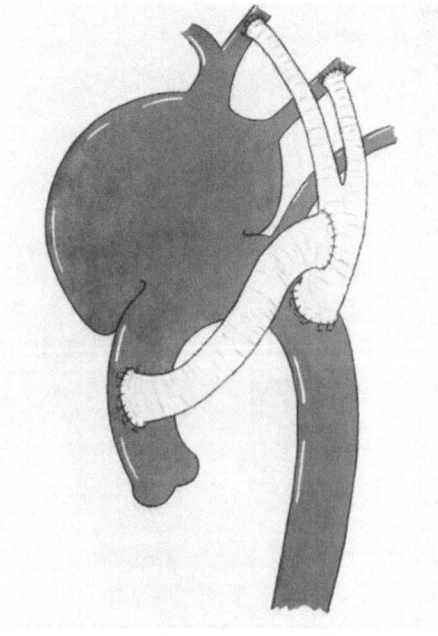

Fig. 13. (C)

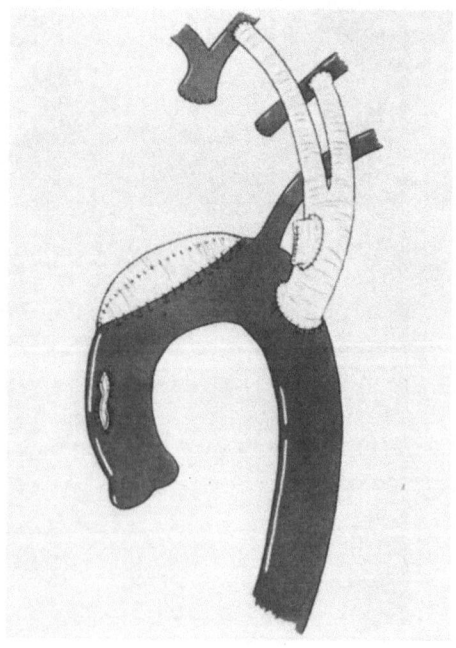

Fig. 13. (D)

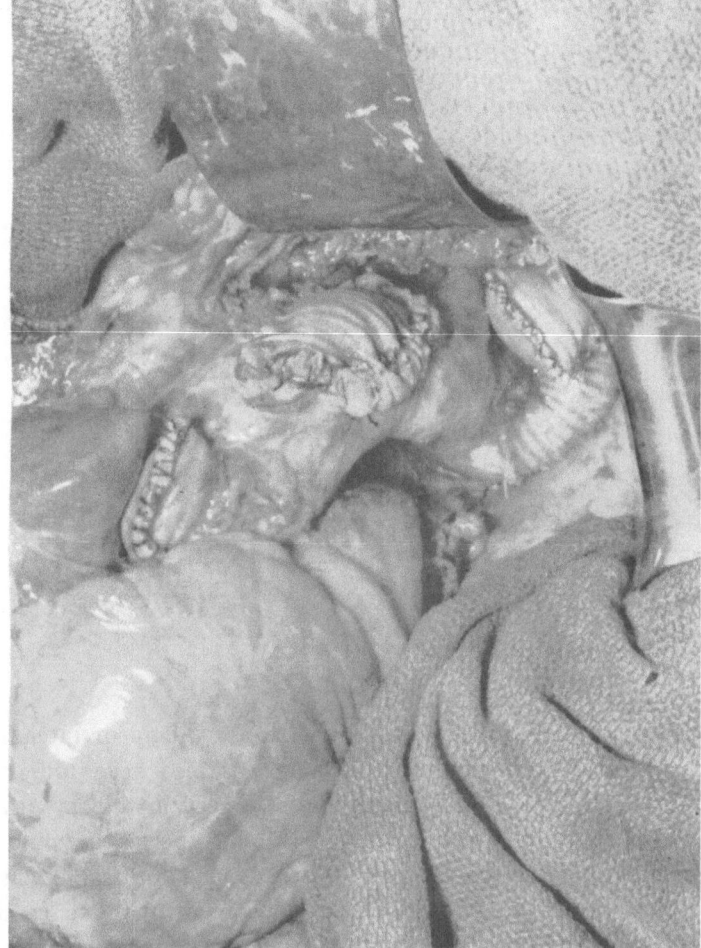

Fig. 13. (E)

Fig. 13. (A) Posterior-anterior roentgenogram of chest and (B) angioaortogram showing extensive aneurysms involving ascending aorta and transverse arch

Fig. 13. (C) Drawing illustrating method of treatment utilizing temporary bypass graft to maintain normal aortic circulation during excision of aneurysm

Fig. 13. (D) Drawing illustrating completed procedure with patch graft angioplasty to repair excised segment of aortic arch and conversion of temporary bypass graft to innominate and left common carotid arteries into the permanent graft

Fig. 13. (E) Photograph made at operation showing completed procedure

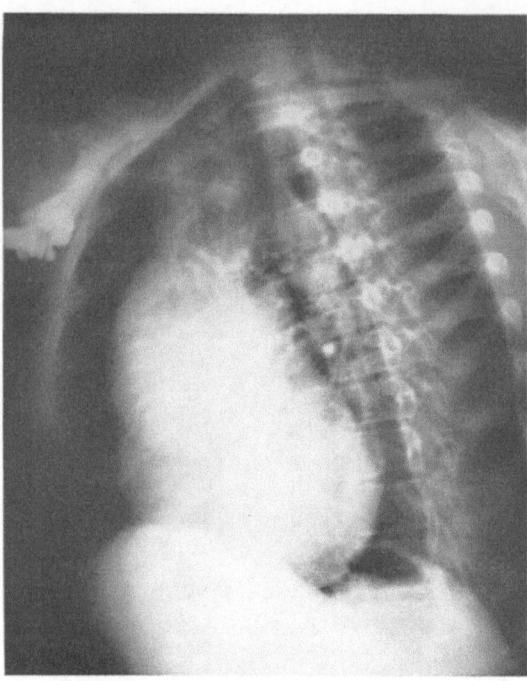

viability and to prevent serious left ventricular strain by maintenance of blood pressure at near normal levels. This method has also been found most useful in the application of excisional therapy for dissecting aneurysms. While such aneurysms may involve any part of the aorta our experience would suggest that those in which surgical treatment is most frequently applicable arise in the descending limb of the aortic arch and the upper segment of the descending thoracic aorta. In such cases the proximal extent of the dissecting process stops at or just below the origin of the left subclavian artery. Distally the dissecting process may be limited to the descending thoracic aorta or may extend down into the abdominal aorta for a variable distance. In the former instance excisional therapy permits removal of the entire dissecting process and the surgical procedure is much the same as that for fusiform aneurysms of this aortic segment (Fig. 16). In the latter circumstances, however, the procedure requires slight modification in management of the distal extent of the dissecting process. Thus after excising the proximal portion of the dissecting aneurysm the false lumen in the distal opening of the aorta is obliterated by suturing the inner and outer walls following which graft anastomosis may be done thus permitting restoration of normal aortic continuity and circulation (Fig. 17). For well localized aneurysms arising distal to the left subclavian artery another method for temporary bypass that may be employed consists in the insertion of a plastic catheter through a small opening in the left subclavian artery proximally and into the descending thoracic aorta distally (Fig. 18). Still another method, which may be used for this purpose and which is applicable in cases in which the aneurysm is well localized to the mid-portion of the descending thoracic aorta, is a temporary internal shunt (Fig. 19). Finally, in more extensive forms of the disease in which the aneurysm involves

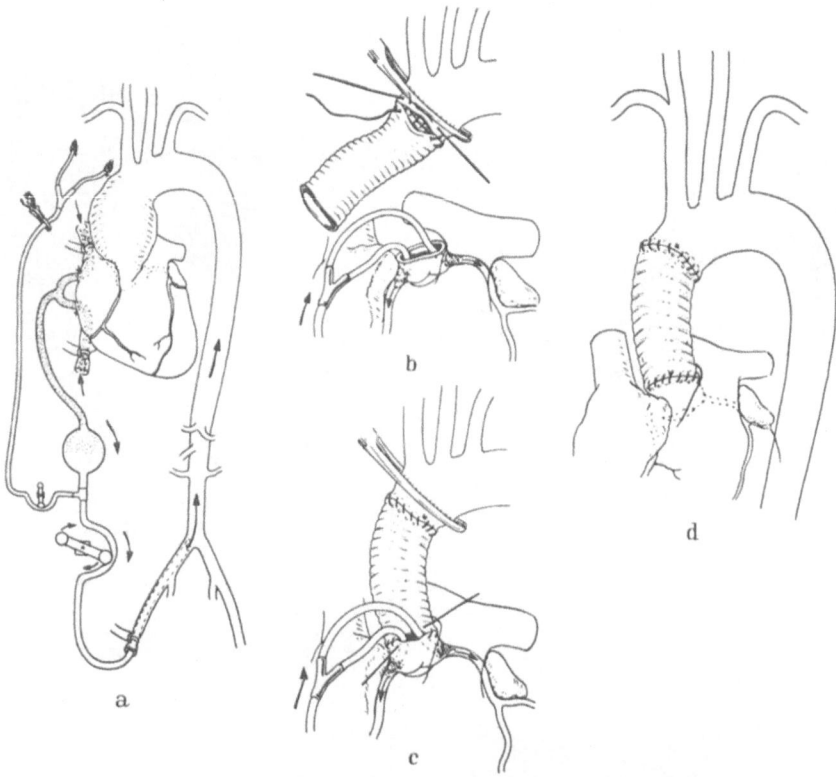

Fig. 14. (B) Drawings illustrating method of treatment in this case utilizing cardiopulmonary bypass with coronary artery perfusion. (a) Method of utilizing artificial heart-lung apparatus with separate pump for coronary artery perfusion. (b) After applying occluding clamp to aorta distal to fusiform aneurysm but proximal to innominate artery, aneurysm is excised and catheters are inserted into ostia of the coronary arteries to provide coronary artery perfusion. Graft is attached to distal anastomosis first. (c) Proximal anastomosis of the graft is then performed leaving a small opening anteriorly to prevent removal of coronary perfusion catheters following which anastomosis is quickly completed and occluding clamp on aorta removed to permit restoration of circulation. (d) Completed replacement of ascending aorta by graft. (In cases in which this method must be employed for aneurysms that involve the proximal segment of aorta but also extend upward to involve the innominate and carotid arteries, additional catheters may be used for separate perfusion of these vessels)

the entire descending thoracic aorta, it may be preferable to employ the principle of conversion of the temporary bypass graft into the permanent graft. This has become possible with the development of the dacron tube as a vascular replacement that may be used first as a temporary bypass graft to maintain circulation during cross-clamping of the aorta and subsequently as the permanent graft replacement for the excised aortic segment (Fig. 20).

This method is particularly applicable for the third category of aneurysms, i.e., those located in the thoraco-abdominal segment of aorta. Owing to the fact that the principal vessels to the abdominal viscera arise from this segment of aorta,

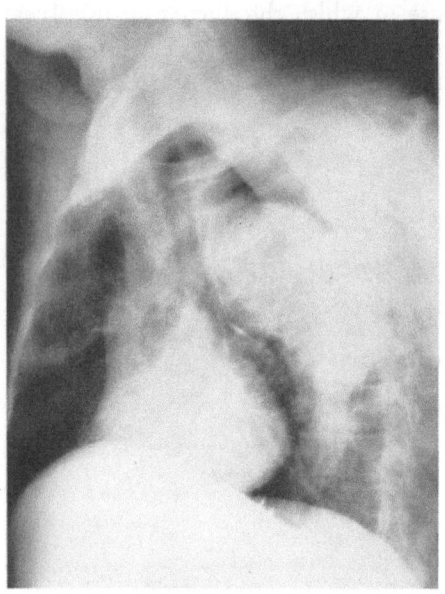

Fig. 15. (A)

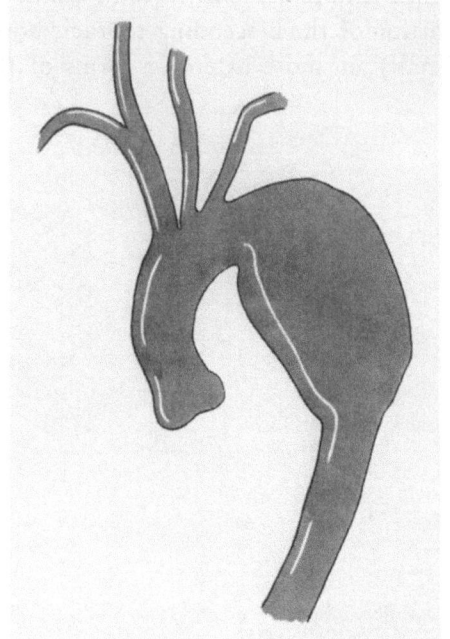

Fig. 15. (B)

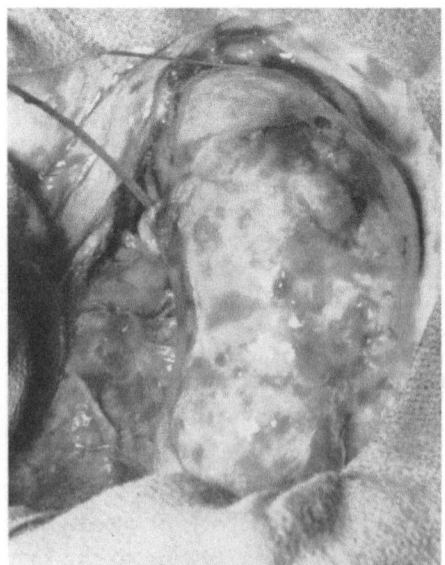

Fig. 15. (C)

Fig. 15. (A) Preoperative angiocardiogram showing large fusiform aneurysm of upper segment of descending thoracic aorta

Fig. 15. (B) Drawing showing location and extent of aneurysm

Fig. 15. (C) Photograph made at operation showing fusiform aneurysm after it has been mobilized from surrounding structures

Fig. 15. (D) Photograph made at operation showing completed replacement of excised segment of
aorta and aneurysm with knitted crimped dacron
graft

Fig. 15. (E) Drawings illustrating method of treatment by excision and graft replacement utilizing
pump-bypass from left auricle to left femoral
artery

Fig. 15. (F) Postoperative angiocardiogram showing normal restoration of aortic circulation

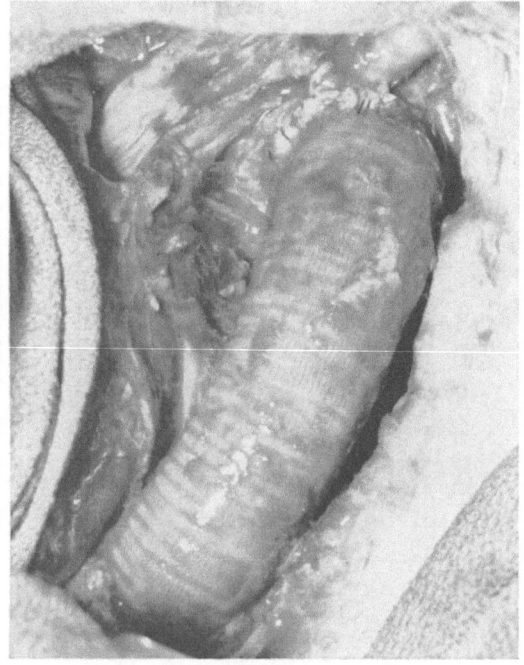

Fig. 15. (D)

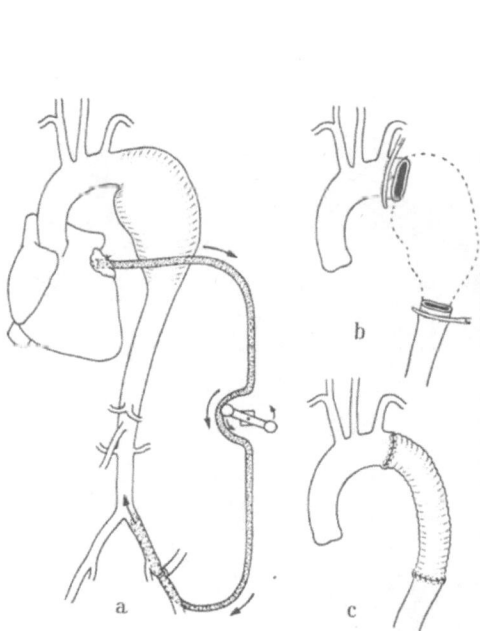
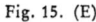

Fig. 15. (E)

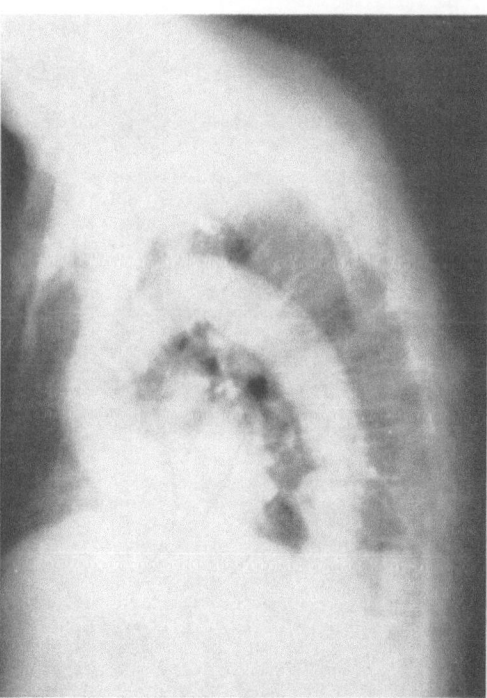

Fig. 15. (F)

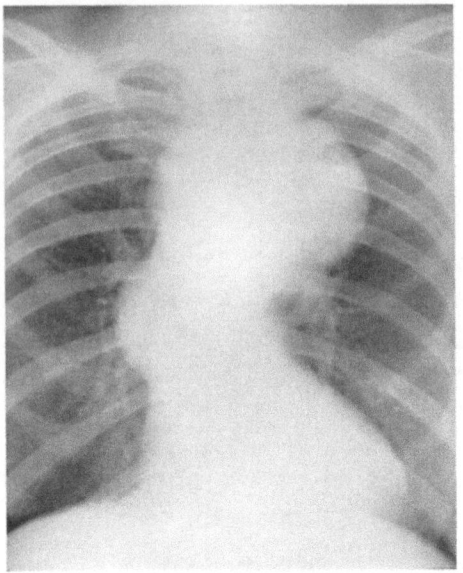

Fig. 16. (A)

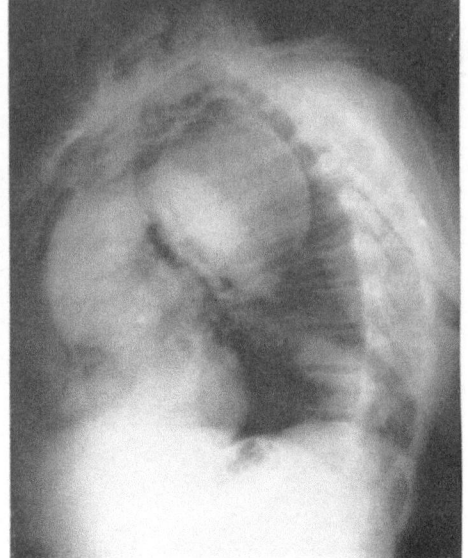

Fig. 16. (B)

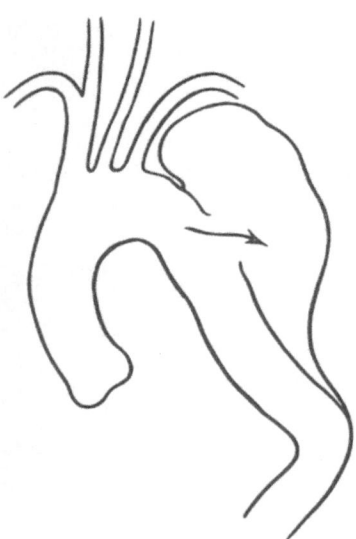

Fig. 16. (C)

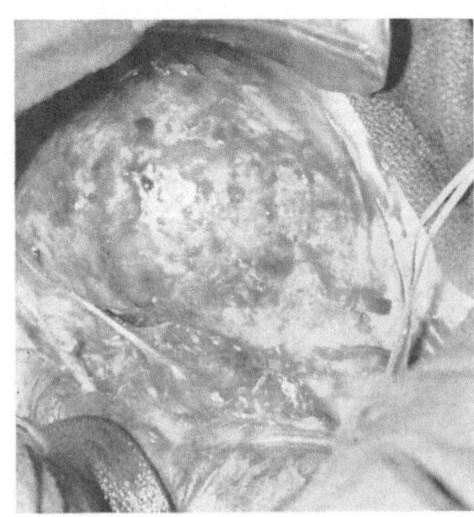

Fig. 16. (D)

Fig. 16. (A) Posterior-anterior roentgenogram of chest
and (B) angiocardiogram showing dissecting aneurysm
of upper segment of descending thoracic aorta

Fig. 16. (C) Drawing illustrating location and extent
of dissecting aneurysm

Fig. 16. (D) Photograph made at operation showing
aneurysm

Fig. 16. (E) Photograph made at operation showing
completed procedure with replacement of excised segment of aorta by dacron graft

Fig. 16. (F) Drawing illustrating method of treatment
by excision and graft replacement

Fig. 16. (G) Postoperative angiocardiogram showing
restoration normal aortic continuity and circulation

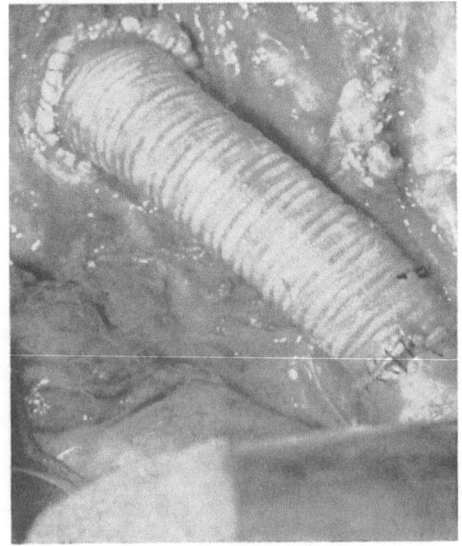

Fig. 16. (E)

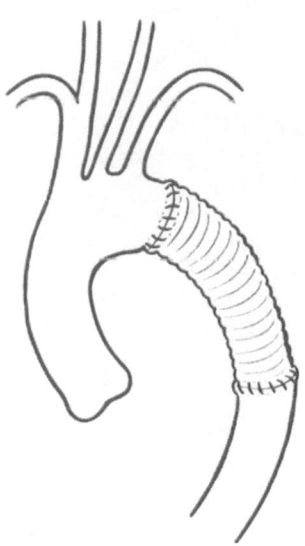

Fig. 16. (F)

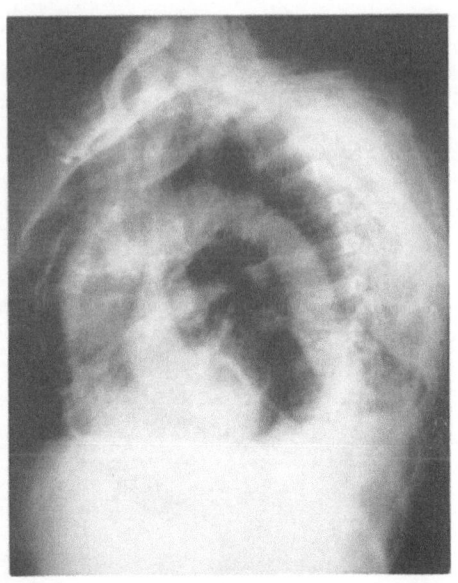

Fig. 16. (G)

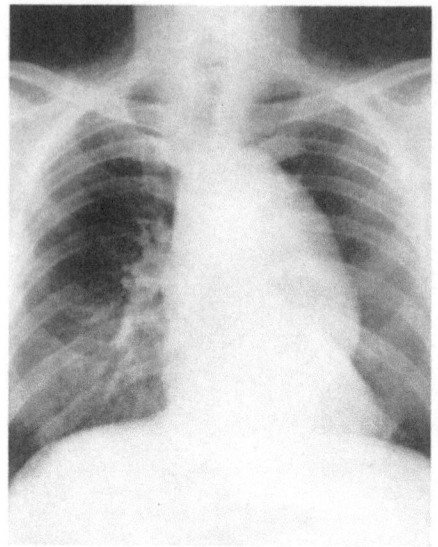

Fig. 17. (A)

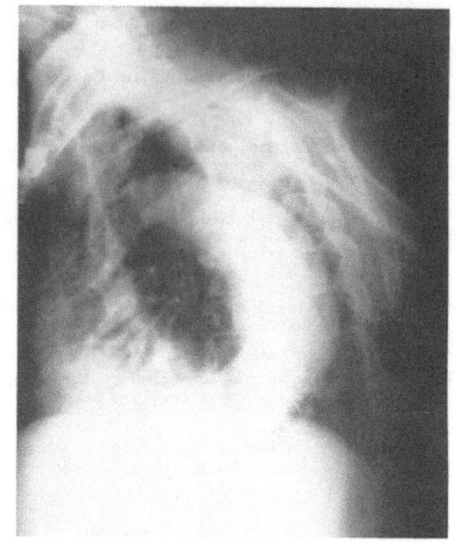

Fig. 17. (B)

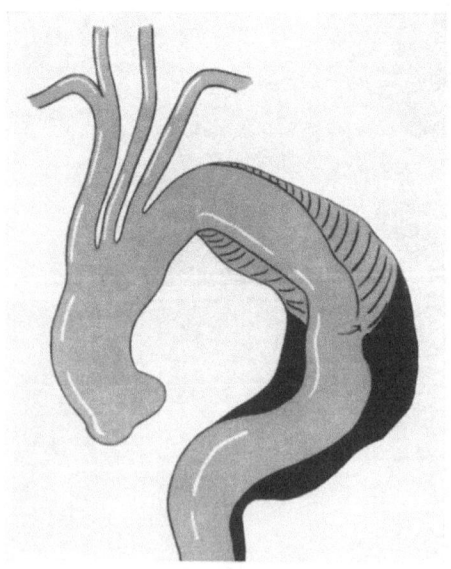

Fig. 17. (C)

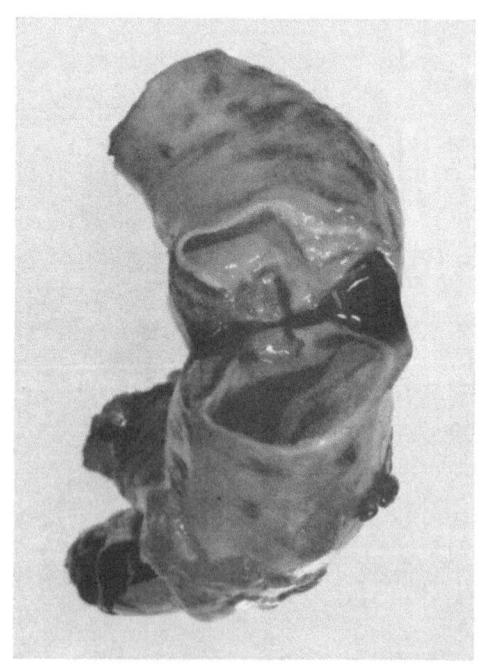

Fig. 17. (D)

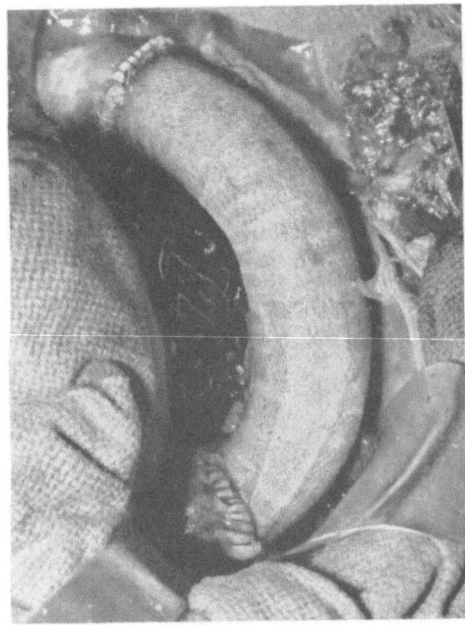

Fig. 17. (E)

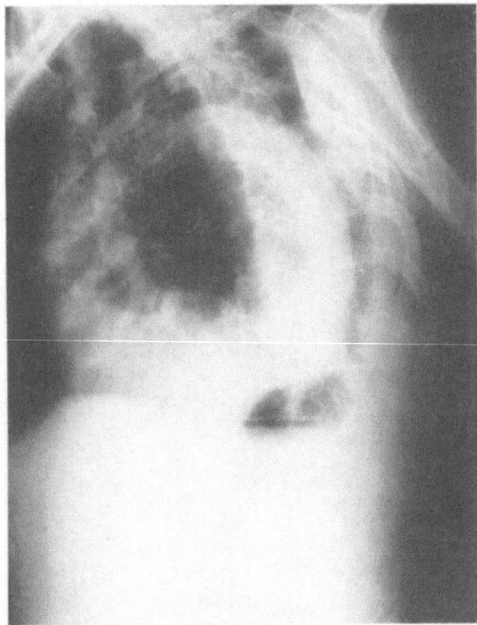

Fig. 17. (F)

Fig. 17. (A) Posterior-anterior roentgenogram of chest and (B) angioaortogram showing extensive dissecting aneurysm of descending thoracic aorta

Fig. 17. (C) Drawing illustrating location and extent of dissecting aneurysm

Fig. 17. (D) Photograph of excised specimen which has been partially transected showing double lumen of dissecting aneurysm with false lumen partly filled with thrombus

Fig. 17. (E) Photograph made at operation showing completed graft replacement of excised segment of dissecting aneurysm

Fig. 17. (F) Postoperative angiocardiogram showing restoration of normal aortic circulation through graft

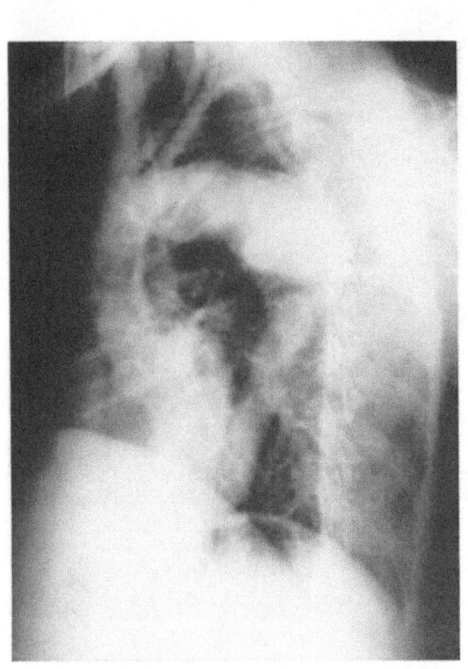

Fig. 18. (A)

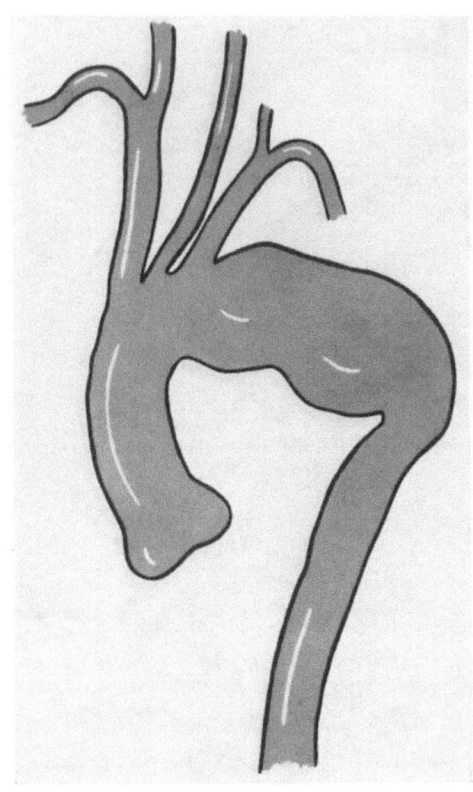

Fig. 18. (B)

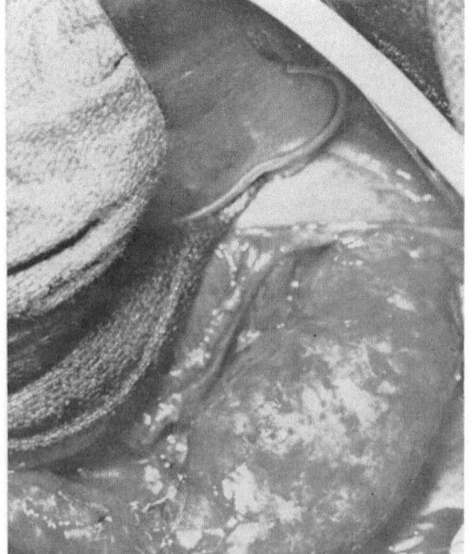

Fig. 18. (C)

Fig. 18. (A) Preoperative angiocardiogram showing fusiform aneurysm of upper segment of descending thoracic aorta

Fig. 18. (B) Drawing illustrating location and extent of aneurysm

Fig. 18. (C) Photograph made at operation showing aneurysm

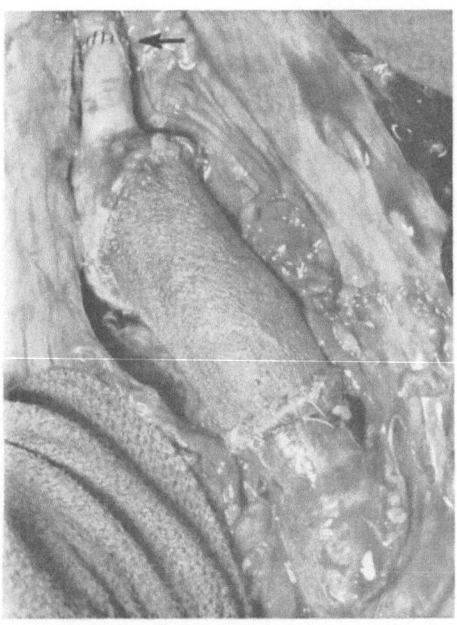

Fig. 18. (D)

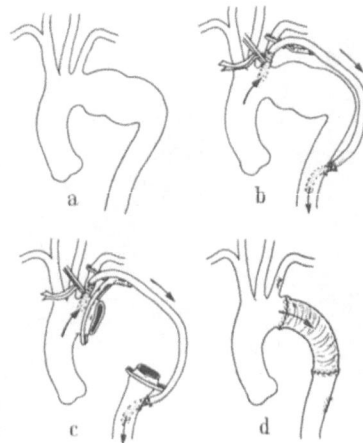

Fig. 18. (E)

Fig. 18. (D) Photograph made at operation showing completed procedure. Note suture repair of left subclavian artery

Fig. 18. (E) Drawing illustrating method of treatment utilizing temporary shunt by means of plastic catheter inserted through left subclavian artery above and into descending thoracic aorta below aneurysm to maintain circulation during procedure of excision and graft replacement

Fig. 18. (F) Postoperative angiocardiogram showing restoration of normal aortic continuity and circulation

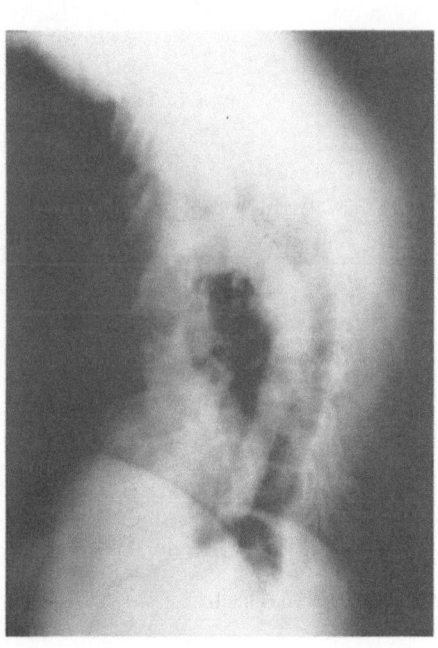

Fig. 18. (F)

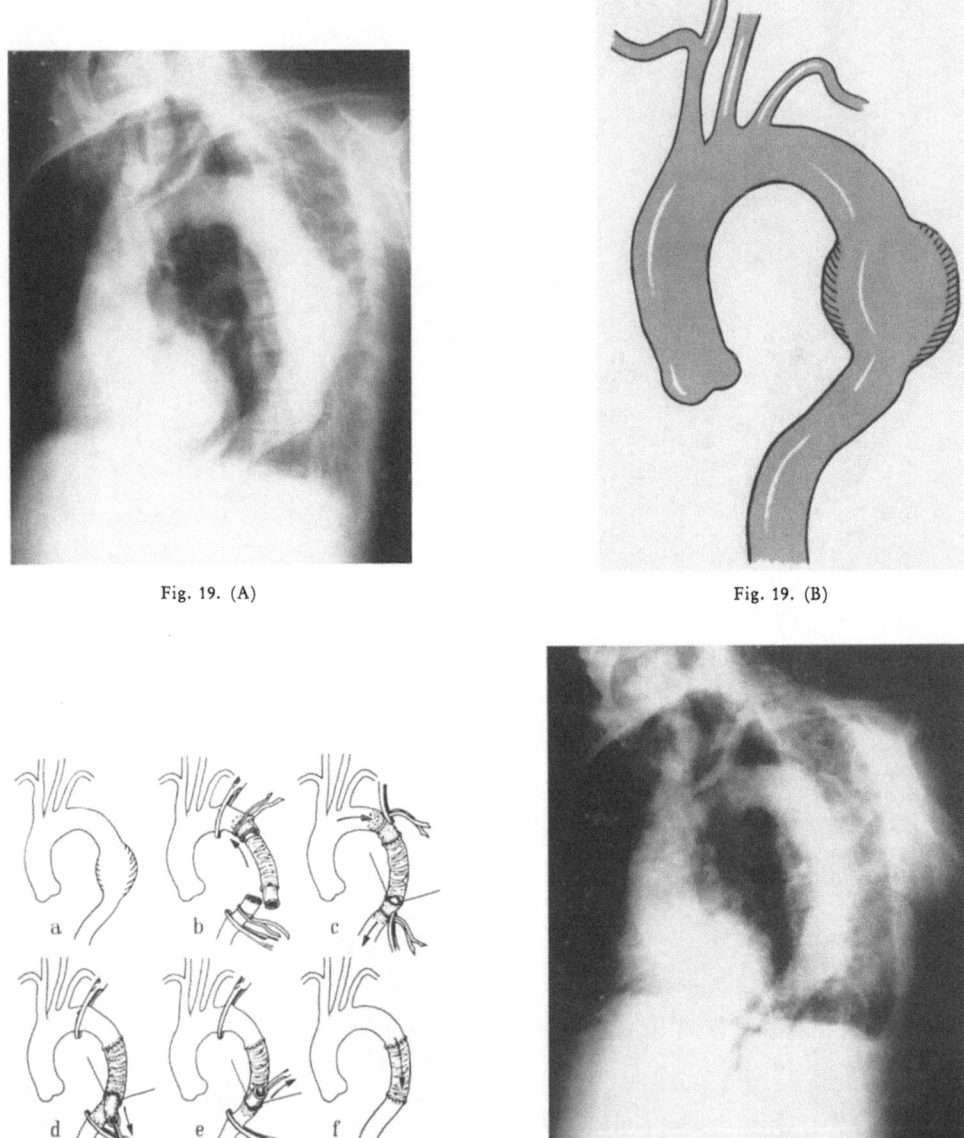

Fig. 19. (A)

Fig. 19. (B)

Fig. 19. (C)

Fig. 19. (D)

Fig. 19. (A) Preoperative angiocardiogram showing well localized fusiform aneurysm of descending thoracic aorta

Fig. 19. (B) Drawing showing location and extent of aneurysm

Fig. 19. (C) Drawings illustrating method of treatment utilizing temporary internal shunt during procedure of excision and graft replacement

Fig. 19. (D) Postoperative angiocardiogram showing normal restoration of aortic continuity and circulation

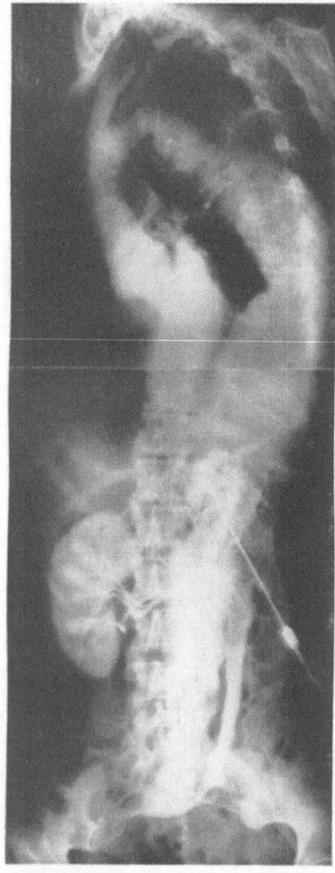

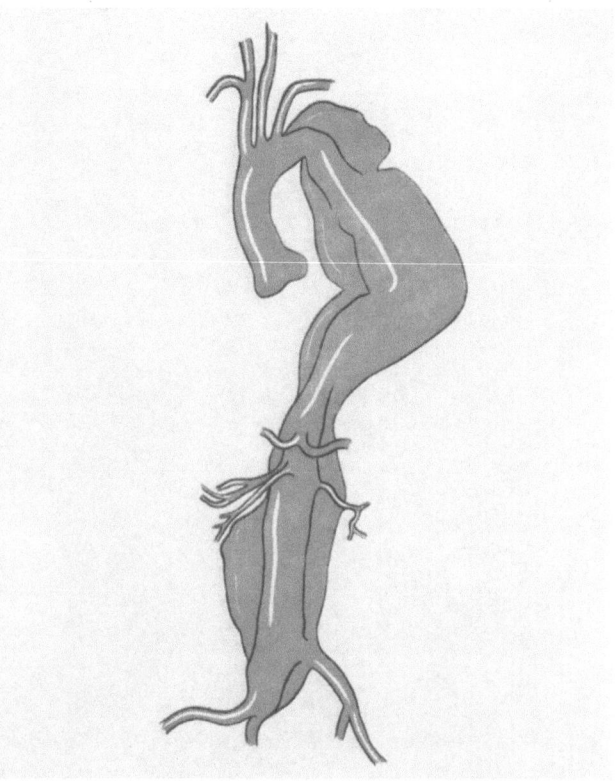

Fig. 20. (A) Preoperative aortogram showing extensive dissecting aneurysm of entire descending thoracic and abdominal aorta

Fig. 20. (B) Drawing illustrating location and extent of aneurysm

there is potential danger of producing fatal ischemic damage to such vital structures as the liver, kidneys, and gastrointestinal tract as a consequence of temporary arrest of circulation during the period of resection and graft replacement. In this connection our experience would suggest that the kidney is the most sensitive organ to ischemia and primary attention should be directed toward this organ in the performance of the procedure. This problem may be satisfactorily met by applying the principle of conversion of the temporary bypass graft into the permanent graft using the dacron tube as a vascular replacement (Fig. 21). By this means the period of arrest of circulation to the kidneys is relatively minimal and should not exceed ten to twenty minutes, which is well within the safe period of tolerance.

It is thus apparent that various technical methods are now available that permit effective means of overcoming the different problems associated with excisional therapy of aortic aneurysms of variable location and extent. Even patients with aneurysms located in both the thoracic and the abdominal aorta

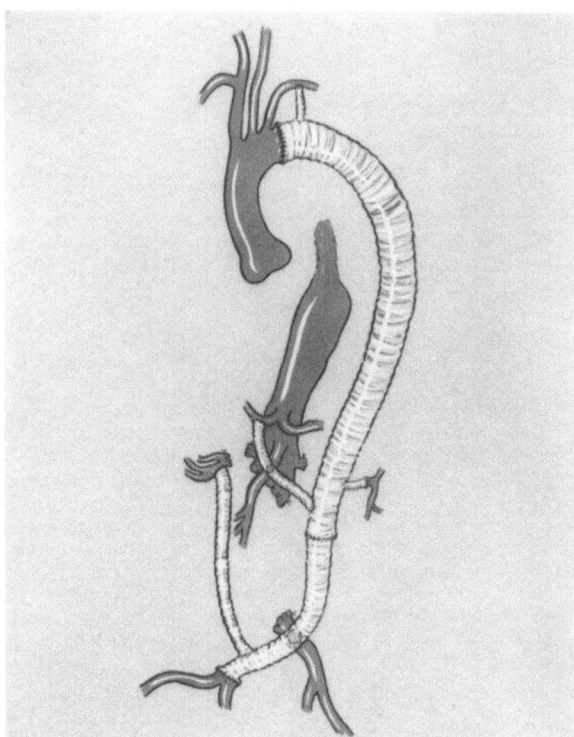

Fig. 20. (C) Drawing illustrating method of surgical treatment by utilizing temporary bypass graft which is subsequently converted into permanent graft. The graft is first attached to left subclavian artery by end-to-side anastomosis and then brought through diaphragm and tunneled through left peritoneal gutter to be attached by side-to-side anastomosis to left common iliac artery and end-to-side anastomosis to right common iliac artery. Three segments of tubular grafts are then attached to this long graft by end-to-side anastomoses, one of which is attached to the left renal artery and another to the right renal artery by end-to-side anastomoses. The remaining segment is attached to the superior mesenteric artery by side-to-side anastomosis and to the hepatic artery by end-to-side anastomosis. With circulation now maintained through the grafts an occluding clamp is applied to the descending thoracic aorta just distal to the left subclavian artery and major portion of descending thoracic aorta is excised and sutured. Major portion of abdominal aortic aneurysm distal to renal arteries is similarly excised and sutured. The proximal opening of descending thoracic aorta is attached to graft by end-to-end anastomosis. Suture closure of both renal arteries, superior mesenteric artery, and celiac axis at their origin proximal to graft anastomosis completes procedure

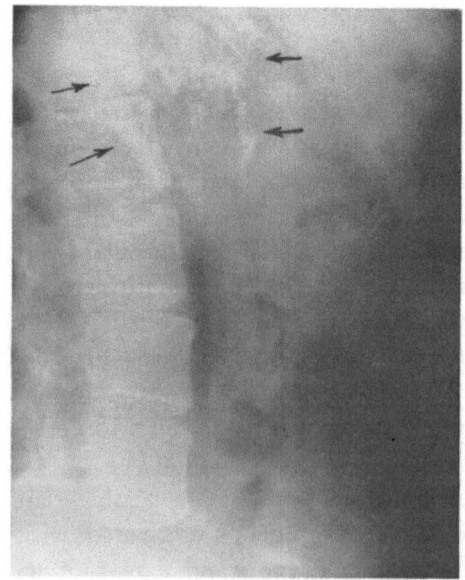

Fig. 21. (A) Preoperative roentgenogram showing thoracoabdominal aneurysm with flecks of calcium outlining wall involving upper segment of abdominal aorta and lower segment of descending thoracic aorta as indicated in (B) drawing illustrating location and extent of aneurysm

Fig. 21. (C) Drawing showing method of surgical treatment of excision and graft replacement utilizing principle of conversion of temporary dacron bypass graft into permanent graft

Fig. 21. (D) Photograph made at operation showing completed replacement of resected segment of aorta with dacron graft including branches to celiac, superior mesenteric, and renal arteries

Fig. 21. (A)

Fig. 21. (E) Postoperative aortogram showing restoration of vascular continuity and circulation through graft

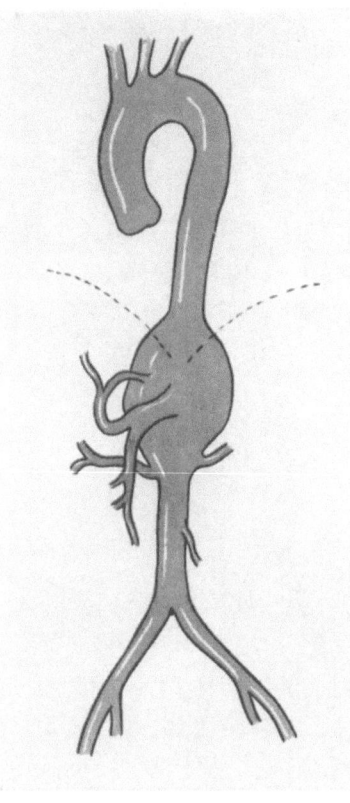

Fig. 21. (B)

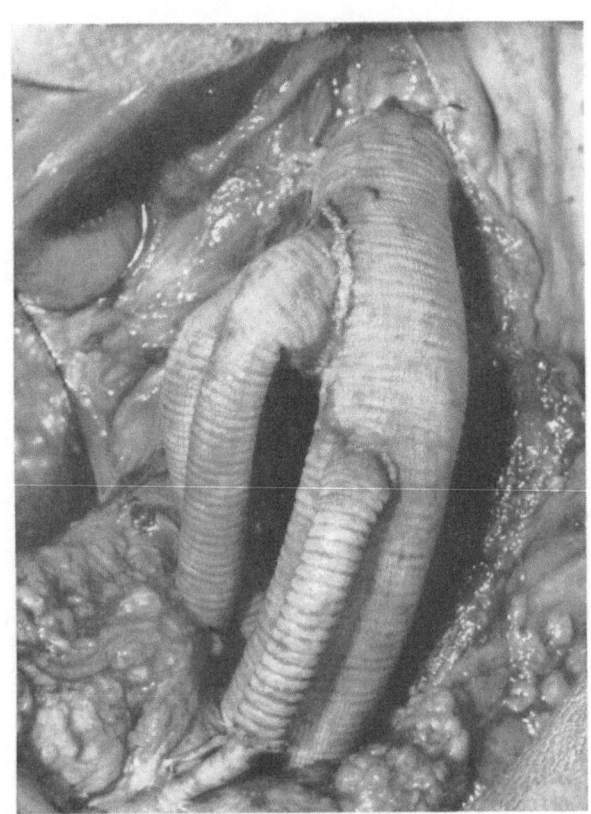

Fig. 21. (D)

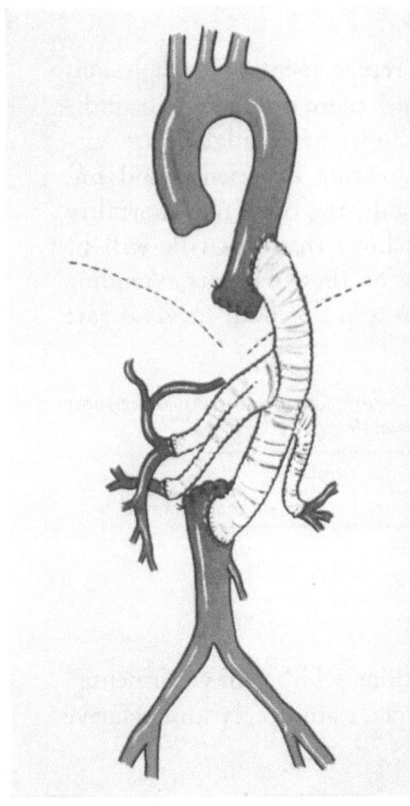

Fig. 21. (C)

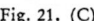

Fig. 21. (E)

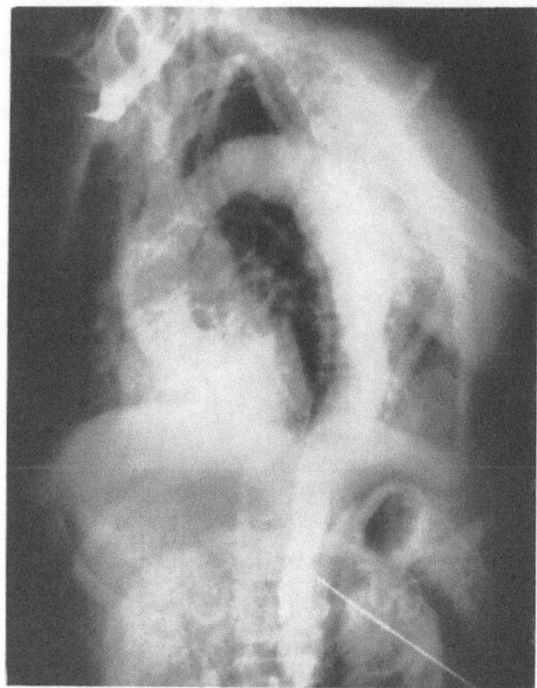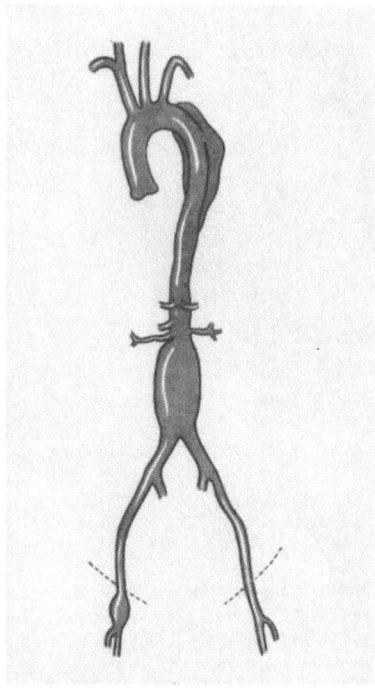

Fig. 22. (A)   Fig. 22. (B)

Fig. 22. (A) Preoperative aortograms showing dissecting aneurysms of descending thoracic and abdominal aorta. In addition, patient had a fusiform aneurysm of right femoral artery

Fig. 22. (B) Drawing showing location and extent of aneurysms

may be successfully treated by excision and graft replacement of both lesions (Fig. 22). Indeed so far as the lesion itself is concerned there are few contraindications to operative treatment since technical methods are available for virtually all forms of the disease. Moreover with increasing experience and improvements in the application of these various methods, the operative mortality has been steadily reduced and there is reason to believe that this risk will be further diminished (Table 6). Follow-up observations on these patients extending well over five years have also been most gratifying in terms of both survival rate and maintenance of normal activities.

Table VI. *Comparison of results of surgical treatment of fusiform aneurysms of descending thoracic aorta in first and second series chronologically*

	No. cases	Deaths	
		No. cases	per cent
First series	33	10	30
Second series	78	13	17
Total	111	23	21

In conclusion let me say that while the observations which I have presented here have been derived largely from our own experience I am deeply appreciative

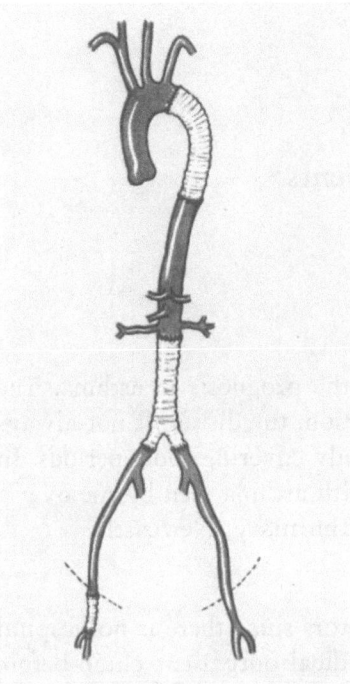

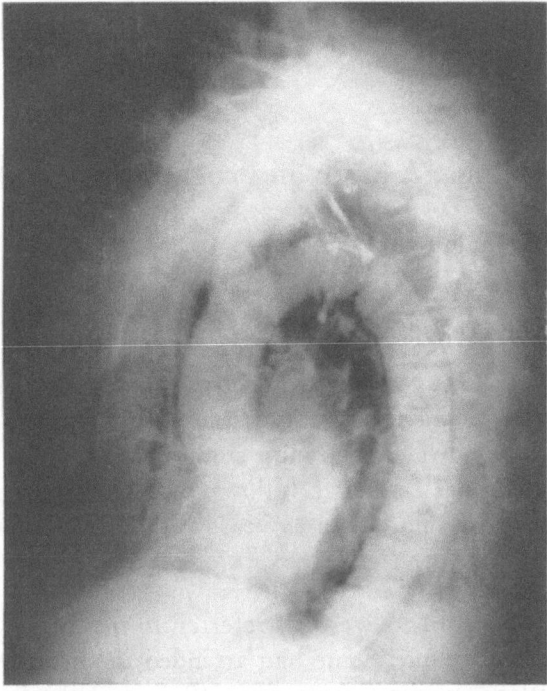

Fig. 22. (C)   Fig. 22. (D)

Fig. 22. (C) Drawing showing method of treatment by resection and graft replacement of aneurysms of descending thoracic and abdominal aorta and right femoral artery. The latter two procedures were done in one stage about three months after the dissecting aneurysm of the thoracic aorta was excised

Fig. 22. (D) Postoperative angiocardiogram showing restoration of normal continuity and circulation in descending thoracic aorta

of the pioneering efforts and the numerous contributions which have been made by a host of investigators throughout the world. Since many of them are present in this audience, it gives me much pleasure to express these sentiments of high tribute. The truly impressive progress that has taken place in the field of cardio-vascular surgery during the past decade provides a brilliant reflection of these efforts.

As is evident from my presentation many of these changing conceptual and technical developments have come from schools of surgery in various countries, and this meeting is a testimonial to the spirit of generous cooperation and warm friendship that pervades the medical scientific world. Wherever we find a dedication to humanitarian purposes and a joining together for the exchange of information, it seems that we also find a key to the preservation of lasting peace among people of different cultures. Here we have had the privilege of personal communication and of providing each other with the most recent knowledge we have gained in our clinics and laboratories. These objectives have, of course, been traditional in the history of medicine, and it is a fact in which we can all take pride because it is the fabric of which peace, understanding, and good will are woven.

Asthma: A Study in Prognosis of 1,000 Patients *

A. G. OGILVIE

The Prognosis in Asthma

It is not easy to find adequate information about the prognosis in asthma. The condition is notoriously liable to spontaneous variation, the disease is not always clearly defined, and most studies have been small, only covering short periods. In this paper I report a follow-up of 1,000 patients with asthma seen by me over a period of more than 25 years at the Royal Victoria Infirmary, Newcastle.

Material

These patients were all referred to me by their doctors since there is no hospital asthma clinic. Some had attended the ordinary medical outpatient clinic before 1935, but most came after 1935, and the first 1,000 who had completed adequately a questionnaire about their present health were chosen. Only those details which were clearly recorded at the initial interview were used in the analysis.

When this series started, specialized psychiatric advice was not readily available. This may have been an advantage since inaccuracies and misleading results might occur if there were a comparison of psychiatric diagnosis in 1935 with psychiatric assessment to-day.

The patients were given an explanation of the disorder, reassurance, and an account of the remedial measures available. Emphasis was placed on the part which an individual patient must play in his or her own treatment and on co-operation in physiotherapeutic procedures, and a reassuring and reasonable attitude was adopted. Parents and relations needed this; it always included "debunking" the asthma bogey, since I dislike the pretence that the condition is not asthma at all. Other remedies, medicinal and specific, were advised as seemed wise and feasible, anti-allergic hygiene was included, and experience alone dictated treatment.

Definitions

Bronchial asthma. — This is a condition characterized by recurrent bouts of wheezing, mainly or entirely expiratory, with an associated variable degree of difficulty in breathing and of expiratory obstruction. Although the intervals between these bouts are often symptom-free, yet a ventilatory defect may

* Published in Thorax **17**, 183 (1962).

sometimes be detected by special methods (ENGSTRÖM, ESCARDO, KARLBERG, and KRAEPELIEN, 1959; STRANG, 1961). If the asthma had symptom-free intervals it was considered intermittent, and if wheezing and dyspnoea persisted it was called continuous. These terms are purely descriptive, and are not intended to carry any particular significance such as is implied in extrinsic and intrinsic asthma (RACKEMANN, 1950).

At an international symposium at the University of Groningen (ORIE and SLUITER, 1961) it was agreed that "asthma refers to the condition of subjects with widespread narrowing of the bronchial airways, which changes its severity over short periods of time either spontaneously or under treatment, and is not due to cardiovascular disease". My definition is similar to this, though I have used clinical language so that intermittent and continuous types can be included. An eosinophilia was not regarded as an essential finding (even though eosinophils are found with greater frequency in the sputum of asthmatics) since its presence did not confirm the diagnosis, and its absence, particularly during broncho-pulmonary infection, did not refute the diagnosis.

Chronic bronchitis. — This is a condition with cough and phlegm persistent throughout the winter or throughout the year, with a minimum duration of two years. The absence of other diseases of the lungs is implicit (OGILVIE and NEWELL, 1957 a; FLETCHER, 1959). In asthmatics a cough is not normally a prominent symptom and occurs only during and after attacks.

Recurrent bronchial infection. — This is a frequently recurrent and febrile chest condition occurring usually in children or adolescents and often associated with asthmatic exacerbation. Such an illness responds well to antibiotic treatment, and the asthmatic reaction is relieved. Here this condition is called "recurrent bronchitis". This is different from "childhood bronchitis" in which bronchopneumonia or a severe attack of bronchitis is followed by a persistent cough with phlegm. There is mild febrile exacerbation, usually without bronchiectasis, but occasionally with a few dilated segmental bronchi. These two groups of recurrent and childhood bronchitis have been included with chronic bronchitis in the initial analysis, but receive special attention later as their prognosis differs from that of the chronic bronchitic.

Allergic sensitivity. — This was recognized as a significant feature if one or both of the following requirements were satisfied:

1. A clear history was given of repeated recurrence or aggravation of symptoms after contact with one or more allergens.

2. A strongly positive skin reaction, i.e., an irregular weal of a diameter of at least 10 mm. associated with erythema, was obtained to the prick or the intradermal administration of a standard testing solution.

Desensitization. — I prefer this name to the less euphonious though more correct term hyposensitization for treatment designed to reduce the sensitivity of an individual to a specific substance or substances.

Age of onset. — This has been variously defined (Fagerberg, 1957; Flensborg, 1945; Baagøe, 1931). Many will accept the onset only when clinically clear-cut asthmatic attacks occur, even though in many patients recurrent respiratory symptoms have been noted for years previously. This seems to me to be unfortunate. Symptoms, particularly in early childhood, often fall short of gross wheezing. There are frequent attacks of "bronchitis", consisting of cough with or without dyspnoea, which last from a few hours to a week. The child is not ill, or "felled" as we call it up here in the north-east. He coughs and may occasionally vomit clear phlegm. There may be a mild rectal pyrexia, the distinction from an attack of acute bronchitis is quite sharp, and an eosinophilia can be found. Wheezing is present, but often only on auscultation.

In my patients, this period of recurrent coughing spells has been noted to precede frank asthma by several years, whilst in adults with continuous asthma a persistent wheeze has sometimes been observed as a mode of onset before the occurrence of obvious asthmatic attacks. The age of onset has been dated from such early symptoms, and it has not been difficult to determine.

Present health. — This was classified into four groups.

A (Good). — Most of these patients had been entirely free from symptoms for at least two years. Other less perfect individuals are included, since I have allowed a few mild asthmatic attacks provided they did not cause disability on more than seven days in the year. Moderate continuous dyspnoea, interfering with the patient's life to a minimal extent, was also permitted, as was a moderate productive cough.

B (Fair). — Patients in this grade suffered constantly or repeatedly from their disorder. They had recurrent asthmatic attacks, which were often severe, about once a month. They were usually, though not necessarily, persistently breathless up to the degree allowed in Fletcher's grade II (Fletcher, 1952). None of the employed persons were allowed to lose more than a total of four weeks' work on average per year. Housewives presented some difficulty, but if ordinary housework could be done, even though by an extra effort, then they were admitted.

C (Poor). — In this grade there was severe recurrent asthma, always continuous between attacks, with breathlessness amounting to grade III or above, and an annual loss of work of more than four weeks. Many patients had been unable to work at all for a number of years, and some were completely disabled. A patient who was maintained on steroid therapy *of necessity* was placed in this grade, even if his condition was reasonably satisfactory.

D (Dead). — These patients had died from status asthmaticus, bronchopneumonia, cor pulmonale, or emphysema. Those in whom the chest condition played no part in the fatal issue, e.g., war casualties, have been excluded entirely from the analysis; two patients who died of carcinoma of the bronchus and one dying of pulmonary tuberculosis have also been excluded.

Method

The record was a four-page folder which was read page by page personally by the author, and the details abstracted in sequence: Only after this was the questionnaire opened, so no subconscious bias should have influenced the analysis. It was annoying when the questionnaire was found to be blank or useless, as it was on less than three dozen occasions: the careful return of a blank questionnaire is an interesting phenomenon.

Results

Table I shows the composition of the series. There are rather more men than women, but this is not likely to be a source of inaccuracy as analyses have shown no significant clinical differences between the sexes. The average duration of male and female cases is similar, as is the average follow-up period.

Table I. *Asthma follow-up: Details of series*

1,000 patients	{	562 males		
		438 females		
Average duration	{	Male 20·6 years	{	Longest 69 years
				Shortest 4 years
		Female 22·3 years	{	Longest 72 years
				Shortest 3 years
Average follow-up	{	Male 11·3 years	{	Longest 33 years
				Shortest 3 years
		Female 10·5 years	{	Longest 33 years
				Shortest 3 years

There is little difference in present health between the sexes (Table II), and such difference as there is is not significant. Since sex did not appear to be a factor in prognosis, and since in all subsequent analyses men and women showed negligible differences, they have been grouped together.

Table II. *Sex in relation to present condition*

Present health	A (Good)	B (Fair)	C (Poor)	D (Dead)	Total
Male	302 (54%)	117 (21%)	99 (18%)	44 (7%)	562
Female . . .	181 (44%)	139 (32%)	90 (20%)	28 (4%)	438
Total	483 (48%)	256 (26%)	189 (19%)	72 (7%)	1.000 (100%)

The outlook in those patients with the onset before 16 years of age is much more favourable than in those with the onset at 16 or over (Table III). This has been noted in other series (RACKEMANN and EDWARDS, 1952; UNGER, 1945; FLENSBORG, 1945).

Table III. *Age of onset in relation to health*

Present health	A (Good)	B (Fair)	C (Poor)	D (Dead)	Total
Under 16 . .	375 (60%)	146 (23%)	87 (14%)	16 (3%)	624
16—	108 (29%)	110 (29%)	102 (27%)	56 (15%)	376
Total	483 (48%)	256 (26%)	189 (19%)	72 (7%)	1.000

The proportion of patients with an early onset in Group A is more than twice as great as those with a later onset. Thereafter there is a steady reversal of this position as we pass from the well, through the poor, to the dead. The percentage of those with late onset who are dead is five times that of those with an early onset. Most authors have recognized a number of onset periods, such as 0 to 5, 6 to 10, and so on, but I thought that a single age limit was likely to show a clearer and more obviously significant result if indeed a difference in prognosis was to appear, and this decision seems to have justified itself.

Table IV shows that four out of five of those with intermittent asthma are affected before 16 years of age, whereas only half of the continuous asthmatics show this early onset. It is evident that intermittent asthma, probably closely resembling RACKEMANN and EDWARDS' (1952) "extrinsic" asthma, is associated with an early onset.

Table IV. *Age of onset in relation to symptoms when first seen*

Symptoms	Intermittent	Continuous	Total
Under 16	320 (81%)	304 (51%)	624 (62%)
16—	85 (19%)	291 (49%)	376 (38%)
Total	405 (40%)	595 (60%)	1,000

Table V shows the present health of the patients, divided into the intermittent and continuous type of asthma, according to their condition when first seen. The outlook is much better in the intermittent group.

Table V. *Clinical type in relation to present health*

Clinical type	A (Good)	B (Fair)	C (Poor)	D (Dead)	Total
Intermittent .	263 (65%)	89 (22%)	43 (10%)	10 (2%)	405 (40%)
Continuous .	220 (37%)	167 (29%)	146 (25%)	62 (9%)	595 (60%)
Total	483 (48%)	256 (26%)	189 (19%)	72 (7%)	1,000

When Tables III and V are placed side by side, the good resemblance is evident.

A further study of the intermittent and continuous asthmatics showed another point of wide difference between them. A negligible proportion of those with bronchitis when first seen were intermittent, while those asthmatics without bronchitis were evenly divided between the intermittent and continuous groups (Table VI).

Table VI. *Incidence of bronchitis in relation to clinical type*

Clinical type	Bronchitis	No. bronchitis
Intermittent	14	391
Continuous	290	305
Total	304	696

The development of bronchitis in an asthmatic tends to convert the intermittent into the continuous type, and this is suggested by the later tables in this series. It is a partial explanation of the high proportion of continuous asthmatics who had bronchitis when first seen, but only a partial explanation, since 52% of continuous asthmatics had no bronchitis. However, the continuous asthmatic is several times more liable to bronchitis than is the intermittent case.

A confirmation of this suggestion is seen when Table VII is studied. This shows those patients, not bronchitic when first seen, who were found to have become bronchitic at follow-up. The number is considerable, and both intermittent and continuous asthmatics are involved. But the continuous asthmatic is more liable to develop bronchitis than is the intermittent (two-thirds against two-fifths).

Table VII. *Pattern of symptoms and development of bronchitis during period of follow-up*

When first seen	At follow-up
Intermittent, non-bronchitic. . . .	43% developed bronchitis
Continuous, non-bronchitic	64% developed bronchitis
Total	53% developed bronchitis

Perhaps the most important figure is the last, which shows that 53% of non-bronchitic asthmatics developed bronchitis over the years. The seriousness of this will be seen when we study the influence of bronchitis on prognosis.

Table VIII. *Incidence of bronchitis initially and at follow-up*

	Bronchitis	No bronchitis
When first seen	304* (30%)	696 (70%)
At follow-up	607 (61%)	393 (39%)

* 113 recurrent and childhood bronchitis.

Table VIII gives the net gain in bronchitis for the whole series and shows that the original position is nearly reversed. Whereas only 30% had bronchitis when first seen, 60% had bronchitis on follow-up.

Table IX shows the final condition at follow-up, comparing the health of the bronchitic directly with that of the non-bronchitic. The difference is a remarkable one. No less than 92% of the non-bronchitics are in good health, as has been defined in this article, whereas only one-fifth of the bronchitics qualified for this grade.

Table IX. *Chronic bronchitis and bronchial infection at follow-up in relation to present condition*

	A (Good)	B (Fair)	C (Poor)	D (Dead)	Total
Bronchitis . .	120 (20%)	228 (38%)	187 (30%)	"72" (12%)*	607 (60%)
No bronchitis	363 (92%)	28 (7%)	2 (19%)	"0" (0%)*	393 (40%)
Total	483 (48%)	256 (26%)	189 (19%)	72 (7%)	1,000 (100%)

* This is referred to in the text.

In column D, all the deaths have been placed in the "bronchitic" box, but this figure is put in inverted commas. Many of these deaths took place years ago, and it has not always been possible to obtain information from the doctor about the patient's health in the years before death or even the exact cause of death. In these circumstances information from relatives has been accepted. Sometimes detailed answers were received which could be accepted as reliable, but at other times all that could be decided was that the patient had been "chesty" for years and that he had died of chest trouble. Since such information is imprecise, all the fatal cases have been put together.

It is known that asthmatics may die of uncomplicated status asthmaticus, and WILLIAMS and LEOPOLD (1959) have reported in detail a series of such cases. WILLIAMS (1953), in a review of 165 cases verified at necropsy (including 25 of his own), concluded that infection was a dominant cause of death in status asthmaticus. A study has been made of the deaths among asthmatic patients in the Royal Victoria Infirmary during the five years 1956 to 1960, together with other series reported in the literature, in all of whom full necropsy reports were available (CARDELL and BRUCE PEARSON, 1959; GAY, 1946; ROBERTSON and SINCLAIR, 1954; THIEME and SHELDON, 1938). The total number is 169, 128 of whom showed clear evidence of bronchopulmonary infection. The remaining 41 showed the changes of status asthmaticus only, and so 25% to 30% of the deaths in these asthmatics were due to uncomplicated asthma, comparable with BULLEN's (1952) series, in which one-third of the 132 necropsies showed death to be due to uncomplicated asthma. If this were the proportion in the present series, from 18 to 24 of the 72 should have been placed in the "no-bronchitis" box. Even so, Table IX suggests that the development of bronchitis has a most unfavourable influence on bronchial asthma.

We now have to consider an important group of cases. Fifty-four patients out of 304 with bronchitis (or bronchial infection) were found on follow-up to have lost their bronchitis; 21 were females and 33 were males. All were in the A (good

health) group with two exceptions; one man and one woman were graded as B
(fair). This result may be compared with Table IX. It is almost identical with that
of the "no bronchitis" group, and suggests that to lose bronchitis is as favourable a
prognostic feature as the development of bronchitis is unfavourable. Table X
shows a breakdown of these patients according to the kind of bronchial infection
which they had when first seen: in only 13 of the 54 was chronic bronchitis of the
adult type present.

Table X. *Patients losing bronchitis during follow-up period*

Initial condition	Total No.	No. losing bronchitis
Chronic bronchitis	191	13
Recurrent and childhood bronchitis . .	113	41
Total	304	54

These 13 patients are of interest since bronchitis is usually thought to be
progressive, and it has been shown in this series to have an unfavourable
prognostic effect in the asthmatic. They represent only 5% of the total who were
bronchitic when first seen and 1.3% of the whole series, but they are significant in
that they indicate that even wellestablished bronchitis can sometimes remit. In a
study of bronchitis in Newcastle upon Tyne (OGILVIE and NEWELL, 1957 b) it was
found that 5% of male and 9% of female bronchitics considered that their health
was improving.

The other 41 patients whose bronchial symptoms had cleared up were all
young and were mostly first seen as children. In 20 of them the condition was one
of recurrent bronchitis (see Definitions). These illnesses are treated nowadays by
antibiotics, and in 12 patients this could have influenced the outcome. The other
21 patients had childhood bronchitis. There were only 113 of these recurrent and
childhood bronchitics in the series, and since 41 improved, the recovery rate is
high (36%), which is unexpected in view of the tendency of the asthmatic person
to develop chronic pulmonary infection, which has been shown so clearly in the
present series.

I attribute it partly to the fact that these patients were all children or
adolescents, and partly to the antibiotic treatment which at least 12 of the
children had, but I think that some other unknown factor or factors also played
a part.

Those with recurrent and childhood bronchitis who did not show this recovery
mostly developed ordinary chronic bronchitis, except for three who acquired
bronchiectasis.

Three hundred and forty-eight of the 1,000 patients showed evidence of
allergic sensitivity (Table XI). This is 35%, and is only a little less than that
observed by RACKEMANN and EDWARDS (1952), who reported 40% in their series
of 688 patients.

Table XI. *Allergic sensitivity in relation to present condition*

	A (Good)	B (Fair)	C (Poor)	D (Dead)	Total
Allergy . . .	196 (56%)	79 (23%)	59 (17%)	14 (4%)	348
No allergy . .	287 (44%)	177 (27%)	130 (20%)	58 (9%)	652
Total	483 (48%)	256 (26%)	189 (19%)	72 (7%)	1,000

This suggests that the criteria of diagnosis in bronchial asthma used in the United States may not differ so widely from those applied in the United Kingdom as is often thought. The prognostic influence of allergic sensitivity is seen to be quite moderate. Those with allergic sensitivity do a little better than the others, but the difference is marginal.

Treatment by desensitization had no effect on long-term prognosis, although usually the immediate result was beneficial (Table XII). This is in line with the experience of McALLEN (1961), who studied the effect of treatment both by the subcutaneous and by the endobronchial routes: those who improved were found to have returned to their original condition in about six months. The conclusion must be that whatever part allergic sensitivity may play in the course of bronchial asthma, it is not a factor of major importance in long-term prognosis. It also seems as if desensitization as a means of treatment plays only a minor role in the determination of the health of the patient in later life, effective though it often is in the short term.

Table XII. *Desensitization of allergic asthmatics in relation to present health*

	A (Good)	B (Fair)	C (Poor)	D (Dead)	Total
Desensitization	64 (53%)	29 (24%)	25 (21%)	3 (2%)	121 (35%)
No desen- sitization .	132 (58%)	50 (22%)	34 (15%)	11 (5%)	227 (65%)
Total	196 (56%)	79 (23%)	59 (17%)	14 (4%)	348 (100%)

Discussion

The chief difficulty in discussing the natural history and outcome of the asthmatic state is the wide variation in approach, in diagnosis, and in classification which is to be found in the extensive literature. I have made reference to the literature only when essential, and many important contributions have been discussed briefly or not at all.

VAUGHAN and BLACK (1954) emphasize the unreliability of insurance and other official analyses, and sum up the prognosis in quite a general way. They recognize "the continuous form and the spasmodic or intermittent", and go on to say that "the life span of the former may be distinctly shorter than that of the latter". This statement, though unsupported by quoted statistical evidence, accords closely with the conclusions of this study. FAGERBERG (1957) emphasizes the importance of the age of onset, which he considers has been too much neglected in the past: my results confirm this view even although the definition of onset is not quite the same as his.

The terms "extrinsic" and "intrinsic", popularized if not actually introduced by RACKEMANN (1950), probably refer to patients similar to those included in my intermittent and continuous groups respectively, but they cannot be regarded as truly identical groups. The comparison which follows is therefore not exact, but the close similarity in the results perhaps excuses it. They followed 688 asthmatic children for 20 years, divided them into two groups, the "allergic" and the "mixed unidentified and bacterial" group. The allergic group (extrinsic) were carefully and meticulously treated on anti-allergic principles, and the others in other ways. The object was to demonstrate the influence of intensive treatment, and the allergic group seem to the best group to take for comparison. It is difficult to be certain that their "cured or relieved", "mild or moderate", and "severe" groups are closely similar to the A, B, and C groups of this series, but assuming that they are, we see how extremely close the result is to that in the Newcastle intermittent cases (Table XIII).

Table XIII. *A comparison of* RACKEMANN *and* EDWARDS' *"allergic" group with the Newcastle "intermittent" cases*

Present health	A (Good)	B (Fair)	C (Poor)	D (Dead)
RACKEMANN and EDWARDS	178 (64%)	78 (27%)	19 (7%)	5 (2%)
Newcastle	263 (65%)	89 (22%)	43 (10%)	10 (2%)

In the classification of VAUGHAN and BLACK (1954) and of UNGER (1945), the terms paroxysmal and chronic seem to be identical with those used in the Newcastle series, but other difficulties in comparison arise.

RACKEMANN and EDWARDS' (1952) mixed group cannot of course be compared with the continuous group. But if we take this whole series and compare it with the 624 Newcastle patients in whom the onset was before the age of 16, Table XIV is the result.

Table XIV. *A comparison of* RACKEMANN *and* EDWARDS' *series with the Newcastle patients whose onset was before age 16*

Present health	A (Good)	B (Fair)	C (Poor)	D (Dead)
RACKEMANN and EDWARDS	337 (50%)	252 (36%)	75 (11%)	24 (3%)
Newcastle	375 (60%)	146 (23%)	87 (14%)	16 (3%)

The result is again similar, once more assuming that the criteria are comparable. Such coincidence between the two series of similar size, though widely separated in time and space and differing in the approach to treatment, is striking. It encourages the view that the development of the asthmatic state in Boston and in Newcastle is not very dissimilar. RYSSING's (1959) follow-up of FLENS-BORG's (1945) series is less easy to compare, although the condition on follow-up appears to be less favourable generally. This series was designed purely as a natural experiment, and no special treatment was given: it is impossible to say how this influenced the results.

In my patients, the more favourable outlook for the asthmatic who begins to have symptoms in childhood is confirmed. When asthma begins before 16 the symptoms are intermittent in four out of five, whereas, when the onset is later, only two out of four are intermittent. The intermittent patient has a considerably more favourable prognosis, and this is a probable explanation of the better prospect in those with an early onset (see Table V). When the intermittent and continuous groups were compared, the incidence of bronchitis was initially much higher in the continuous group, and was almost negligible in the intermittent (see Table VI). The incidence of bronchitis and bronchial infection in the whole series (30%) is close to the estimate of COOKE (1947), whose figure was 35%.

Although 53% of all patients had developed bronchitis during the follow-up period, this tendency was much greater in the continuous group. Only 43% of the intermittent asthmatics, non-bronchitic initially, developed bronchitis, as against 64% of the continuous non-bronchitic asthmatics. This means that there is a significant tendency among asthmatics to develop bronchitis, and this tendency is greater in the patient with continuous symptoms. Table IX shows that this constitutes a major factor in prognosis. Of the 393 patients still not bronchitic on follow-up, 92% qualified for the A or good health label: whereas of the 607 bronchitics only 20% so qualified.

Fortunately, bronchial infection need not necessarily lead to deterioration, although it usually does so. There were 54 patients with bronchitis and bronchial infection who were found on follow-up to have lost their bronchitis, and with two exceptions these were in the A or good health group. The proportion is 98%, as high as, or higher than, in those who did not develop bronchitis at all (see Table VIII).

A breakdown of these "bronchitis losers" shows that in 41 the condition was recurrent or childhood bronchitis. These 41 recoveries in 113 cases of bronchitis in young persons support the view that the outlook is better at this age than when bronchitis develops later in life. Antibiotic treatment was intensively applied in 12 out of the 41 and may have contributed to their recovery, though this does not affect the conclusion since antibiotic treatment was given to numbers of the chronic bronchitics also. Table XIII shows also that even from chronic bronchitis itself recovery is possible, though it is infrequent. Neither allergic sensitivity nor the desensitization treatment given seemed to affect the long-term prognosis (Tables XI and XII).

This study suggests that if we can prevent the development of bronchitis in an asthmatic patient or can relieve him of it should he acquire it, we shall do more for the patient than can be done in any other way.

Summary

One thousand unselected patients with bronchial asthma have been followed up for an average period of 11 years, with extremes of 33 years and three years. The average period from the first symptoms to the date of follow-up was 20.6 years in the 562 males and 22.3 years in the 438 females, with extremes of 72 years and three years. Since throughout the analysis no differences were found between the sexes, they have been grouped together.

Terms used, such as asthma, chronic bronchitis, childhood bronchitis, age of onset, etc., have been carefully defined, as have the descriptions of intermittent and continuous asthma. The present state of the patients has been classified as A (good), B (fair), C (poor), and D (dead).

Early age of onset (before 16) and intermittent asthma were associated and had a more favourable prognosis, while the childhood bronchitic had a better outlook than the adult bronchitic. Intermittent and continuous asthma have been compared. The incidence of bronchitis initially was higher in the continuous group, and the tendency to develop bronchitis over the years (present in all asthmatics) was also greater in the continuous group. Those with bronchitis were in much poorer health on follow-up than those without.

This suggests that the presence or development of bronchitis in an asthmatic is a serious complication of unfavourable prognostic significance, and conversely that the lesser tendency to bronchitis which has been found in patients with early onset, and in intermittent asthma, is the reason for their better prognosis.

The presence or absence of demonstrable allergic sensitivity and of specific desensitization treatment has no obvious important influence on long-term prognosis.

Of 113 patients with recurrent and childhood bronchitis initially, 41 were found to have lost their bronchitis on follow-up, whereas of 191 with chronic bronchitis, 13 had lost their bronchitis. Fifty-two of these 54 "bronchitis losers" were in good health on follow-up, suggesting that the loss of bronchitis is as favourable a feature as the development of bronchitis is unfavourable.

A chief object of management in bronchial asthma should be the prevention of bronchitis, and the chief aim of treatment should be to rid the patient of bronchitis should he develop it. Other factors are secondary, though important.

References

BAAGØE, K. H.: Ugeskr. Laeg. 93, 79 (1931). Quoted by Fagerberg.
BULLEN, S. S.: J. Allergy 23, 193 (1952).
CARDELL, B. S., and R. S. BRUCE PEARSON: Thorax 14, 341 (1959).
COOKE, R. A.: Allergy in Theory and Practice. Philadelphia: Saunders 1947.
ENGSTRÖM, I., F. E. ESCARDO, P. KARLBERG, and S. KRAEPELIEN: Acta paediat. (Uppsala) 48, 114 (1959).
FAGERBERG, E.: Acta allerg. (Kbh.) 11, 293 (1957).
FLENSBORG, E. W.: Acta paediat. (Uppsala) 33, 4 (1945).

FLETCHER, C. M.: Proc. roy. Med. **45**, 577 (1952).
— Thorax **14**, 286 (1959).
GAY, L. H.: The Diagnosis and Treatment of Bronchial Asthma. London: Baillière, Tindall and Cox 1946.
MCALLEN, MONICA K.: Thorax **16**, 30 (1961).
OGILVIE, A. G., and D. J. NEWELL: Chronic Bronchitis in Newcastle upon Tyne, p. 13. Edinburgh: Livingstone 1957 a.
— — Chronic Bronchitis in Newcastle upon Tyne, p. 97, E. 10. Edinburgh: Livingstone 1957 b.
ORIE, N. G. M., and H. J. SLUITER: Bronchitis, p. 281. Assen, Netherlands: Royal vangorcum 1961.
RACKEMANN, F. M.: J. Amer. med. Ass. **142**, 534 (1950).
—, and MARY C. EDWARDS: New Engl. J. Med. **246**, 815, 858 (1952).
ROBERTSON, C. K., and K. SINCLAIR: Brit. med. J. **1**, 187 (1954).
RYSSING, E.: Acta Paediat. (Uppsala) **48**, 255 (1959).
STRANG, L. B.: M. D. Thesis. University of Durham 1961.
THIEME, E. T., and J. M. SHELDON: J. Allergy **9**, 246 (1938).
UNGER, L.: Bronchial Asthma, p. 38. Springfield, Ill.: Thomas 1945.
VAUGHAN, W. T., and J. H. BLACK: Practice of Allergy, 3rd ed. St. Louis: Mosby 1954.
WILLIAMS, D. A.: Thorax **8**, 137 (1953).
—, and J. G. LEOPOLD: Acta allerg. (Kbh.) **14**, 83 (1959).

Choice and Limitations of the Various Operations for the Surgical Treatment of Lung Cancer

GIANFRANCO FEGIZ, M.D.

The total number of patients who have undergone operations for cancer of the lung is by now large enough to permit statistical evaluation of the immediate and long-term results that have been obtained. Particular importance attaches to the long-term results, since from a comparative examination of the results obtained with different techniques it should be possible to draw conclusions that will enable us to select our therapeutic approach for the future. The immediate results are less important: they are shown by all the available statistics to be improving, and the reasons for such improvement are to be found in the greater degree of perfection of surgical techniques and the wider experience accumulated by surgeons, and of course advances in anaesthesia and reanimation. In view of the high technical standards that have been achieved today it is unlikely that these results will undergo much change in future years.

More may legitimately be expected of the long-term results, especially since the experience acquired to date and further research into the causes of long-term failures (the majority of which involve tumour recurrence) should allow us to form conclusions that may in some way modify our present therapeutic approach. The urgent need for such conclusions is reflected by the large number of published articles concerning certain unresolved questions: whether pulmonary excision should be total or partial, whether excision should be accompanied by systematic lymphadenectomy or not, and whether or not intrathoracic or extrathoracic structures invaded by the tumour should be extensively removed.

It is generally accepted that excision is today the treatment of choice for lung cancer; numerous definitive cures recorded in published case histories more than justify the risk involved, while no other physical or drug therapy can show results that are in any way comparable with those obtained by surgery.

On this assumption let us now briefly examine the technical aspects of the various surgical operations, investigate the respects in which they differ, and evaluate the results obtained as recorded in our own and other case reports so as to obtain as reliable evidence as possible of the advantages that any one type of operation may have over others.

Operations for cancer of the lung

Total excision

a) Simple pneumonectomy. This operation entails removal of the lung only, i.e. without systematic excision of the mediastinal lymph nodes.

This operation is more simple and rapid than the radical pneumonectomy discussed below. It will naturally be unacceptable, at least theoretically, to those surgeons who demand for every carcinoma, wherever located, the total removal of the tumour and of its dependent lymph nodes. Certain surgeons maintain that systematic removal of the mediastinal lymph nodes is useless; for reasons given below, we disagree with this hypothesis.

b) Radical pneumonectomy. This operation differs from the preceding in that it entails the removal not only of the lung but also of the whole of its dependent lymph nodes, of the mediastinal pleura that invests it, and of the surrounding fatty tissue. In some cases, if the operation is to be really radical, the pericardium must be opened up and the vessels ligatured intrapericardially; in other cases resection of the pericardium (for neoplastic infiltration) and of the phrenic and vagus nerves may be necessary.

Certain authors who are advocates of systematic radical pneumonectomy have maintained the necessity of evacuating the mediastinum, involving the skeletisation of the vena cava, the trachea, the oesophagus, and the pulmonary vessels from the base of the neck to the diaphragm. This can be done only by the removal en bloc of a portion of the pericardium and of the phrenic nerve that passes over its surface and the ligaturing of the vessels within the pericardial sac itself (WATSON, ALLISON).

In actual fact most surgeons who favour radical pneumonectomy, considering simple pneumonectomy inadequate, confine the operation to mediastinal lymphadenectomy. This entails removal of the fatty and fibrous tissue, together with the lymph nodes it contains, in the space between the superior vena cava and the trachea (above, behind, and beneath the azygos vein), around the main bronchus, beneath the carina, in the pulmonary ligament behind the vena cava inferior, beneath the latter, and along the oesophagus.

This radical operation should not of course be confined only to cases showing unmistakable lymph node metastasis, but should be carried out systematically, that is, even in cases where no such invasion has taken place at least as far can be determined macroscopically.

c) Extended pneumonectomy. By this is meant pneumonectomy extended to the resection of ribs, of parts of the chest wall of the angle of the carina, of the diaphragm, of the atrial wall, of the vena cava, as dictated by the neoplastic invasion of these areas.

As stated above, this operation of extended pneumonectomy is carried out for the most part in cases of localised invasion of the areas listed and when the surgeon considers it is possible to combine pneumonectomy with total removal of the invaded areas.

The results obtained by this type of operation are considered below in the light of published case histories. In certain cases, however, the removal of the extrapulmonary structures or organs mentioned is dictated not by neoplastic invasion but by indirect causes. Thus surgeons have, though actually without spectacular success, treated Pancoast's syndrome by the removal en bloc of the lung together with the invaded chest wall and the related vascular and nervous structures, resulting inevitably in interscapulohumeral disarticulation.

d) Palliative or "noncurative" (Ruggieri) pneumonectomy. This includes operations that do not fall under the "radical" heading and that are performed for contingent reasons, e.g. the desire to treat the symptom (very severe cough, pains, haemorrhage, infection) and not the disease as such, or for reasons of a technical nature (haemorrhage following laceration of a pulmonary bloodvessel caused by exploratory measures and necessitating sacrifice of the lung without the possibility of removing all the neoplasm or all the invaded lymph nodes).

Such operations are the exception and exceed the scope of the present article.

Partial excision

a) Simple lobectomy or bilobectomy. The principle reason for performing lobectomy, particularly for cancer, is one of economy, i.e. a desire to preserve healthy lung tissue. In the opinion of certain surgeons it should be performed in all cases, i.e. even when preoperative examination indicates that the patient is well able to support total pneumonectomy; others consider that this operation should be carried out only where the patient would not survive removal of the whole lung. The former include CHURCHILL, SWEET, SCANNEL and WILKINS; other surgeons take a similar view, though preferring to limit lobectomy to certain welldefined cases (NISSEN, CHRISTIANSEN, SMITH and OTHEEN, BOYD et al.).

These are the arguments most generally accepted (the present author applies similar principles); they are opposed by certain authors (OCHSNER, DOUBLER and BLALOCK) who maintain that lobectomy should be regarded as an operation that is not in fact radical or (LATREILLE and LATARJET) that is should be confined to cases of purely peripheral neoplasia. Those who consider that lobectomy is inadequate can be said to share the opinion of those who maintain that lymphadenectomy is essential to the radicality of the operation. That is to say, they may be regarded as advocates of the following type of operation.

b) Radical lobectomy or bilobectomy. By this is meant lobectomy accompanied by systematic lymphadenectomy of "all" the lymph nodes that are recognised as being the typical sites of tumorous metastasis; thus removal of the lymph nodes of the basis and hilus of the lobe is not enough; it will also be necessary to remove the mediastinal connective tissue together with the lymph nodes situated in the areas that would be removed in radical pneumonectomy. It is thus clear that the criticisms directed against lobectomy may be justified by the difficulty of performing a genuinely radical operation when it is necessary to remove lymph nodes that remain covered by vascular and bronchial structures that cannot be sacrificed in lobectomy.

The answer that may be given to the critics of lobectomy for cancer is that the forms exhibiting marked metastatic involvement of the lymph nodes are naturally not good indications for lobectomy, and that on the other hand if precise operative techniques and tactics are employed, i.e. when the surgeon has an adequate measure of experience at his disposal, it is possible to achieve radicality in cases that are not so extreme as those mentioned.

Lobectomy is of course contraindicated if the tumour is located too close to the line of section on the bronchus, yet this is true not only for radical lobectomy but for all types of excisions for tumour.

c) Extended lobectomy. This entails the combination of lobectomy or bilobectomy with the removal of proximal anatomical structures such as ribs, diaphragm, pericardium. These operations, involving more than pulmonary excision pure and simple, correspond exactly to the extended pneumonectomy already referred to. The limitations of this type of operation are governed by considerations of its true effectiveness, based particularly on evaluation of the long-term results, which are for the most part very poor.

This category includes the operation of sleeve resection, consisting in the resection of a segment of bronchial wall beyond the lobar bronchus corresponding to the removed lobe. This operation may, if necessary, be accompanied by resection of segments of pulmonary artery and followed by suturing to repair the loss of tracheobronchial substance or by

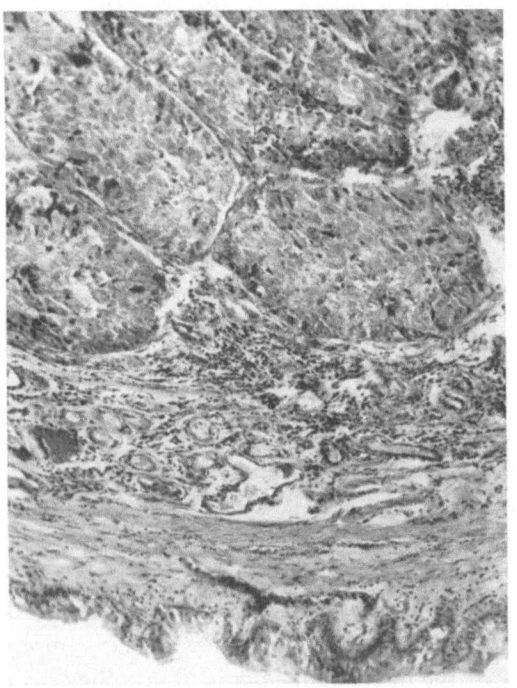

Fig. 1. Neoplastic infiltration beneath bronchial mucosa, which appears normal

reimplantation of the main bronchus. Operations of this type are naturally performed in exceptional circumstances; their advocates include JOHNSTON and JONES, PRICE-THOMAS, MATHEY, and PAULSON and SHAW. In our own opinion, the opportunities for performing operations of this type are rare indeed in view of the amount of bronchial tissue that must be removed proximal to the macroscopic edge of the tumour to achieve true radicality (Fig. 1); although in theory the operation may offer considerable promise it is much less acceptable from the doctrinal and practical points of view. Nevertheless, a number of case reports (JOHNSTON and JONES, PAULSON and SHAW, PRICE-THOMAS, MATHEY) record the survival of patients for several years after undergoing this type of operation and would thus appear to bear out the arguments on which it is based. PRICE-THOMAS, in fact (1960), has found a higher percentage of survivals after lobectomy accompanied by sleeve resection than after lobectomy not so accompanied.

d) Segmental resection. It is clear in the light of the most commonly accepted precepts of cancerology that operations of this type cannot be indicated, except in the event of diagnostic error, other than in cases where the respiratory surface of the patient has been so severely reduced that lobectomy would appear to be excessive.

Nevertheless, cases have been occasionally recorded of patients surviving for several years after undergoing such an operation, an operation that is so little in accordance with the fundamental principles of cancer therapy (THOMPSON: 11 and 5 years respectively). The only comment that can be made is that these cases, clearly fortuitous ones, obviously exhibited the characteristics of "carcinoma in situ", the typical behaviour of which is well known.

Choice of operation

It will be seen from the above review that the different types of surgical treatment that enter into consideration are the following:

(1) Simple pneumonectomy
(2) Radical pneumonectomy (with systematic lymphadenectomy)
(3) Simple lobectomy
(4) Radical lobectomy (with systematic lymphadenectomy),

and, in special cases:

(5) Extended pneumonectomy
(6) Extended lobectomy
(7) Segmental resection.

Certain surgeons would allow two further possibilities:

(8) Palliative pneumonectomy (performed in order to treat the symptom rather than the disease in cases where the radical operation is not possible)

(9) Noncurative pneumonectomy (performed, also where the radical operation is impossible, in cases of emergency, e.g. for intraoperative haemorrhage that cannot be controlled otherwise).

One further possible type of operation, discussed in greater detail below, may be added:

(10) Implantation of radioactive isotopes with or without pulmonary excision.

The technical aspects of these operations have already been covered, and mention has also been made of some of the more authoritative opinions on the subject. Valid conclusions can clearly be drawn only by making a comparative study of the results that are obtainable with the aid of these various methods. This is easier to do on the theoretical plane than on the practical. Each surgeon naturally bases his own conclusions on factual data that must be regarded as objective; without casting doubt on the results reported, however, we must bear in mind that in many cases the data given by various workers are dissimilar and often confusing. Thus some authors do not distinguish between radical operations and simple excision, others carry out total lymphadenectomy only in rare cases, and others fail to distinguish between pneumonectomy and lobectomy when publishing their long-term results. Furthermore, not all of them give percentage figures of precise statistical significances, considering only those patients whom they have been able to follow up and omitting those who for one reason or another have been lost from sight: if the latter represent a large fraction it is clear that the figures recorded lose much of their value.

Let us, however, give some figures selected from reports covering large numbers of cases, and afterwards our own. (See Table I.)

Table I. *Operative mortality after lobectomy and pneumonectomy*

	Lobectomy %	Pneumonectomy %
BROCK	4	21.6
BURFORD *et al.*	12	13
CECCARELLI.	4.8	18
CHRISTIANSEN and SMITH	10	20
CHURCHILL *et al.*	6.4	10
GIFFORD and WADDINGTON	14.7	26
JENNY	11.3	13.6
JOHNSTON	13	7
JONES	1	6.6
RUGGIERI.	10.7	19.2
SANTY *et al.*	7	18
SAUVAGE *et al.*.	4.5	11.8
SELLORS	9	24
SHAW	3	9
WIKLUND.	9	16

It should be pointed out that the operative mortality is influenced to a considerable degree by the age of the patient: thus NISSEN found a mortality of 60% in pneumonectomy and of 20% in lobectomy for patients aged 70 and over.

The site of the neoplasm also has a certain influence on the operative risk. Thus it is generally admitted that the postoperative mortality is higher in removal of the right lung than in that of the left (NÈGRE *et al.*, GIFFORD *et al.*, BIGNALL *et al.*).

As far as the long-term results of the different types of operation are concerned, the following table summarises some of the more significant figures given by various authors.

Table II. *Survival five years after operation*

	Pneumon-ectomy (unspec-ified) %	Pneumon-ectomy (without system-atic lymph-aden-ectomy) %	Pneumon-ectomy (radical) %	Lobec-tomy (unspec-ified) %	Lobec-tomy (simple) %	Lobec-tomy (radical) %	Excision (unspec-ified) %
BELCHER	29			38			
BIANCALANA . . .		16	0		10		
BROCK		30	40			44	
CHRISTIANSEN and SMITH . . .	20			18			
CHURCHILL and SWEET . . .			24			33	
JENNY		26			25		
OVERHOLT and BOUGAS . . .		24			27		
RUGGIERI		31			17.6		
THOMPSON							27.3
VOSSSCHULTE . . .							11.2
WATSON		22	27		25		
WIKLUND							25

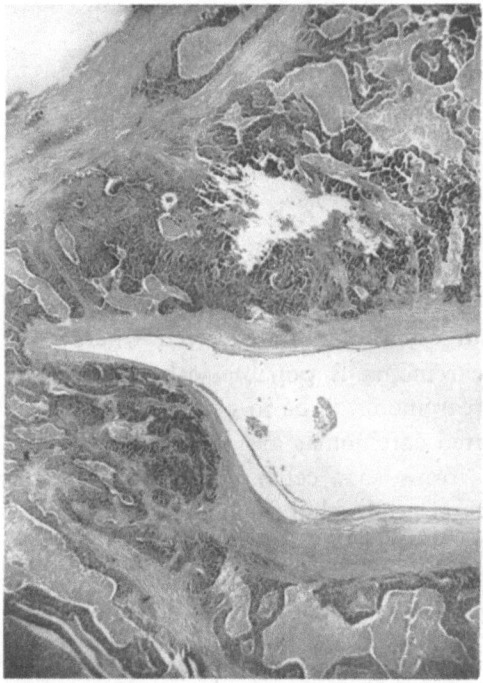

Fig. 2. Neoplastic invasion of the wall of a branch of the pulmonary artery

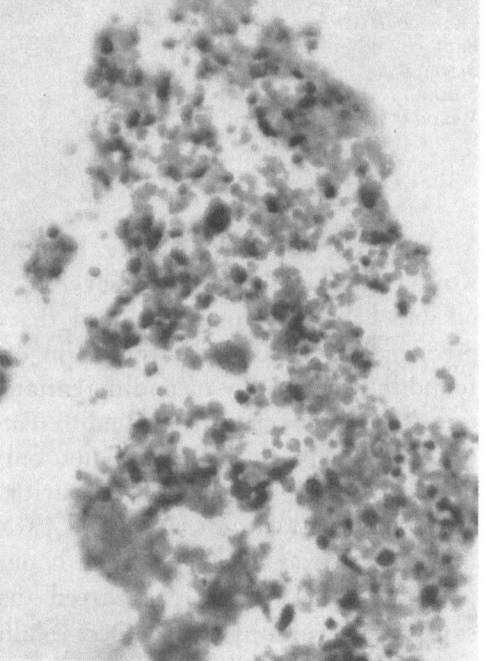

Fig. 3. Neoplastic cells in the lumen of a pulmonary vessel (same case)

One question of undisputed interest is that of vascular invasion by the tumour. Clearly the prognosis of cases with vascular invasion will be very much poorer than when no invasion is present (see Figs. 2 and 3). MAGGI and GNAVI found that out of 125 patients this condition was present in 51%; it reached its maximum (60%) in undifferentiated carcinoma and minimum in epidermoid (45%). Survival after five years in cases where neoplastic invasion of the vessels was found in the removed part was 2%, as against 18% in cases where no such invasion was found. JOHNSTON, KIRBY and BLAKEMORE found that the percentage of cases exhibiting vascular invasion was as high as 71% (100% in the undifferentiated forms). The five-year survival rate was 6% in these cases and 75% in the others. NOHL found a survival rate of 44% in cases without vascular invasion and 30% in cases where invasion was present.

The relationship between histological type and long-term survival is shown in the following table:

Table III. *Survival after 5 years with reference to histological type*

	Epidermoid carcinoma %	Adenocarcinoma %	Undifferentiated carcinoma %
BELCHER	32	53	37
BIGNALL and MOON	36	41	26
CHRISTIANSEN and SMITH	13		
GIBBON, TEMPLETON and NEALON. . . .	24		13
GIFFORD and WADDINGTON	38	0	19
DE BEAGEAU and PAPILLON	16		
OCHSNER *et al.*	21	7	11
PAULSON and SHAW	17	22	0
SANTY *et al.*			5
SIDDONS	39	42	34
VALDONI (1957)	41.6	33.3	33.3 (survival nil in oat cell carcinoma)

Different conclusions have been drawn from these data. Whereas some workers have noted that the survival of undifferentiated carcinoma patients is nil and have therefore concluded that surgery should be deferred wherever a preoperative diagnosis of this form of carcinoma is possible, others have not found the malignancy of undifferentiated carcinoma to be so great. The explanation is a simple one: not all undifferentiated carcinomas are of the same degree of malignancy; thus we find not only forms (oat cells) whose prognosis is decidedly poor but also forms with large cells that are considerably less malignant (KIRKLIN, MCDONALD, CLAGETT, MOERSCH and CAGE). This difference in behaviour was clearly apparent in our own series of cases.

Almost all workers are agreed that epidermoid carcinoma represents the category in which by far the best results are to be expected from surgery. These are the forms in which certain surgeons, opposed to systematic lymphadenectomy in other forms, insist that the operation be rendered as radical as circumstances will allow (WATSON).

A particularly interesting aspect of the subject, with regard to the question of whether systematic lymphadenectomy should be carried out or not, is the percentage survival in cases with and without metastatic invasion of the lymph nodes removed during surgery. See the following table.

Table IV. *Survival five years after excision*

	Invasion of lymph nodes %		No invasion of lymph nodes %	
	Pneum.	Lob.	Pneum.	Lob.
BIANCALANA	2.4		12	
CHURCHILL *et al.*	16	20	46	35
JOHNSTON *et al.*	15		43	
NOHL	18		55	
OCHSNER *et al.*	14		38	

Case statistics of the institute of surgery of the University of Rome (Professor PIETRO VALDONI).

Evaluation of the long-term results of lung cancer operations performed in the Institute was undertaken as early as 1957. The findings were collected by CAPPELLINI and OLIVA and published in detail, and were later brought up to date by VALDONI in 1959 and 1961.

In order to have still more complete and up-to-date figures available for the present article, we carried out a fresh examination of the data, reviewing all patients admitted to the Institute and following up discharged patients. Of the figures obtained in this manner we give below the ones most relevant to our subject.

Table V. *Institute of Surgery University of Rome (Professor P. VALDONI)*
Lung cancer

	No. of admissions	Not operated	Thoracotomy	Excision	Postoperative mortality (number of deaths)	Discharged cured
1946—1959	876	387	169	320	104	216
1959—1962	280	147	36	97	8	89
Total	1156	534	205	417	112	305

It will be seen from the above figures that the number of patients judged inoperable on the basis of clinical examination has increased, while the percentage of patients subjected to explorative thoracotomy has diminished. A further observation of greater practical interest is that the operative mortality has dropped to 8.2%.

It was found during the previous investigation carried out in the Institute that the survival rate three years after the operation was virtually identical with that five years after, and it was therefore concluded that if a patient who has undergone excision reaches his third year after the operation he has an excellent chance of surviving the full five years that are traditionally required before his cancer can be regarded as cured. The findings of the 1957 enquiry showed that

36.8% of the patients dismissed as cured were still alive after three years and 35.7% after five.

In view of these findings, which are in fact borne out by other figures published in the literature, a fresh investigation was carried out covering all patients dismissed from the Institute up to December 1959. We were then able to determine the survival rate of these patients after three years.

Our findings are given in tabular form below.

Table VI. *Survival after operation for lung cancer (191 patients)*

6 months	1 year	2 years	3 years
132	100	74	67
69.9%	52.3%	38.7%	35.07%

It will be observed from the above table that the percentage of patients surviving three years after the operation is almost exactly the same as that found in the previous enquiry carried out five years ago.

The following diagram gives some idea of what can be expected to happen in one hundred cases of lung cancer.

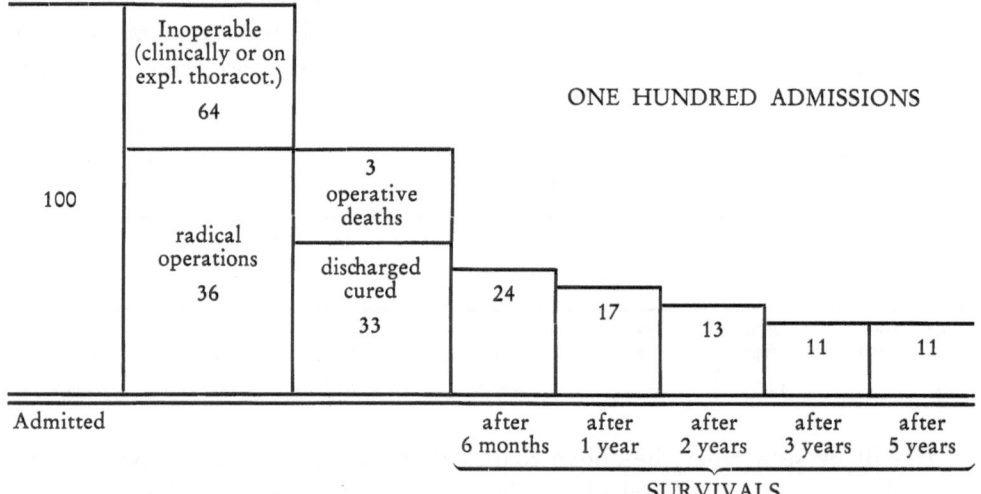

Fig. 4. Lung cancer. One hundred admissions

The risk involved in operations for lung cancer was found statistically to be 8.2% for the period 1959 to 1962. This mortality figure is lower than the corresponding figure for the previous period (for reasons that it is purposeless to describe in detail since they will be familiar to all who are engaged in this type of surgery).

The following two tables show the percentages of postoperative deaths and of three year survivals respectively.

Table VII. *Postoperative deaths (last three years)*

Pneumonectomy	12%
Lobectomy	4.2%

Table VIII. *Survival rate three years after operation (320 patients)*

	No. of patients	Dismissed cured	Followed up	3-year survivals
Pneumonectomy	269	180	160	51
Lobectomy	51	36	31	16
Total	320	216	191	67

At this point it is necessary to add one or two comments regarding the significance of some of these figures.

The relatively high mortality for lobectomy in the first period can be explained by the fact that this operation was in most cases carried out not because it was indicated by the site or diffusion of the tumour but because the advanced age, the very deteriorated general condition, and, more particularly, the impaired circulatory and respiratory situation of the patient necessitated this more economical procedure. If, in fact, we re-examine the cases subjected to lobectomy during this period we find that the early deaths included four cases of thoracectomy, three in which the age of the patient was over 65, and two with severe emphysema.

In recent years, as a consequence of the fact that we are now favourably inclined to lobectomy accompanied by lymphadenectomy in cases where such an operation would appear to be genuinely radical, the percentage of lobectomies has increased with respect to that of pneumonectomies, and at the same time the mortality for the former has dropped to 4.2%.

The following table gives the percentage survival rates:

Table IX. *Survival rate three years after operation (as percentage of cases followed up after being dismissed as cured)*

Pneumonectomy	31.8%
Lobectomy	51.6%
(Total	35%)

Our own case histories show, more clearly in this respect than those of other workers, that the long-term survival after lobectomy is considerably greater than after pneumonectomy.

Finally, to complete the statistical data that must be considered essential for the purposes of this article (i.e. leaving out of consideration other, equally important, figures that are not immediately relevant to the subject under discussion), we give below a table illustrating the survival rate as a function of the lymphatic invasion of the tumour.

Table X. *Survival rate three years after surgery as a function of lymph node metastasis (191 cases)*

No. of cases	Metastatic invasion of lymph nodes removed during surgery	Survival rate
127	absent	44.8%
64	present	15.6%

Comments and conclusions

The choice and the limitations of the various operations that may be performed for bronchopulmonary carcinoma are affected by numerous factors that must always be taken into account. The most important of these factors are the age of the patient, his general and, in particular, cardiorespiratory condition, and the site and extent of the tumour.

If, however, we ignore extreme cases in which the advanced age of the patient or his poor general condition oblige us to resort to less extensive procedures, what should be our attitude when we are confronted with a choice between lobectomy and radical pneumonectomy? And, in either case, what importance should be attached to systematic lymphadenectomy?

Starting with the assumption that the main criterion on which the choice should be based is provided by the long-term results of the various operations, we have carried out a careful evaluation of the survival figures recorded in our own case histories, which cover 1,156 patients.

In this manner we have ascertained that the three-year survival rate (from which the five-year rate does not differ significantly) is 31.8% for radical pneumonectomy and 51.6% for lobectomy. Since, moreover, the operative mortality is 12% for pneumonectomy and 4.2% for lobectomy, it may be deduced from our own case histories that preference should wherever possible be given to lobectomy.

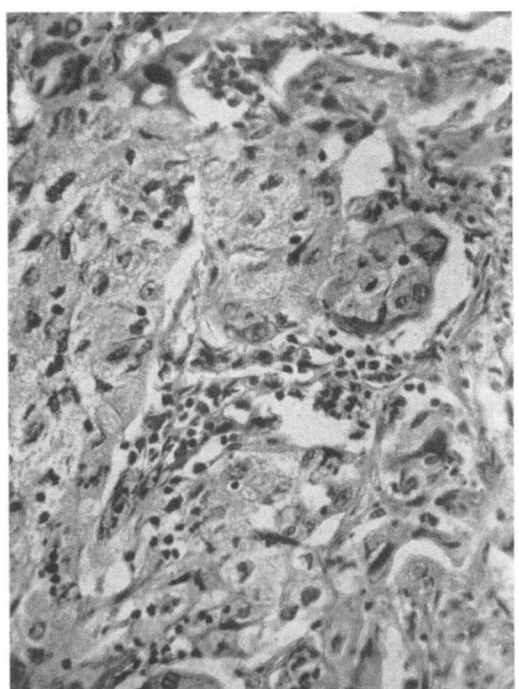

Fig. 5. S. Italo: Undifferentiated carcinoma of the apex of the right lung with invasion of wall and Pancoast's syndrome, treated by segmentary resection and implantation of Au[198]

The doubts expressed by certain surgeons regarding the radical nature of lobectomy may therefore be dismissed in the light of the above results.

We must on the other hand acknowledge that pneumonectomy is of great therapeutic value in cases in which it is indicated; this is borne out by the long-term survival rate even in elderly patients and also by the observation that the general condition of the patient and his capacity for work are not greatly affected.

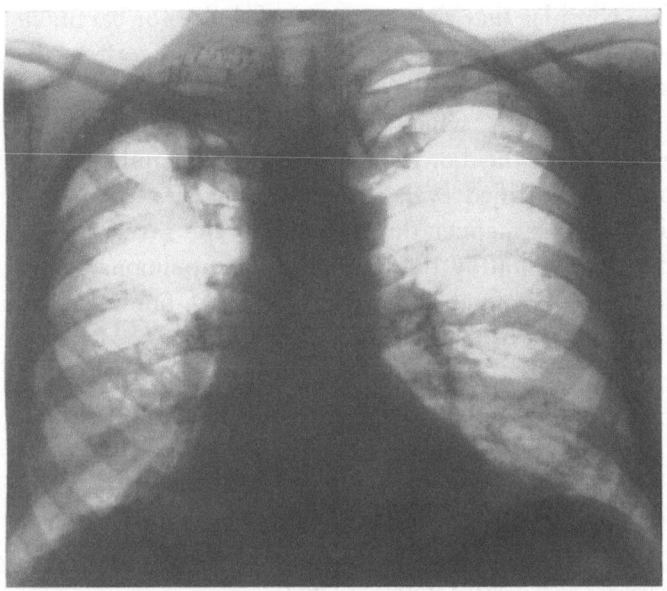

Fig. 6. S. Italo: X-ray of chest 3 years later; the general condition of the patient is excellent, the painful symptoms have vanished completely, and there are no signs of tumour recurrence

Whether pneumonectomy or lobectomy is performed we feel it essential that systematic lymphadenectomy be carried out in order to ensure that the operation is truly radical. Support for this opinion can be found in the figures tabulated above relating to the long-term survival of patients operated on in this manner and also the observation that in one third of these cases metastases were found in the lymph nodes removed during the operation. In this context we would emphasise that the long-term survival rate was distinctly higher for those cases in which no metastases were found (44.8%) than in those in which lymph node invasion was observed (15.6%). These figures bear witness to the value of lymphadenectomy, which, we repeat, should be done systematically, even in cases in which the hilar and mediastinal lymph nodes appear normal.

The indications for operation are highly disputable in cases exhibiting invasion by the tumour of extrapulmonary structures such as the chest wall, the diaphragm, the pericardium and the recurrent and phrenic nerves.

In cases such as these the operation of extended excision may resolve the basic problem of removing the tumour completely; the long-term results are, however, very poor.

The most promising of the various operations performed for neoplasm exhibiting invasion of this type would appear on the basis of our case histories to be pulmonary excision accompanied by the implantation of radioactive gold in the walls; using this method, we have obtained survivals of more than three years in cases of tumour of the apex of the lung with Pancoast's syndrome (Figs. 5 and 6).

We therefore consider that the treatment of choice for carcinoma of the apex of the lung with Pancoast's syndrome is resection of the affected segment or of the upper lobe and implantation of Au^{198} in the wall.

Apart from these results, which are fairly reassuring, we are of the opinion that in many cases on the borderline between operability and inoperability surgery is more than justified even though the chances of a final cure may be very slight, since in this manner the patient may be saved the pains, generally very severe, due to invasion by the tumour of extrapulmonary structures and at the same time hope of a final cure (which, even if minimal, should never be denied to the patient) can be maintained.

References

University of Rome. Institute of surgery

ALATI, E., U. MILANI, e G. CAPPELLINI: Note clinico-statistiche in rapporto alla etiopatologia del cancro del polmone. Arch. Chir. Torace 1, 1 (1957).

BIOCCA, P.: Alcune considerazioni sui tumori maligni primitivi del polmone. Sperimentale 99, 1 (1946).

— Sui tumori maligni primitivi del polmone. Arch. Chir. Torace 2, 57 (1947).

— Pneumonectomies and lobectomies: a statistical review. Proc. VI. Congr. Int. Coll. of Surgeons, Rome 1949.

— Ricerche sulla funzionalità cardio-circolatoria dopo pneumonectomia e lobectomia. Arch. Chir. Torace 5, 3 (1949).

BOLAFFIO, G.: Frequenza, aspetti formali e significato dei fenomeni rigenerativi e metaplasici dell'epitelio bronchiale in caso di carcinoma del polmone. Arch. Chir. Torace 7, 273 (1952).

CAPPELLINI, G., e M. MAURIZI: Necrosi e suppurazioni in corso di carcinoma polmonare. Arch. Chir. Torace 3, 449 (1958).

—, e G. OLIVA: Considerazioni sui risultati a distanza del trattamento chirurgico del cancro del polmone. Arch. Chir. Torace 1, 51 (1957).

CARBONI, R., e M. BALBI: Le calcificazioni nelle ombre rotonde del polmone. Recentia med. (Roma) 24, 4 (1959).

CORTESINI, R., R. CARBONI, e F. VIRNO: Studio sperimentale della funzionalità respiratoria dopo interruzione dell'arteria e delle vene polmonari. Archivio ed Atti Soc. It. Chir., Vol. II, LXI Congr., Rome 1959.

DARDI, M.: Contributo clinico alla pneumonectomia allargata per cancro del polmone. Rass. giul. Med. 10, 3 (1954).

DELLA PENNA, G., e M. BALBI: La distribuzione segmentaria dei tumori del polmone. Atti VI° Congr. Naz. Chir. Torace 3, 513 (1958).

FARACO, P., e G. OLIVA: Le metastasi contro-laterali nel cancro del polmone. Atti VI° Congr. Naz. Chir. Torace, Vol. II, 1958.

FEGIZ, G.: Il cancro del polmone a lungo decorso. Progr. med. (Napoli) 17, 3 (1961).

Fegiz, G., A. Leggeri, G. Cappellini, e M. di Paola: Contributo allo studio della patologia segmentaria del polmone. Arch. Chir. Torace 4, 193 (1960).

Ficari, A., M. Mele, e I. Baschieri: Trattamento chirurgico associato con infissione di isotopi radioattivi nel carcinoma polmonare: alcuni risultati a distanza. Boll. Accad. med. Roma, 30 June 1961.

— Le metastasi linfonodali nel carcinoma bronco-polmonare. Riv. Tuberc. 7, 448 (1959).

Maurizi Enrici, M., e G. Cappellini: Comportamento atipico di carcinoma bronchiale. Casi rari dell'apparato respiratorio. Ed. Minerva med. 1958.

Oliva, G.: La tracheostomia nel trattamento dell'insufficienza respiratoria in chirurgia toracica. Arch. ed Atti Soc. It. Chir., Vol. II, LXII Congr., Naples, 1960.

Pesci, A., G. Cappellini, e G. Oliva: La diffusione ai grossi vasi nel cancro del polmone. Arch. Chir. Torace 633, 7 (1950).

Provenzale, L.: Valore e limiti degli studi di funzione respiratoria nella moderna chirurgia del torace. Arch. Chir. Torace 633, 7 (1950).

—, e S. Tagliacozzo: L'esplorazione funzionale del circolo polmonare nella chirurgia di exeresi del polmone. Arch. Chir. Torace 1, 1 (1957).

Ricceri, R., S. Tagliacozzo, e P. Biocca: Ricerche sulla ventilazione polmonare in pazienti sottoposti a lobectomia e pneumonectomia. Arch. Chir. Torace 6, 437 (1953).

Smareglia, M., e P. Malatesta: Il cancro asintomatico del polmone. Recentia med. (Roma) 6, 1 (1959).

Sposito, M., P. Biocca, e B. Masini: Rilievi elettrocardiografici dopo lobectomia e pneumonectomia. Comunicaz. Academia Medica di Roma 21, 2 (1948).

Stipa, V.: La diffusione linfatica del carcinoma bronco-polmonare. Arch. Chir. Torace 1, 181 (1962).

Tagliacozzo, S., e A. Pesci: L'invasione della parete toracica nel cancro del polmone. Arch. ed Atti. Soc. It. Chir., LIX Congr. Turin, 1957.

— — L'invasione della parete toracica nel cancro del polmone. Aspetti anatomici, istologici e clinici esaminati attraverso una serie di correlazioni convergenti in un criterio selettivo di operabilità. Gazz. int. Med. Chir. 67, 1 (1957).

Tonelli, L.: Aspetti Clinici, quadro anatomico e problema istogenetico del carcinoma alveolare del polmone. Arch. Chir. Torace 3, 261 (1948).

Valdoni, P.: Considerazioni sulla diagnosi dei tumori del polmone. Boll. Soc. Med. Livornese 1, 1 (1946).

— Cancro del polmone. G. Med. milit. 97, 1 (1950).

— Alcuni dati statistici nello studio del cancro del polmone. I problemi del servizio sociale, 4, 1950.

— Cancro del polmone. Paper presented at 52nd Congr. Soc. It. Surg., Montecatini, 1950.

— Cancro del polmone. Atti IV⁰ Congr. Naz. Lega It. Contro i Tumori, 1950.

— Debe operarse el cáncer de pulmón? Séptimas Jornadas Argentinas de Cirugia Torácica, 1955.

— Si deve operare il cancro del polmone? Lezioni sui tumori, III corso aggiornamento, Vol. I, Udine, 1956.

— Cancro del polmone. Boll. Ooncol. 31, 2 (1957).

— Risutati lontani degli interventi chirurgici per cancro del polmone. Proc. Int. Med. Conf. Verona, October 1959.

— Criteri attuali di operabilità del cancro del polmone. Progr. med. (Napoli) 16, 73 (1960).

Venturini, A.: Compressione della vena cava superiore da tumori mediastinici e polmonari. Atti V congr. Naz. Chir. Torace, Vol. II, Ischia, 1956.

Zannini, G.: Osservazioni sulla funzionalità cardio-circolatoria dopo pneumonectomia. Il comportamento della pressione venosa. Policlinico, Sez. prat. 55, 3 (1948).

(Further Bibliography)

Abbott, O.: Experiences with surgical resection of the human carina, tracheal wall and contro-lateral bronchial wall in cases of right total pneumonectomy. J. thorac. Surg. 19, 906 (1950).

Allison, P. R.: Intrapericardial approach to the lung root in the treatment of bronchial carcinoma by dissection pneumonectomy. J. thorac. Surg. 15, 99 (1946).

ALLISON, P. R.: Discussion of surgical management of carcinoma of the lung. J. thorac. 20, 349 (1950).

BELCHER, J.: Lobectomy for bronchial carcinoma. Lancet 7104, 639 (1959).

BIANCALANA, L.: Risultati del trattamento chirurgico del carcinoma bronchiale. Paper presented to IVth Int. Med. Conf., Verona, 1959.

BIGNALL, J.: Carcinoma of the lung. London: Publ. Livingstone 1958.

—, and A. MOON: Survival after lung resection for bronchial carcinoma. Thorax 10, 183 (1955).

BISHOP quoted by RUGGIERI, V. inf.

BLALOCK quoted by RUGGIERI, V. inf.

BOYD, D.: Choice of operation for bronchogenic carcinoma. Surg. Clin. N. Amer. 41, 755 (1961).

BROCK, R.: Radical pneumonectomy. Thorax 15, 7 (1960).

BURFORD, T., T. FERGUSON, and H. SPJUT: Results in the treatment of bronchogenic carcinoma. J. thorac. Surg. 36, 316 (1958).

CECCARELLI, G.: Sulla terapia chirurgica del cancro del polmone. Proc. IVth Int. Med. Conf., Verona, 1959.

CHRISTIANSEN, K., and D. E. SMITH: Bronchogenic carcinoma: a sixteen years study. J. thorac. cardiovasc. Surg. 43, 267 (1962).

CHURCHILL, E., R. SWEET, J. SCANNEL, and E. WILKINS: Further studies in the surgical management of carcinoma of the lung. J. thorac. Surg. 36, 301 (1958).

GIFFORD, J., and J. WADDINGTON: Review of 464 cases of carcinoma of the lung treated by resection. Brit. med. J. 5021, 723 (1957).

GORDON, W.: Lymphatic spread in the surgical treatment of lung cancer. Amer. J. Surg. 104, 866 (1962).

JENNY, R.: Operative Probleme beim Bronchialcarcinom. Thoraxchirurgie 10, 134 (1962).

JOHNSTON, J., C. KIRBY, and W. BLAKEMORE: Should we insist on radical pneumonectomy as a routine procedure in the treatment of carcinoma of the lung? J. thorac. Surg. 36, 309 (1958).

—, and P. JONES: The treatment of bronchial carcinoma by lobectomy and sleeve resection of the main bronchus. Thorax 14, 48 (1959).

KIRKLIN, J., J. McDONALD, O. CLAGETT, H. MOERSCH, and R. CAGE: Bronchogenic carcinoma: cell type and other factors relating to prognosis. Surg. Gynec. Obstet. 100, 429 (1955).

LATREILLE, R., et M. LATARJET: Ou en est le traitement chirurgicale du cancer primitif du poumon? Lyon Chir. 56, 656 (1960).

MAGGI, G., e M. GNAVI: Frequenza e significato prognostico dell'invasione vascolare nel carcinoma bronchiale. Cancro 13, 487 (1960).

MATHEY, J.: Les résultats de la résection bronchique dans le cancer bronchopulmonaire primitif. Proc. IVth Int. Med. Conf., Verona, 1959.

NEGRE, E., H. PUJOL e A. THEVENET: Bilan de 119 interventions pour cancers broncho-pulmonaires. Ann. Chir. 15, 549 (1961).

NISSEN, R.: publ. in RICHTER, v. inf.

NOHL, H.: The value of scalene node biopsy in intrathoracic diseases. Brit. J. Tuberc. 52, 266 (1958).

OCHSNER, A., A. OCHSNER JR., H. DOUBLER, and J. BLALOCK: Carcinoma of the lung. LVIII Congress Int. Surg. Soc., Munich 1959.

OVERHOLT, R., and J. BOUGAS: Fifty-one cases of lung cancer with five years survival. J. Amer. med. Ass. 161, 961 (1956).

— Surgical benefits in pulmonary carcinoma. VIth Int. Congr. Dis. Thor., Vienna 1960.

PAULSON, D., and R. SHAW: Results of broncho-plastic procedures for bronchogenic carcinoma. Amer. Surg. 151, 729 (1960).

PRICE-THOMAS, C.: The present position relating to cancer of the lung. Thorax 15, 9 (1960).

RICHTER, G.: Behandlungsergebnisse beim Bronchialcarcinom. Thoraxchirurgie 10, 161 (1962).

ROUVIERE, H.: Anatomie des lymphatiques de l'homme. Paris: Publ. Masson 1934.

RUGGIERI, E.: Cancro del polmone. Paper presented to VIII Nat. Congr. Thor. Surg., Venice 1962.

SANTY, P., P. GALY, M. LATARJET, et P. JAUBERT DE BEAGEAU: Résultats et indications des traitements des cancers bronco-pulmonaires. À propos de 900 observations. Bronchi 9, 318 (1959).

SAUVAGE, R., H. LE BRIGAND, et M. MERLIER: Analyse d'une série de 557 interventions pour cancer bronchique. Mém. Acad. Chir. 85, 811 (1959).

SCHEININ, M.: Pulmonary cancer and circulating cancer cells. Acta Chir. Gynec. Finn. 51, 1 (1963).

SIDDONS, A.: Cell type in the choice of cases of carcinoma of the bronchus for surgery. Thorax 17, 308 (1962).

SMITH, R.: The results of raising the resectability rate in operations for lung carcinoma. Thorax 12, 79 (1957).

SPJHUT, H., C. ROPER, and A. BUTCHER: Pulmonary cancer and its prognosis. Cancer 14, 1251 (1961).

THOMAS, C.: The present position relating to cancer of the lung. Lobectomy with sleeve resection. Thorax 15, 9 (1960).

THOMPSON, V.: The present position relating to cancer of the lung. Results of resection. Thorax 15, 5 (1960).

VOSSSCHULTE, K.: Indications et résultats thérapeutiques dans les carcinomes primitives des bronches. Bronchi 9, 336 (1959).

WATSON, V.: Radical surgery for lung cancer. Cancer 9, 1167 (1956).

WIKLUND, TH.: Indications et résultats du traitement chirurgical des cancers bronchiques. Bronchi 9, 350 (1959).

Author index